IMMUNOSUPPRESSIVE DISEASES OF POULTRY

Warning:
Veterinary science is constantly evolving, as are pharmacology and the other sciences. Inevitably, it is therefore the responsibility of the veterinary clinician to determine and verify the dosage, the method of administration, the duration of treatment and any possible contraindications to the treatments given to each individual patient, based on his or her professional experience. Neither the publisher nor the author can be held liable for any damage or harm caused to people, animals or properties resulting from the correct or incorrect application of the information contained in this book.

Plaza Antonio Beltrán Martínez nº 1, planta 8 - letra I
(Centro empresarial El Trovador)
50002 Zaragoza - Spain

Design and layout:
Servet editorial - Grupo Asís Biomedia, S.L.
www.grupoasis.com

Printing:
Grupo Milán, S.L.
Pol. Alcoz Bajo, C/ Paraíso 5 dpdo., Nave B
50410 Cuarte de Huerva
Zaragoza - Spain

ISBN: 978-84-941389-5-9
D.L.: Z 1507-2013

Printed in Spain

IMMUNOSUPPRESSIVE DISEASES OF POULTRY

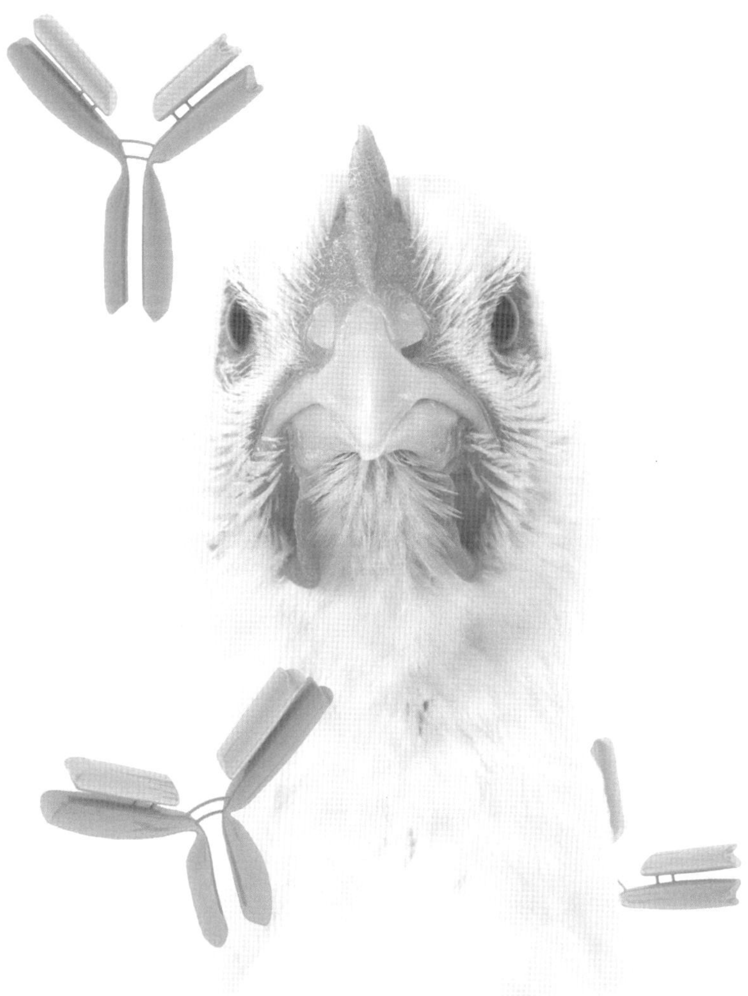

Edited by

Isabel M. Gimeno

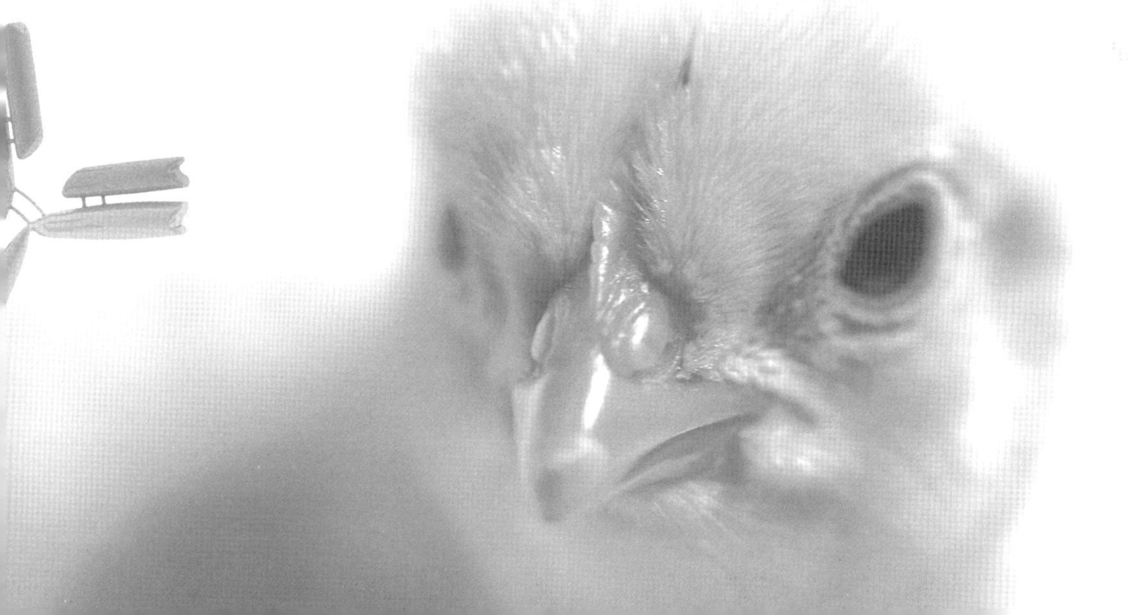

SERVET

Dedicated to the memory of my father
Dr. Luis Gimeno Sacristán

ACKNOWLEDGMENTS

Authors thank Dr. Tatiana Blasco and the editorial staff in Grupo Asís for assisting in the preparation of this book. We would also like to acknowledge Drs. David Ledoux (University of Missouri, Columbia, MO, USA) and William Huff (USDA/ARS-Poultry Center of Excellence for Poultry Science, University of Arkansas, Fayetteville, AR, USA) for providing photographs of mycotoxin lesions.

AUTHORS

Isabel M. Gimeno (Editor)

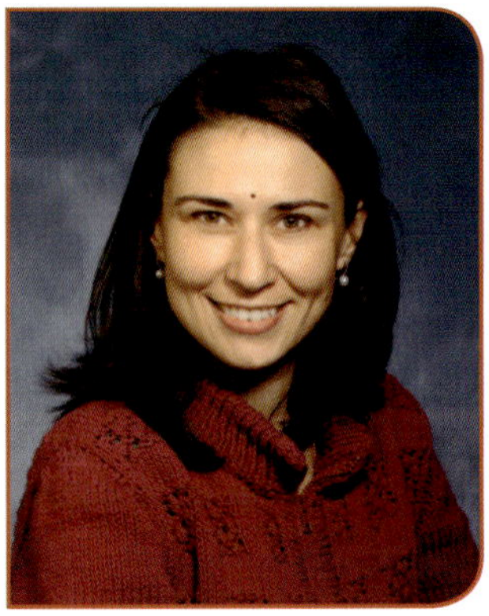

Dr. Isabel M. Gimeno received her Veterinary Degree (1995), MS (1996), and PhD (1999) from *Universidad Complutense de Madrid*, Spain. She is a Diplomate of the American College of Poultry Veterinarians since 2002. She conducted postdoctoral research in *Centro de Investigación en Sanidad Animal* (CISA), Spain and in the USDA-ARS Avian Disease and Oncology Laboratory (ADOL), East Lansing, MI, USA. She is currently an associate professor in the College of Veterinary Medicine, North Carolina State University. Since 1994, her main area of research is Marek's disease focusing on pathogenesis, diagnosis, and control. She has authored or co-authored over 40 peer reviewed publications, 5 book chapters, over 60 other publications, and has given 28 invited presentations in various countries. She has been supporting the poultry industry with Marek's disease diagnosis and control strategies throughout her professional career.

Roser Dolz Pascual

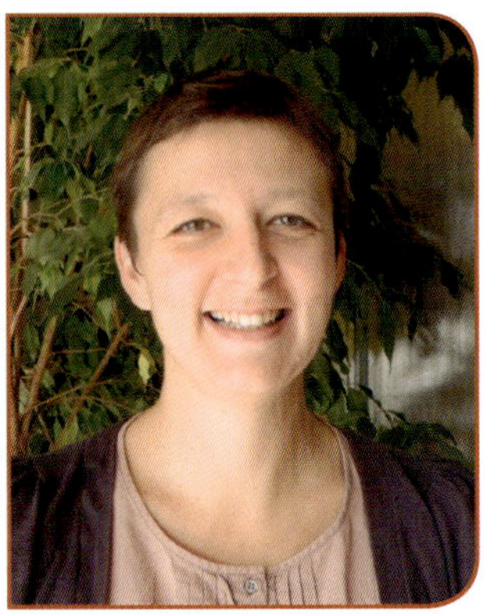

Dr. Roser Dolz Pascual received her Veterinary Degree (2001), MS (2004), and PhD (2007) from *Universitat Autònoma de Barcelona*, Spain. She is currently a researcher in *Centre de Recerca en Sanitat Animal* (CReSA). Her main areas of research are focused on molecular epidemiology and pathogenesis of avian viral diseases, mainly Infectious Bursal Disease, Avian Infectious Bronchitis and Avian Influenza. Currently, she is also involved in several projects aimed to study risk factors and colonization dynamics of *Campylobacter* on poultry flocks. She has authored and co-authored over 20 peer reviewed publications and one book, and has given 10 invited presentations in Spain and other countries.

Oscar J. Fletcher

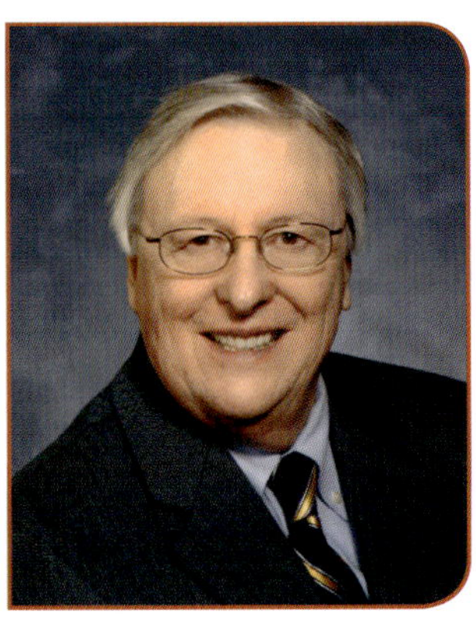

Dr. Oscar J. Fletcher has a BS degree from Wofford College (1960), DVM (1964) and MS (1965) degrees from the University of Georgia, and PhD from the University of Wisconsin, Madison (1968). In 1972, Dr. Fletcher moved to the Department of Avian Medicine in the College of Veterinary Medicine at the University of Georgia, where he devoted his professional efforts to avian pathology. He currently is a Professor in the Department of Population Health and Pathobiology at NC State University. He is also a member of the American Association of Avian Pathologists, member of the Editorial Board of Avian Diseases, Editor of the third edition of the Avian Histopathology Manual, Diplomate of the American College of Veterinary Pathologists and a founder diplomate of the American College of Poultry Veterinarians. He is author or co-author of over 140 publications in refereed journals, 14 book chapters, over 60 other publications, and has given 27 invited presentations in the US and other countries.

Natàlia Majó Masferrer

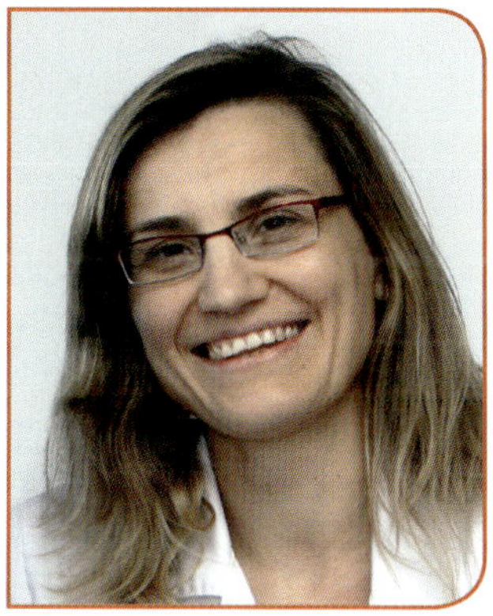

Dr. Natàlia Majó Masferrer obtained her Veterinary Degree (1992) and PhD (1996) from *Universitat Autònoma de Barcelona*, Spain. She is also a Diplomate of the European College of Veterinary Pathologists since 2000. She is currently assistant professor at the Veterinary School in the *Universitat Autònoma de Barcelona*. In 2002, she joined CReSA (Research centre in animal health) and, since then, all her research activity has been carried out in this institution where she is responsible of the research group on avian viruses. Her main task as responsible of this group is to write and execute research projects and contracts funded by public bodies or external private companies and mainly related with viral diseases of poultry (avian influenza, infectious bronchitis virus and infectious bursal disease virus). She has published more than 60 peer reviewed scientific papers and has more than 150 contributions to national and international congresses.

Enrique Montiel

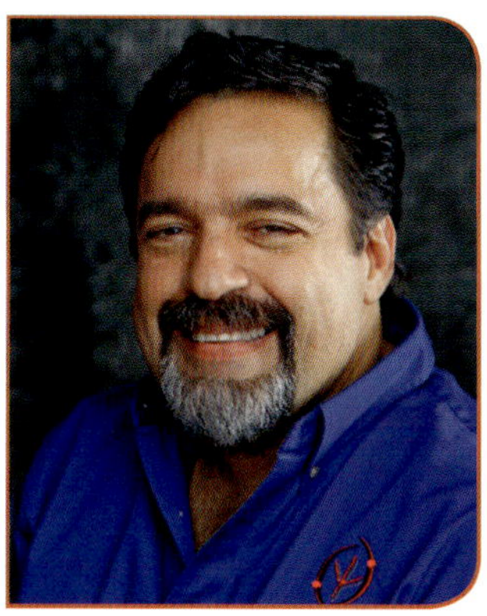

Dr. Enrique Montiel obtained his Veterinary Degree from the *Universidad del Zulia* in Maracaibo, Venezuela, in 1985. In 1995 he received a Master of Science degree from the University of Delaware in Newark DE, USA, working with Dr. J.K. Rosenberger on Marek's disease and other immunosuppressive diseases of poultry. He became a Diplomate of the American College of Poultry Veterinarians in 1997. Dr. Montiel has worked in the poultry industry around the world for more than 25 years and made contributions to research on various subjects, especially Marek's disease and Avian influenza. He is an adjunct faculty on various graduate poultry programs in the US and internationally. He currently works as a Senior Veterinarian for Merial Select in Gainesville, GA, USA.

Orlando Osuna

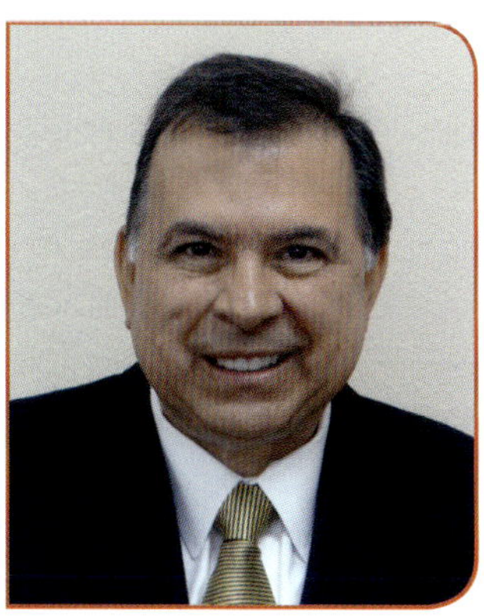

Dr. Orlando Osuna obtained his Doctor Degree in Veterinary Medicine at the National University of Colombia in 1969. Later, in United States, he received his Master of Science and PhD degree at the University of Florida. He is a Diplomate of the American College of Poultry Veterinarians and has worked as a Visiting Professor at the University of Florida, Texas A&M University, and Tokyo University. Upon his return to Colombia, he developed 5-year collaborative research grant with the Japan International Cooperation Agency and the National University of Colombia on the evaluation of fishmeal quality and the toxic effects of gizzerosine in poultry. He also acted as President of AMEVEA, International Association of Poultry Specialists, from 1989 until 1998. At present, Dr. Osuna is the Director of the Health Science Division of Milwhite, Inc. in Brownsville, Texas, where he has the responsibility to provide technical service in Toxicology to Asia and Latin America.

Arun R. Pandiri

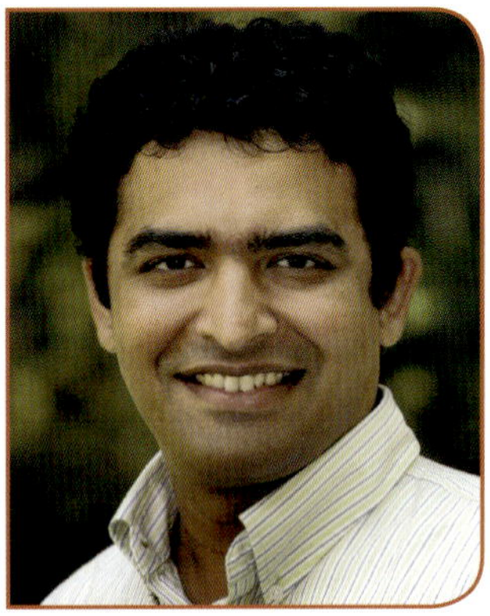

Dr. Arun R. Pandiri received his Veterinary Medical degree from ANGR Agricultural University, Hyderabad, India in 1998; MS from the University of Arkansas, Fayetteville, AR in 2000; and PhD from Michigan State University, East Lansing, MI in 2005. He completed his pathology residency at North Carolina State University, Raleigh, NC and is a Diplomate of the American College of Veterinary Pathologists since 2008. He is currently a pathologist at the Experimental Pathology Laboratories, Inc., in Research Triangle Park, NC. His research interests include tumorigenesis, and avian pathology. Most of his research on tumor viral diseases has been conducted at the USDA-ARS Avian Disease and Oncology Laboratory, East Lansing, MI and North Carolina State University. He is currently the Chair of the Tumor Virus Committee at the American Association of Avian Pathologists.

K.A. (Ton) Schat

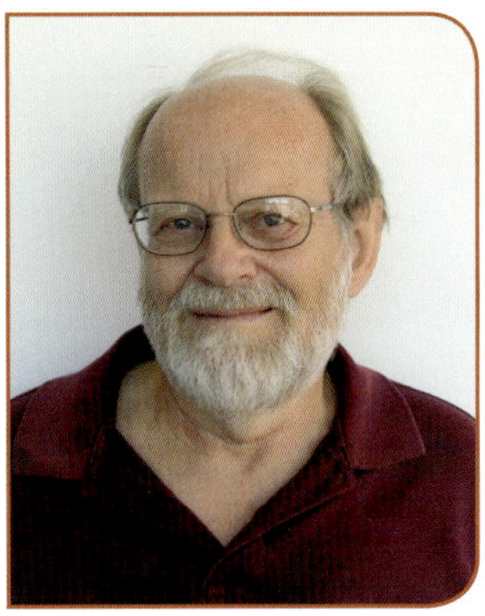

Professor Emeritus K.A. (Ton) Schat received his Veterinary Degree from the University of Utrecht, The Netherlands, in 1970, and his PhD degree in Virology from Cornell University, Ithaca, New York, in 1978. He joined the faculty at the College of Veterinary Medicine, Cornell University in 1978, where he remained until his retirement in 2011. His research focused on the immunology and pathogenesis of viral diseases of poultry, especially Marek's disease and chicken infectious anemia. He has published over 170 papers in peer-reviewed journals and more than 30 book chapters. His contributions to avian disease research were recently recognized by his induction as a founding member of the Hall of Honour of the World Veterinary Poultry Association.

Joan A. Smyth

Dr. Joan A. Smyth received her Veterinary Degree (with honors) from University College Dublin, Ireland, in 1980 and her PhD in 1988 from Queens University Belfast, N. Ireland, for studies on Egg Drop Syndrome '76 (EDS) of laying hens. She is a diplomate of the European College of Veterinary Pathologists. She has over 30 years experience in animal disease investigation and research, and has a particular interest and specialist skills in avian diseases. She worked for 24 years in the Veterinary Sciences Division, Department of Agriculture, Stormont, N. Ireland, and is currently a professor in Department of Pathobiology and Veterinary Science, University of Connecticut. In addition to her early work on EDS, she has carried out research on several major diseases of poultry including chicken infectious anemia, enteric diseases including necrotic enteritis of chickens, as well as emerging avian circoviral infections. She was an Editor with the journal Avian Pathology for 13 years and for many years was a member and committee member of the British Poultry Veterinary Association, and a member of the Poultry Association of N. Ireland. She is author or co-author of 89 peer reviewed articles in scientific journals, has written reviews and book chapters on poultry diseases, and has spoken at many local, national and international conferences on her research.

Guillermo Zavala

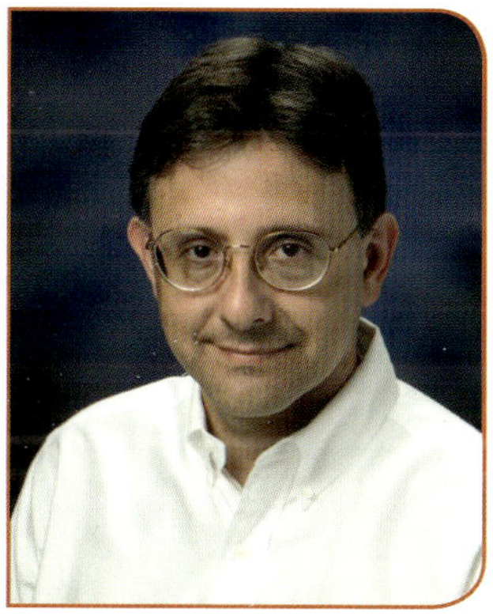

Dr. Guillermo Zavala received his Veterinary Degree from the National Autonomous University of Mexico (UNAM), a Master of Avian Medicine from the University of Georgia, and a MSc and PhD on Medical Microbiology, from the same University. He has participated in projects on Molecular Virology of Retroviruses in the University of Georgia and on Eradication of Oncogenic Avian retroviruses in the University of Melbourne (Australia). He has also worked as a veterinarian in several laboratories, always within the Poultry Division, and currently works as an associate professor at the University of Georgia, United States, where he is responsible for the clinical poultry service. Moreover, he often works in multiple countries of the Americas, Europe, North Africa and Asia. His research interests focus on Applied clinical virology, Control of infectious diseases, Interactions between management and disease, Oncogenic viruses, Infectious Laryngotracheitis, Enteric viruses, Clinical virology and Viral pathogenesis.

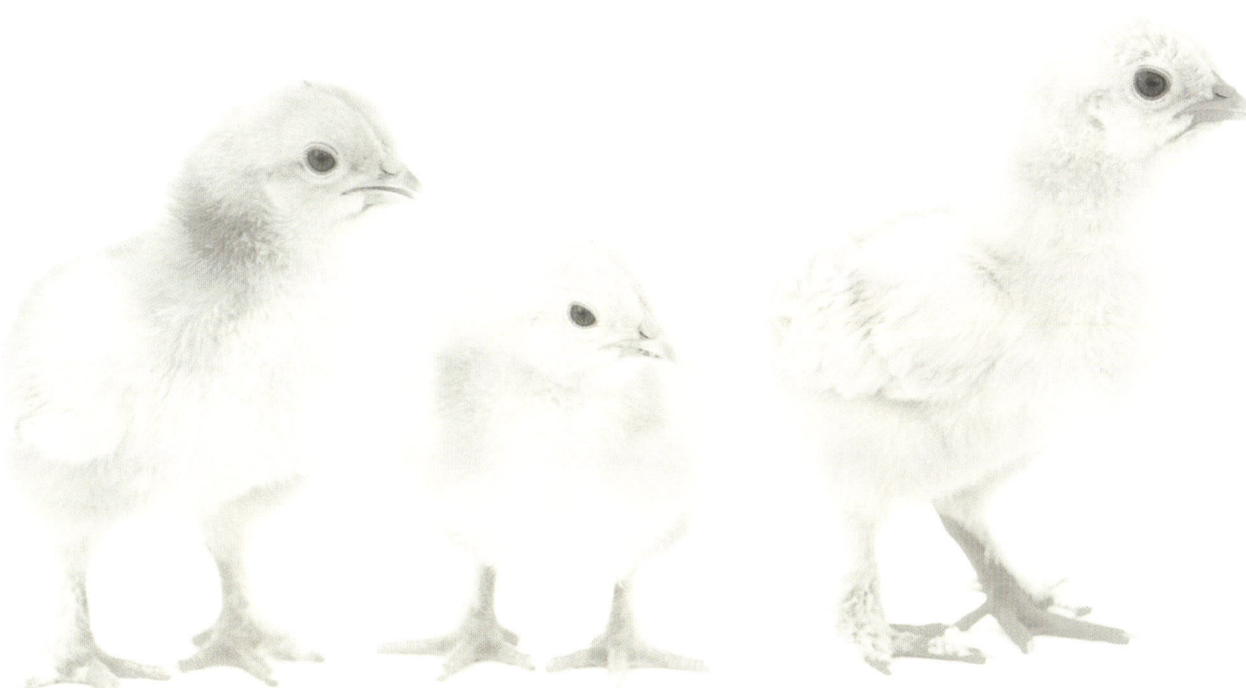

PREFACE

Healthy poultry with a competent immune system is the key for success in the poultry industry. However, the chicken immune system is target of a variety of infectious and non-infectious factors leading to immunosuppression. Immunosuppression is often overlooked since it may not be accompanied by specific clinical signs or lesions but nevertheless its negative effects are seen in production. The mechanisms behind the immunosuppression are complex and may depend on a single etiology or a synergistic combination of etiologies contributing to the immunosuppressive status. Immunosuppression is a complex disease comprised of innate, cell mediated and humoral immune response. Under field conditions, serology (humoral immune response) is commonly used to monitor the health status of poultry that may implicate specific infectious causes for decreased production. However, other aspects of the immune response are not monitored under field conditions due to the lack of proper methods of assessment of the immune function, and as a result immunosuppression in poultry cannot be easily diagnosed or quantified. This book attempts to compile the current knowledge on the most common immunosuppressive diseases of chickens. Immunosuppressive diseases of turkeys and other poultry species are not covered in this book. It is the intention of the authors to provide guidance for the diagnosis of immunosuppressive diseases, and examine the challenges that a diagnostician may face in confirming a diagnosis of immunosuppression. It is the aim of the authors to also emphasize those areas that require more research for a proper diagnosis and control of immunosuppressive diseases. This book features an extensive collection of color photographs depicting the gross and microscopic images, and the text provides background information and practical tips in identifying immunosuppression in poultry under laboratory and field conditions.

The authors of various chapters in this book are recognized leaders in their respective areas of research. I would like to acknowledge their contributions as well as their advice and expertise in the planning and execution of this book. The poultry industry is global and for the benefit of wider audience, this book will be published simultaneously in English and Spanish. The efforts of all the bilingual authors to ensure an accurate translation are greatly appreciated. I finally want to thank Prof. Pedro Villegas for writing the foreword of this book. Prof. Villegas have dedicated his entire career to study poultry diseases both in the laboratory and in the field and his kind words in the foreword are highly appreciated.

Isabel Gimeno

Editor

FOREWORD

It is an honor to be invited to write the foreword of this book dealing with the Immunosuppressive Diseases of Poultry. The Editor, Dr. Isabel Gimeno, has done an excellent job selecting the topics and the authors for each of the chapters in this book.

The chapter on histopathology of immunosuppressive diseases, written by Dr. Oscar Fletcher, is an excellent teaching illustration of the appropriate way to approach the diagnosis of these diseases. The lesion scoring system used to evaluate the microscopic lesions produced by several avian viruses is very useful and hopefully will help to standardize the numerical scale used by avian histopathologists worldwide. Dr. Fletcher also emphasizes the lack of actual and practical methods to measure immunosuppression, therefore we predict and make presumptive diagnoses of immunosuppression based on several morphological changes in tissues, mainly the decrease in the number of lymphocytes and the damage that is observed (necrosis, apoptosis). The description of changes observed in tissues such as bursa of Fabricius, thymus, spleen, and liver are very helpful to differentiate diseases such as Marek's disease, lymphoid leucosis, reticuloendotheliosis, chicken infectious anemia and, of course, infectious bursal disease. To arrive at a useful final diagnosis, it is emphasized that proper collection and selection of tissues is very important to avoid postmortem tissue artifacts. This chapter in avian histopathology is a "real useful jewel" that should be consulted and carefully reviewed to properly understand the efforts that avian histopathologists go through to arrive at a final diagnosis.

Among the noninfectious factors that play major roles on the immune system, the mycotoxins and stress factors are very well described in chapter 2. Dr. Orlando Osuna indicates that approximately 25 % of the world grain supply is contaminated with mycotoxins that are the most dietary immunosuppressive factors. Each mycotoxin is described along with their respective manifestations and clinical signs, as well as their effect on the chicken's immune system. Field diagnosis of mycotoxins is very difficult even when there is full expression of the condition. Moreover, their main effects are subclinical diseases that are even more difficult to diagnose.

The effect of stress induced by environmental conditions on the immune system is less understood, as described by Dr. Enrique Montiel in chapter 2. It is known that stress will affect the immune and endocrine systems but, again, the methods to evaluate these effects are still not practical to be used routinely by the poultry industry. The use of additives or products such as antioxidants, probiotics, vitamins and minerals is common in the industry in an attempt to ameliorate some deficiencies that may result from stress conditions. Again, the methods to evaluate stress-induced immunosuppression are listed and can be used to observe the decrease of antibody levels, heterophil/lymphocyte ratio, relative lymphoid organ weights, and others, but as indicated before, these are indirect methods that allow us to predict immunosuppression.

Infectious bursal disease virus (IBDV) has always been associated with immunosuppression due to its effect on the lymphocytes and "disarrangement of the chicken immune system", to use the words described by the authors, Drs. Natàlia Majó and Roser Dolz. The viruses classified in serotype 1 infect chickens and their virulence varies from mild to very virulent strains. The variant strains are also included in this serotype. The authors describe the genetic diversity of the virus, indicating that the VP1 protein seems to play a significant role in pathogenicity; however, the routine diagnosis of IBDV is based on VP2 sequences. The differential diagnosis of the disease is presented in a table that shows the lesions observed in various other avian diseases. Images of macro and microscopic lesions are also included, and the list of references includes both peer and non peer reviewed publications.

Chapter 4 on chicken infectious anemia (CIAV), written by Drs. Joan Smyth and Ton Schat, is a complete and updated review of this important immunosuppressive disease. Contrary to infectious bursal disease, B cells are considered not susceptible to infection with CIAV. The resistance of this virus to high temperatures and many chemical agents, added to the ability to transmit both vertically and horizontally, and the suggestion that the virus can remain latent, help explain its worldwide presence. The VP3 protein or apoptin has gained importance due to its ability to induce apoptosis in mammalian transformed cells but not in normal cells making it a potential anticancer agent in the future. The control of this disease is currently done by vaccination of the breeding stock during the growing period. Several vaccines are available and so far there is only one serotype and one genotype.

Chapter 5 on Marek's disease infection, written by Drs. Isabel Gimeno and Arun Pandiri, describes the infection and its associated syndromes (lymphomas, neurological, lymphoproliferative, arteriosclerosis). The authors should be commended for organizing the material included in the tables regarding virus-host cell interactions, pathogenesis of the infection, differential diagnosis of tumor viral diseases, and sequence of critical events for immunization. This is also true for the images and illustrations included in the chapter. Each section is updated and well written. The evolution of this virus with the increase of virulence seen with some strains, their ability to break the protection provided by the vaccines, their increase immunosuppressive potential requires more research to be able to properly control this disease.

Chapter 6 on reticuloendotheliosis (RE) and other immunosuppressive viruses, written by Dr. Guillermo Zavala, includes probably the most complete and updated description of the reticuloendotheliosis virus (REV). The author summarizes the important features in REV pathogenesis: the infection can be transmitted vertically, horizontally or iatrogenically; there is persistent or intermittent viremia; transformation of B or T cells; and, of course, severe immunosuppression. RE outbreaks are not commonly seen and the disease is difficult to diagnose since gross and microscopic pathology are not enough to accurately arrive at a diagnoses. Other viruses described as immunosuppressive include reovirus, adenovirus, lymphoid leukosis and fowlpox (when proviral sequences of REV are inserted).

In summary, the recent and updated information presented in this book is and will be a very good contribution to the knowledge in the control of avian diseases in general. The Editor and the authors are all experts in their respective fields and took time from their busy schedules to organize and present excellent information that will be very useful for the readers. This is a very good initial edition that should be reviewed and updated in future years.

Pedro Villegas
Professor Emeritus, University of Georgia,
United States of America

TABLE OF CONTENTS

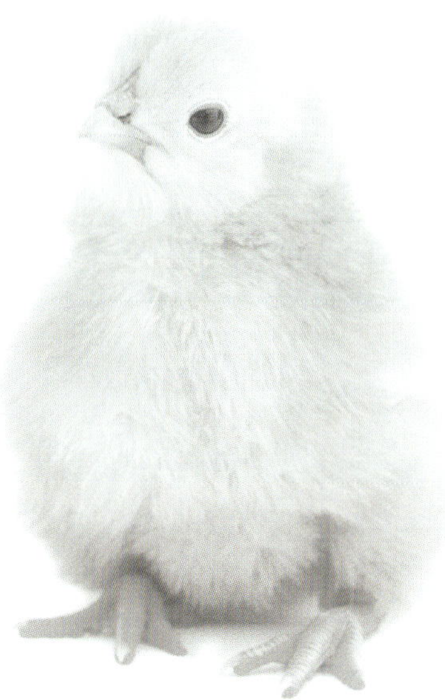

CHAPTER 1

INTRODUCTION: HISTOPATHOLOGY OF IMMUNOSUPPRESSION IN CHICKENS

Oscar J. Fletcher

Introduction

Histologic lesions in lymphoid organs of chickens are associated with immunosuppression. This hypothesis is supported by at least three broad areas of documentation showing correlations between lesions in the bursa of Fabricius (BF), thymus, spleen, and other peripheral collections of lymphocytes with failure to respond to antigenic stimulation by circulating antibody production and/or cell-mediated immunity. These areas of research and/or clinical case reports are:

1. Experimental studies showing immunosuppression following removal or damage to lymphoid organs. Examples are the effects of bursectomy on antibody production described in the classic paper published in 1956 by Glick, Chang, and Jaap [21], research done by Warner et al. on the separation of functions of thymus and BF [71,72], and the studies by Cooper et al. on surgical removal of the BF and/or thymus followed by X irradiation. [11] Readers are referred to several reviews [9,20,62] among the many available.
2. Reports documenting lesions in lymphoid organs and failures of immune system responses in chickens with spontaneous or experimentally induced diseases including infectious bursal disease (IBD), chicken anemia virus (CAV), avian leukosis [45], Marek's disease (MD) [5], aflatoxicosis [27], vitamin A deficiency [4], and stress. [15] Associations between diseases, lesions in lymphoid organs, and immunosuppression were reviewed by Hoerr [27] and Pope. [47,48]
3. Systematic evaluation with subjective scoring of lesions in lymphoid organs in chickens submitted to a state diagnostic laboratory for diagnosis of spontaneous diseases and/or health monitoring allowed temporal associations to be made between lymphoid organ lesions early in life followed by a variety of disease conditions in older chickens. [27] Reports by Toro et al. [66,67] provide examples.

It is important to note that histopathology does not provide direct measurement of immune function. Antibody and cell mediated immune responses to antigenic stimulation are not measured by observation of tissue changes. Reliable, rapid tests for measuring immune function on poultry farms are not available yet; thus, indirect assessments that include gross examination, organ and body weight measurements, and collection of tissues for histopathology are the standard methods used currently.

Histopathology is not enough by itself for assessing immune function. Further tests are required.

It is reasonable, based on the broad lines of evidence presented above, to assume that lesions in lymphoid organs may result in immunosuppression. As an example, Calnek et al. [8] included necrosis and atrophy of BF, thymus, and spleen among the criteria used to assess immunosuppression in MD. However, there will be cases in which immunosuppression is present with no appreciable lesions in lymphoid organs, see Cooper et al. [11] for an example, and there will be cases in which lymphoid organ lesions are not associated with measurable loss of immune function. [54]

Lesions in the major lymphoid organs –BF, thymus, and spleen– are described and illustrated in this chapter. Lesions may be present in other nodular and diffuse collections of lymphocytes including the head-associated lymphoid tissue (HALT) –that includes the conjunctival-associated lymphoid tissue (CALT) and the Harderian gland–, the bronchial-associated lymphoid tissue (BALT), and the gut-associated lymphoid tissue (GALT). These secondary collections should be examined, but are not part of routine protocols.

Apart from the lesions described, lymphocyte infiltration and hyperplasia as part of an inflammatory response occurs, but is very difficult to evaluate in the major lymphoid organs. Increased numbers of lymphocytes in the interfollicular tissue of the BF is one example of lymphocytic inflammation that can be visualized with hematoxylin and eosin stains (H&E). Death of lymphocytes often is followed by atrophy of the major lymphoid organs. IBD,

CAV and MD, as well as the mycotoxins, are of major importance because the causative agents/toxins are so widespread and there is extensive documentation to support their ability to cause immunosuppression. So, they need to be considered in the differential diagnosis when early lesions –lymphocyte loss, inflammation, and reticular hyperplasia– are present.

Readers are referred to the following sections for more detailed descriptions and additional illustrations of lesions associated with the specific entities.

LESIONS COMMON TO THE THREE MAJOR LYMPHOID ORGANS (BF, THYMUS AND SPLEEN)

- Loss of lymphocytes.
- Inflammation including presence of heterophils.
- Increased numbers of macrophages or histiocytes.
- Hyperplasia of reticular cells.
- Fibrosis.

Lesion scoring

Histopathology on standard H&E stained sections of BF, thymus, and spleen is an important component of methods for lymphoid system evaluation and is usually accompanied by subjective scoring of lesions. There are a number of reports on scoring systems and a selected subset are referenced here. [17,25,26,28,42,53,67]

Lesion scoring is any system in which descriptive terms are converted to numbers. The number reflects a subjective judgment, but is reasonably repeatable, especially between mild and severe lesions and when done by one with experience in evaluating avian tissues. Agreement between different pathologists evaluating the same BF sections was less than ideal [43] and is indicative of the need to improve criteria for subjective scoring methods.

It is important that the criteria for each number used in the scoring system be stated clearly. Systems have used 0 or 1 to equal normal or no lesions. A 1 to 4 scale [53] (Table 1) is used commonly for scoring lesions in the BF. The regular pattern of lymphoid follicles within the plicae of the BF provides an excellent organ for lesion scoring. A scoring system with normal = 1, mild loss of lymphocytes = 2; moderate loss of lymphocytes = 3 and severe or diffuse loss of lymphocytes = 4 is used often for scoring of lesions in the thymus. The same general method of scoring can be used to report spleen lesions. The spleen is the most difficult of the three major lymphoid organs to score because of the more complex microanatomy and overall response of the spleen to injury.

In general, ease of use and reproducibility are better if the scoring system is made as simple as possible; thus, using one number for one single item is preferred. Combining multiple lesions into one number is more complicated, harder to reproduce, and confusing. One must consider the time spent doing lesion scoring to the benefit gained ratio and remember that lesion scores are not direct measurements of immune system function. Subjective scores require nonparametric statistics for analysis because the data is ordinal.

Specific recommendations to set up and apply lesion scoring systems*:

- Use a number to represent a morphologic description or specific lesion.
- Assign numbers to each specific item or response of interest rather than combining multiple responses into one score.
- Develop a scoring scale for each organ of interest because each organ has its own unique histology that is likely to influence the patterns of injury.

As an example, estimates of loss of lymphocytes due to either increased apoptosis or necrosis are made by using a number to represent the subjective judgment of the pathologist as to extent of the loss. Thus, no apparent loss is assigned a value of 1; mild loss assigned a value of 2; moderate loss a value of 3; and severe loss a value of 4. The lesion pattern is scored using 2 to equal focal; 3 for mutifocal; and 4 for diffuse. Accounting for multiple lesions can be made easy to apply by assigning a number to each specific lesion of interest. Absence of the lesion is given a score of 1 and presence of the lesion given a score of 2. Summed lesion scores for the organ are then multiplied by the overall extent score to give the total score for the organ. A comparison of an overall subjective method and a multiple lesion evaluation method is provided (Table 1).

Examples of scoring methods for each major lymphoid organ are given below. The lesions listed for each organ are those routinely considered to be of interest. However, additional lesions can be added as desired and the minimum and maximum score adjusted accordingly.

* These suggestions are based on a number of years of experience in evaluating responses to injury in both experimentally controlled conditions and in field case material.

Bursa of Fabricius

The easiest and simplest approach uses the overall subjective impression method (Table 1) with a 1 to 4 (or 0 to 4) scale to reflect the extent of follicular damage.

The multiple lesions method scores the absence (score = 1) or presence (score = 2) of the lesions listed below. Extent is recorded using a 2, 3, or 4 scale.

The multiple lesions method evaluates the following lesions of interest in BF:

- Necrosis or increased apoptosis of follicular lymphocytes.
- Expansion of interfollicular tissue.
- Epithelial hyperplasia.
- Heterophils.
- Edema and/or fibrin.
- Hemorrhage.
- Macrophages.
- Cysts.
- Atrophy of follicles.

The total score per section is the sum of the individual lesion scores multiplied by the overall extent score. The minimum score = 9 (9 x 1) using the lesions listed above and represents a normal BF. The maximum score = 72 (18 x 4) and represents severe damage.

Thymus

The overall subjective impression method (Table 1) uses a 1 to 4 (or 0 to 4) scale to score lymphocyte loss. A score can be recorded for cortex and for medulla, but usually loss of lymphocytes in both cortex and medulla is combined and reported as one score.

The multiple lesions method evaluates the following lesions of interest in thymus:

- Increased apoptosis or necrosis of lymphocytes.
- Hemorrhage.
- Macrophages.
- Atrophy.

Extent is then scored using 2 = focal, 3 = multifocal, and 4 = diffuse. The sum of the lesion scores is multiplied by the extent score to generate the total score for the section. Cortex and medulla can be scored separately, but it is more efficient to generate one score. The minimum score (normal) for the lesions listed is 4 and the maximum is 32 (severe).

Table1. Summary of two general methods for lesion scoring.

A. SINGLE NUMBER OR OVERALL SUBJECTIVE IMPRESSION METHOD		
NUMBER ASSIGNED (Preferred by author)	NUMBER ASSIGNED (Alternative approach and used frequently)	CRITERIA
1	0	• Normal • No lesions
2	1	• Focal • < 25 % of follicles involved
3	2	• Multifocal • 25-50 % of follicles involved
4	3	• Diffuse • > 50 % of follicles involved
	4 (optional)	• Diffuse • Acute necrosis

B. MULTIPLE LESIONS METHOD			
NUMBER ASSIGNED TO EACH LESION OF INTEREST	CRITERIA	DISTRIBUTION OR EXTENT (NUMBER ASSIGNED)	CRITERIA
1	• Not present	2	• Focal
2	• Present	3	• Multifocal
		4	• Diffuse

Spleen

The impression of overall lymphocyte loss is reported using the 1-4 (0-4) scale in the overall subjective impression method (Table 1).

The multiple lesions method evaluates the following lesions of interest in spleen:

- Apoptosis or necrosis of lymphocytes.
- Increase in reticular cells (histiocytes).
- Accumulation of fibrin or fibrinoid necrosis.
- Proliferation of neoplastic lymphocytes.

Scores for Periarteriolar Lymphoid Sheath (PALS) and Periellipsoidal Lymphoid Sheath (PELS) can be reported separately, but this is not done routinely. The minimum score for this example of splenic lesion scoring is 4 (normal) and the maximum lesion is 32 (severe).

Morphometry

Histomorphometry provides objective data based on measurements of selected components of the lymphoid system such as diameter of bursal follicles, thickness of thymic cortex, or relative percent of dark and light stained cells in bursal follicles. [52,53,66] Determination of the mean gray value for selected areas of BF is another approach with theoretical promise. Mean gray value is based on measuring the gray value along a line or in a region of interest for each pixel using the 0 (black) to 255 (white) continuous scale. A major disadvantage of this approach is that the gray values of cells such as histiocytes or reticular cells that replace lost lymphocytes are very similar to lymphocytes.

Bursa of Fabricius (BF)

The normal BF (Fig. 1) has multiple plicae or folds covered by epithelial cells and filled with lymphoid follicles. The plical epithelium is regular (Fig. 1b) with few, if any, folds. A specialized region of more flattened plical epithelium may be seen in close association with individual follicles. Follicles have distinct cortical and medullary compartments that are separated by thin bands of interfollicular connective tissue (Figs. 1c-f). Pyknotic cells are scattered in the cortex and medulla and are remnants of cells undergoing apoptosis or programmed cell death. Evaluation of increased apoptosis is a difficult assessment and differentiation between apoptotic cells and cells undergoing necrosis is not possible unless special techniques are used. The regular pattern of follicle distribution and relatively uniform size of follicles in normal bursae makes lesion scoring of the BF easier than scoring of either thymic or spleen lesions.

Variations of follicle size and mild expansion of interfollicular tissue are encountered frequently. A lesion score of 2 using the 1 to 4 scale described above is illustrated in Figures 2a, c and e. Bursae may have uniform, but small, follicles (Figs. 2b, d and f). In relatively young chickens (14 days in Figure 2), this observation probably represents hypoplasia rather than atrophy. An example of focal bursal atrophy with score = 2 on a 1 to 4 scale is illustrated in figure 3. This is a common observation, is not disease specific, and likely not associated with immunosuppression.

Focal to multifocal necrosis of lymphocytes in the cortex and medulla of bursal follicles (Fig. 4) is observed frequently. These lesions are not disease specific, but infection with MDV [8] is one differential. There are several possibilities for a lesion score in this example. The patchy distribution with relatively few affected follicles would justify a score of 2 (1-4 scale). The presence of acute necrosis (score = 2) and presence of some heterophils (score = 2) (Fig. 4d) would justify a score of 8 if using the multiple lesions method with a score 2 for focal distribution (2 + (2 x 2) = 8). This approach provides for differentiation between focal atrophy (Fig. 3) and focal acute necrosis with some inflammation (Fig. 4).

IBD is a well documented and classic example of an immunosuppressive disease in which the primary target cells are lymphocytes in the BF. [16,37,38,56,61] Responses of the BF to injury are illustrated by the range of lesions caused by IBDV. [19,56,57,63,70,73] Field isolates [19,39,50,63] and vaccine stains of IBDV vary in ability to cause bursal lesions and immunosuppression. [39,50] IBD is characterized by necrosis of lymphocytes in both the medulla and cortex of bursal follicles, expansion of the interfollicular connective tissue by edema, fibrin, heterophils, and macrophages (Fig. 5) and, in some cases, erythrocytes. Diffuse lesions (Figs. 5-7) are typical of classical lesions of IBD, but may be focal or multifocal (Fig. 8). Hyperplasia of plical epithelium (Fig. 5) is common. Some follicles may become cystic (Fig. 9). Cysts may persist in mutifocal areas. Spared or regenerating follicles [35] are prominent (Fig. 10) among the smaller atrophic follicles in many cases of IBD. Acute lesions are followed by atrophy of follicles and fibrosis of the interfollicular tissue (Figs. 11-14).

Severe, diffuse epithelial hyperplasia with intralesional protozoa is characteristic of bursal cryptosporidiosis [7,18,22,49,51] (Fig. 15). Diffuse atrophy (score = 4) is also commonly associated with bursal cryptosporidiosis. It is uncertain if bursal atrophy preceded infection by cryptosporidia.

Expansion of the interfollicular connective tissue by neoplastic lymphocytes (Fig. 16) is characteristic of lymphomas of MD. This location of proliferating tumor cells is, in contrast to the intrafollicular lymphoid neoplasia of lymphoid leukosis (LL) [10,12,14,46] and lymphoid tumors in the BF, caused by reticuloendotheliosis virus (REV). [2,44] MD lymphoma in the BF is associated with loss of cortical and medullary lymphocytes and atrophy of BF follicles (Figs. 16d-f).

Bursal lesions typical of clinical case submissions are illustrated in Figure 17. Lesions range from none (score = 1) (Fig. 17b), through focal (score = 2) (Fig. 17c), multifocal or moderate (score = 3) (Fig. 17d) to diffuse or severe (score = 4) (Figs. 17e and f). On the basis of this range of lesions, one could predict that such a flock would have immunosuppression. Prediction of immunosuppression is just a prediction without actual measurements of immune system function. Increased incidence of diseases as the flock ages provides support for the theory of immunosuppression. The lesions illustrated in Figure 17 are not disease specific, but are consistent with IBD.

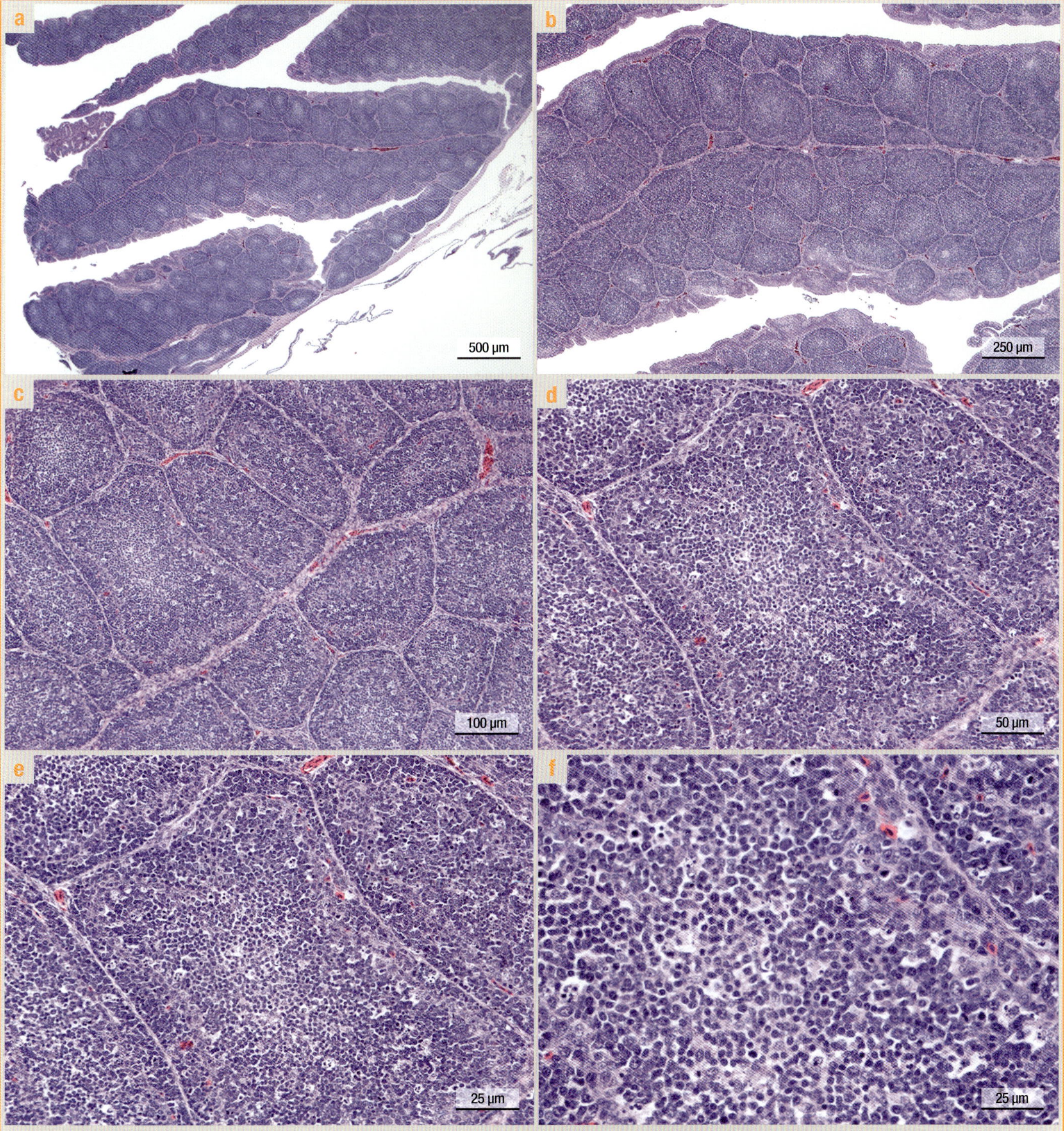

Fig. 1 Normal bursa of Fabricius from a 14 day-old broiler chicken shows plicae filled with relatively uniform follicles. Cortex and medulla are shown in higher magnifications. Interfollicular connective tissue is thin. (a) Bar = 500 μm. (b) Bar = 250 μm. (c) Bar = 100 μm. (d) Bar = 50 μm. (e) Bar = 25 μm. (f). Bar = 25 μm.

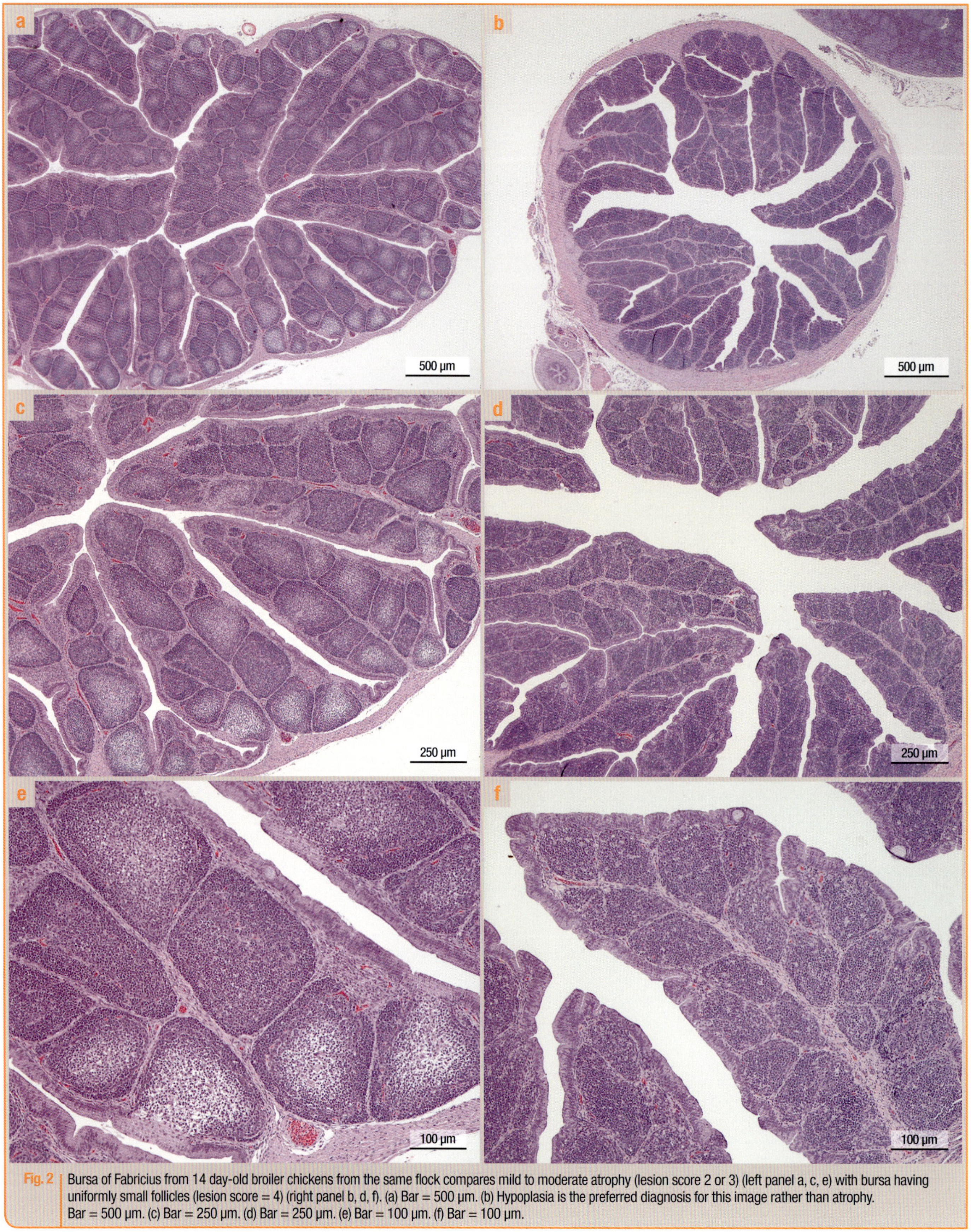

Fig. 2 Bursa of Fabricius from 14 day-old broiler chickens from the same flock compares mild to moderate atrophy (lesion score 2 or 3) (left panel a, c, e) with bursa having uniformly small follicles (lesion score = 4) (right panel b, d, f). (a) Bar = 500 µm. (b) Hypoplasia is the preferred diagnosis for this image rather than atrophy. Bar = 500 µm. (c) Bar = 250 µm. (d) Bar = 250 µm. (e) Bar = 100 µm. (f) Bar = 100 µm.

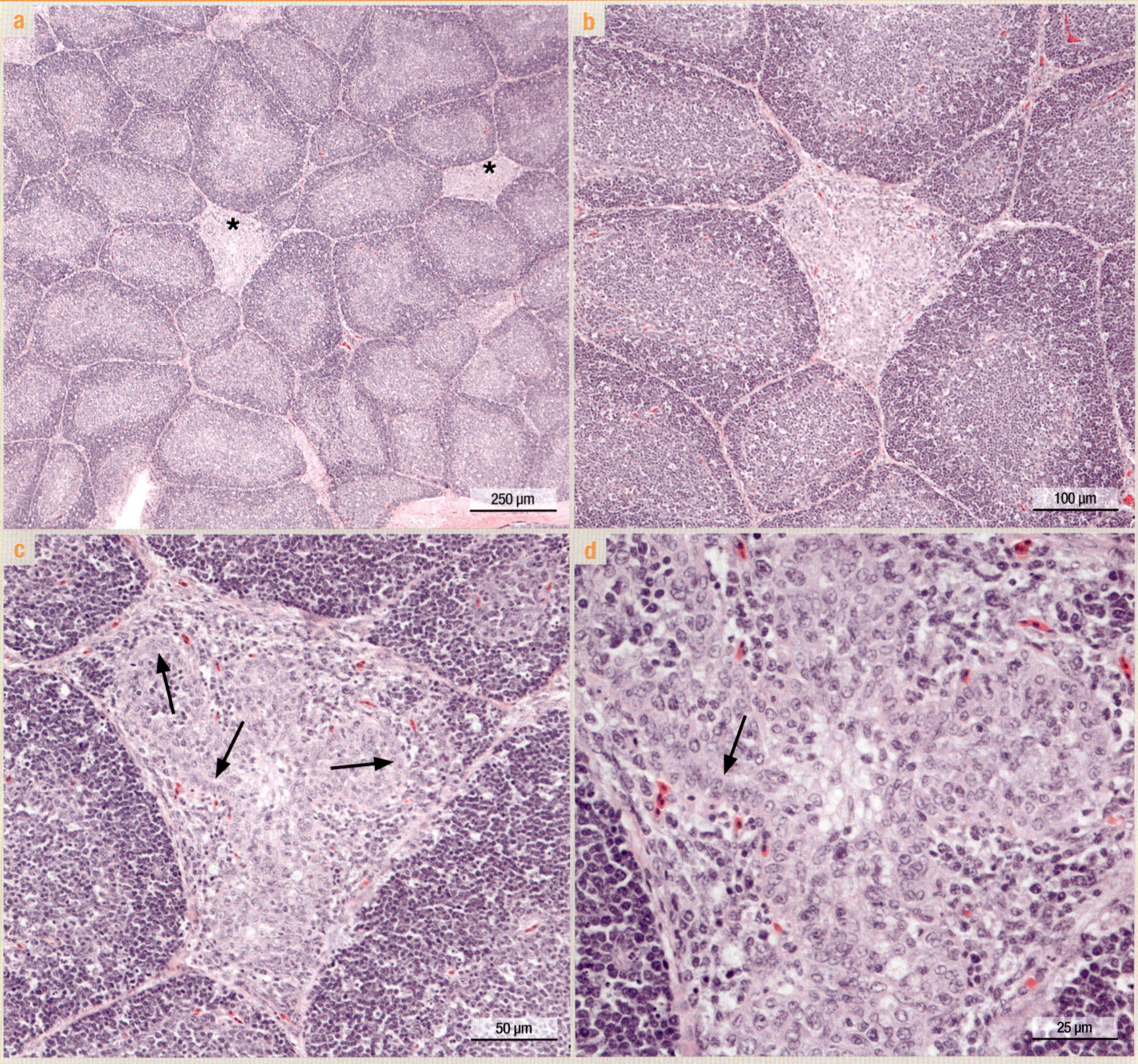

Fig. 3 Bursa of Fabricius from a 34 day-old broiler shows few atrophic follicles scattered among relatively uniform follicles. This is an example of focal atrophy and the lesion score is 2. (a) Asterisks identify atrophic follicles. Bar = 250 µm. (b) Bar = 100 µm. (c) Arrows identify the layer of epithelial cells separating medulla from cortex. Bar = 50 µm. (d) Arrow identifies epithelial cells separating medulla from cortex. Bar = 25 µm.

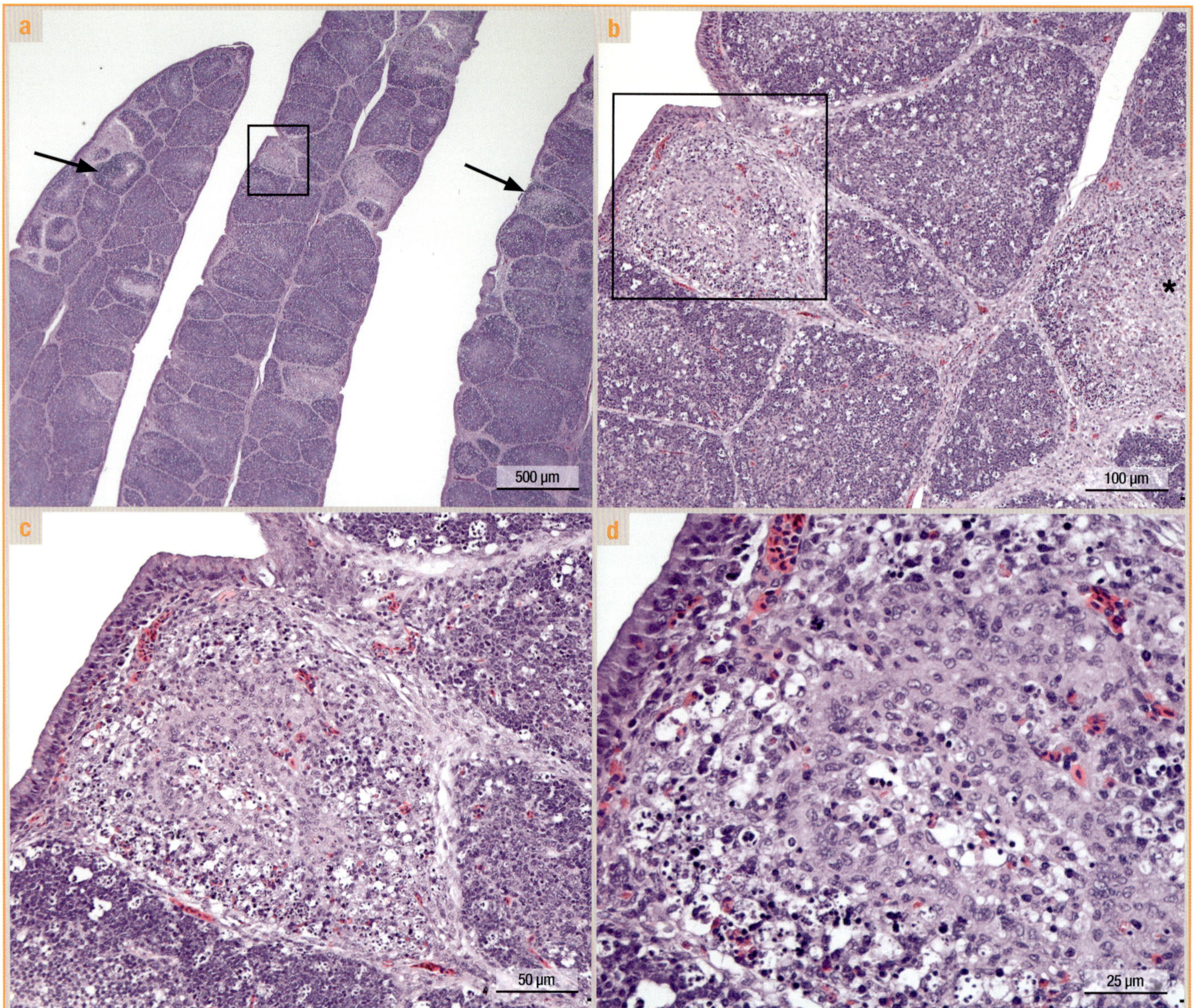

Fig. 4 Bursa of Fabricius from a 21 day-old broiler chicken shows multifocal necrosis (arrows) and loss of cortical and medullary lymphocytes. The lesion score 2 is using the single number, subjective impression method, and 8 is using the multiple lesions method. Box shows follicle with lesions. (a) Bar = 500 µm. (b) Follicle (box) has loss of lymphocytes with acute necrosis and scattered heterophils. Adjacent follicle (*) has diffuse loss of lymphocytes in medulla and severe loss in cortex. Bar = 100 µm. (c) Bar = 50 µm. (d) Bar = 25 µm.

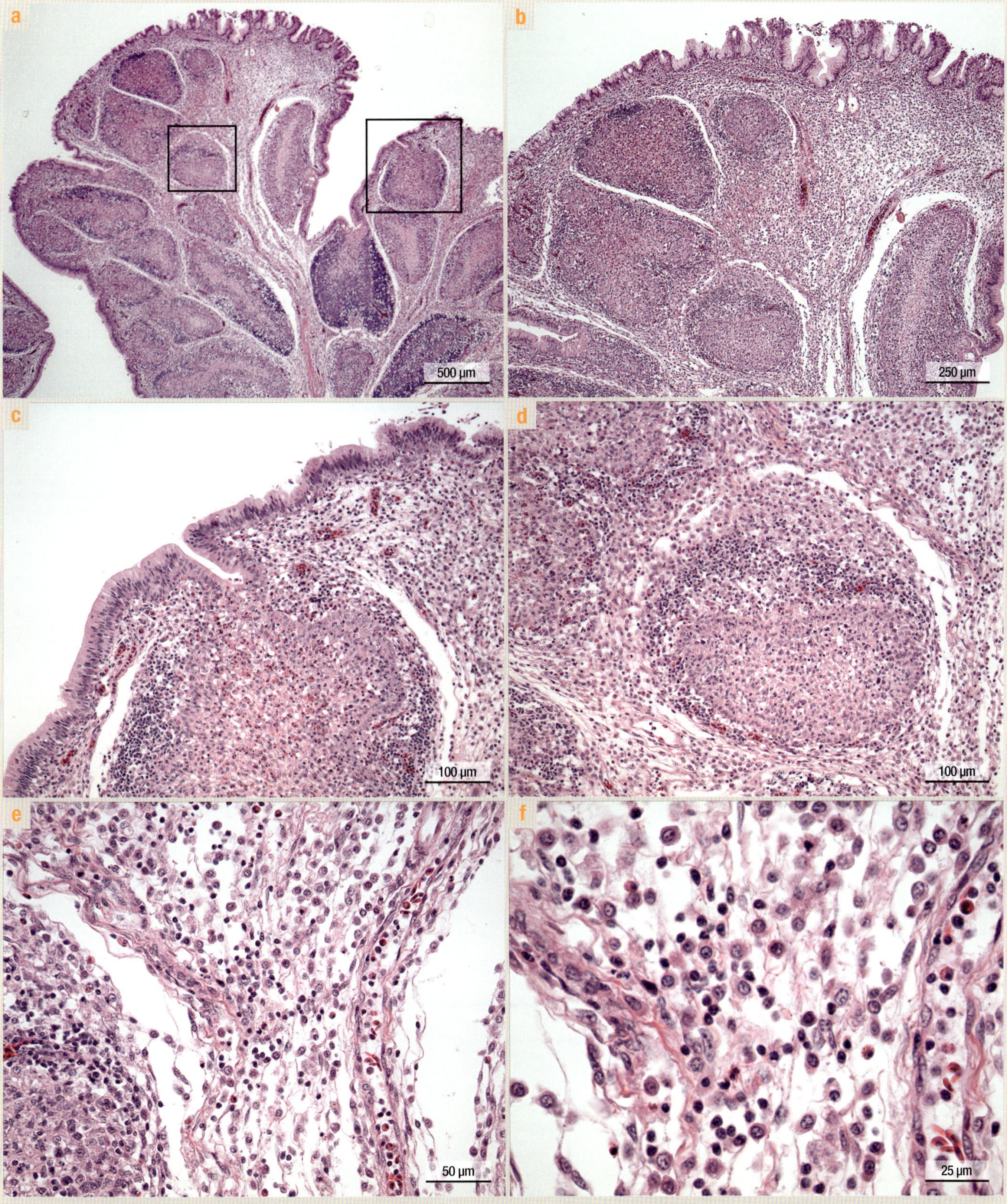

Fig. 5 Bursa of Fabricius from a chicken; age and type not known. Lesions are typical of IBD and illustrate diffuse necrosis of bursal lymphocytes accompanied by expansion of the interfollicular connective tissue due to edema and inflammatory cell infiltration. Plical epithelium is irregular with many small folds. Lesion score is 4.
(a) Regions in the boxes are shown in higher magnifications in (b) and (d). Bar = 500 µm. (b) Bar = 250 µm. (c) Bar = 100 µm. (d) Bar = 100 µm.
(e) Expanded interfollicular tissue. Bar = 50 µm. (f) Edema and inflammatory cells are in this expanded interfollicular region. Bar = 25 µm.

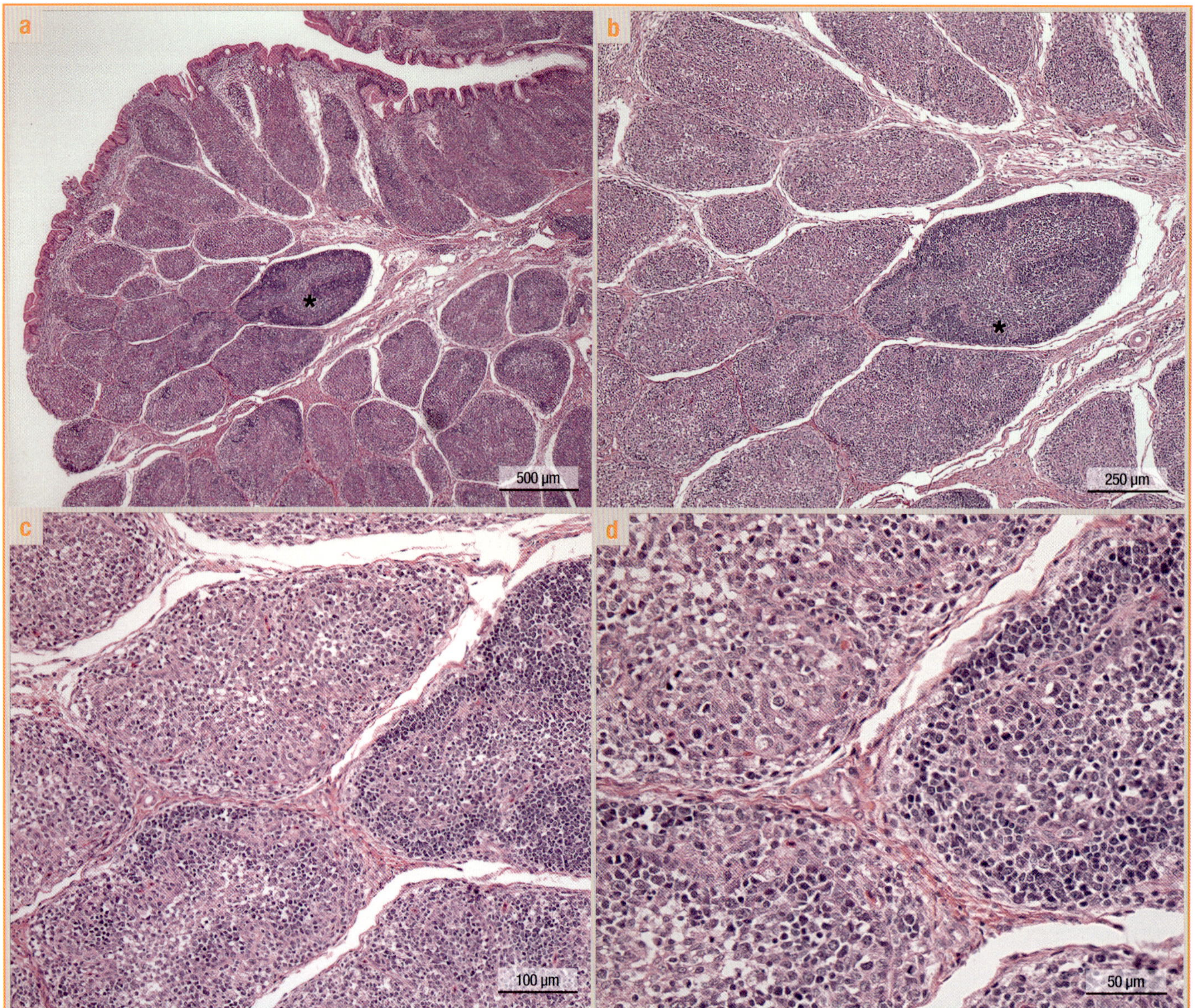

Fig. 6 Bursa of Fabricius from a chicken; age and type unknown; shows lesions of infectious bursal disease (IBD). Lesion score is 4. One relatively normal follicle remains (compared to the other follicles in this figure). It does have cortical atrophy (asterisk). (a) Bar = 500 µm. (b) Bar = 250 µm. (c) Bar = 100 µm. (d) The large follicle has loss of lymphocytes in cortex and medulla. Bar = 50 µm.

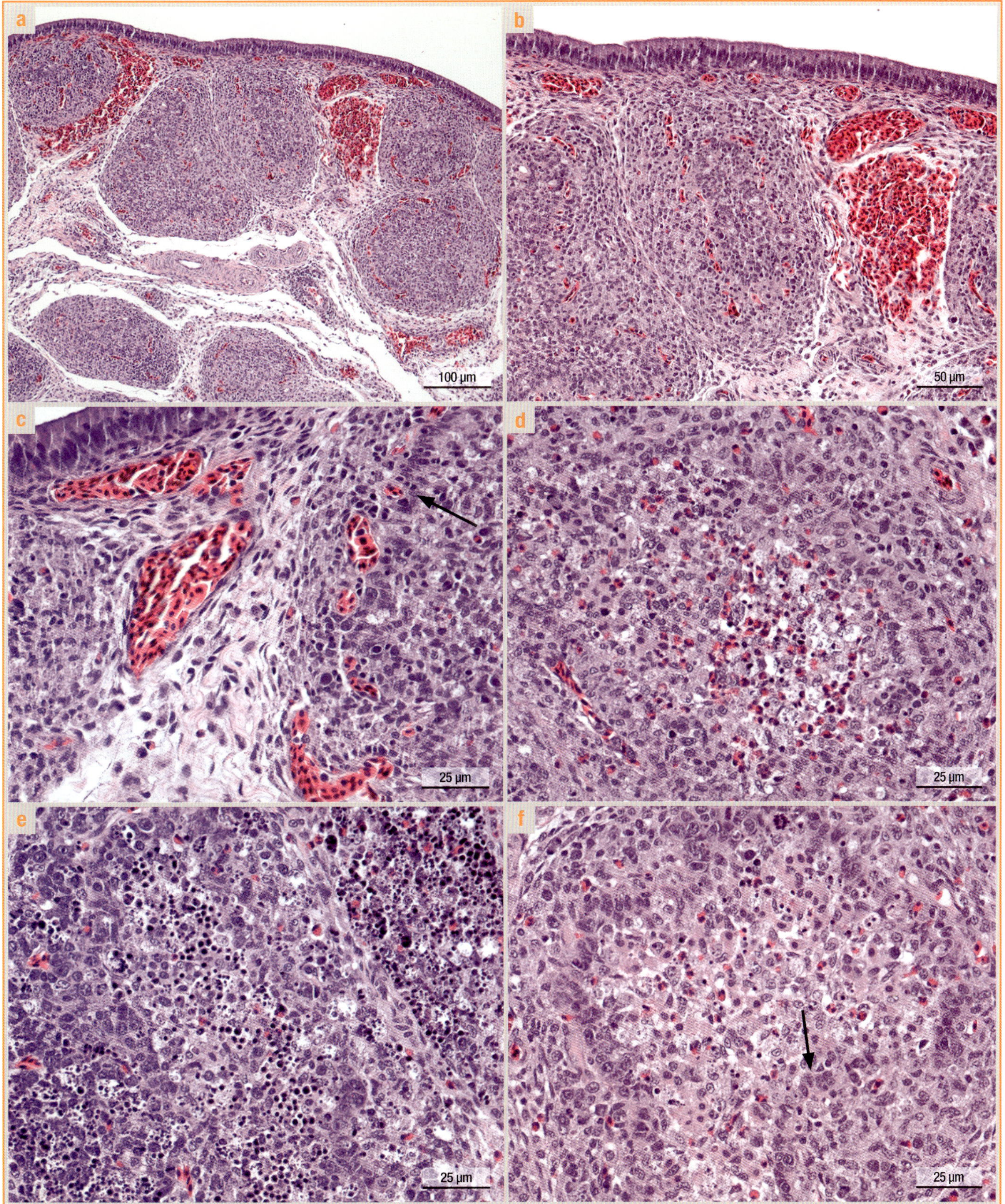

Fig. 7 Bursa of Fabricius from a 30 day-old broiler chicken shows lesions of infectious bursal disease (IBD). Lesion score is 4. (a) Bar = 100 µm. (b) Bar = 50 µm. (c) Epithelial cells separating medulla from cortex (arrow). Bar = 25 µm. (d) Bar = 25 µm. (e) Follicle has diffuse loss of lymphocytes with many pyknotic nuclei present. Bar = 25 µm. (f) Higher magnification of epithelial cells separating the medulla from the cortex (arrow). There is diffuse loss of lymphocytes. Bar = 25 µm.

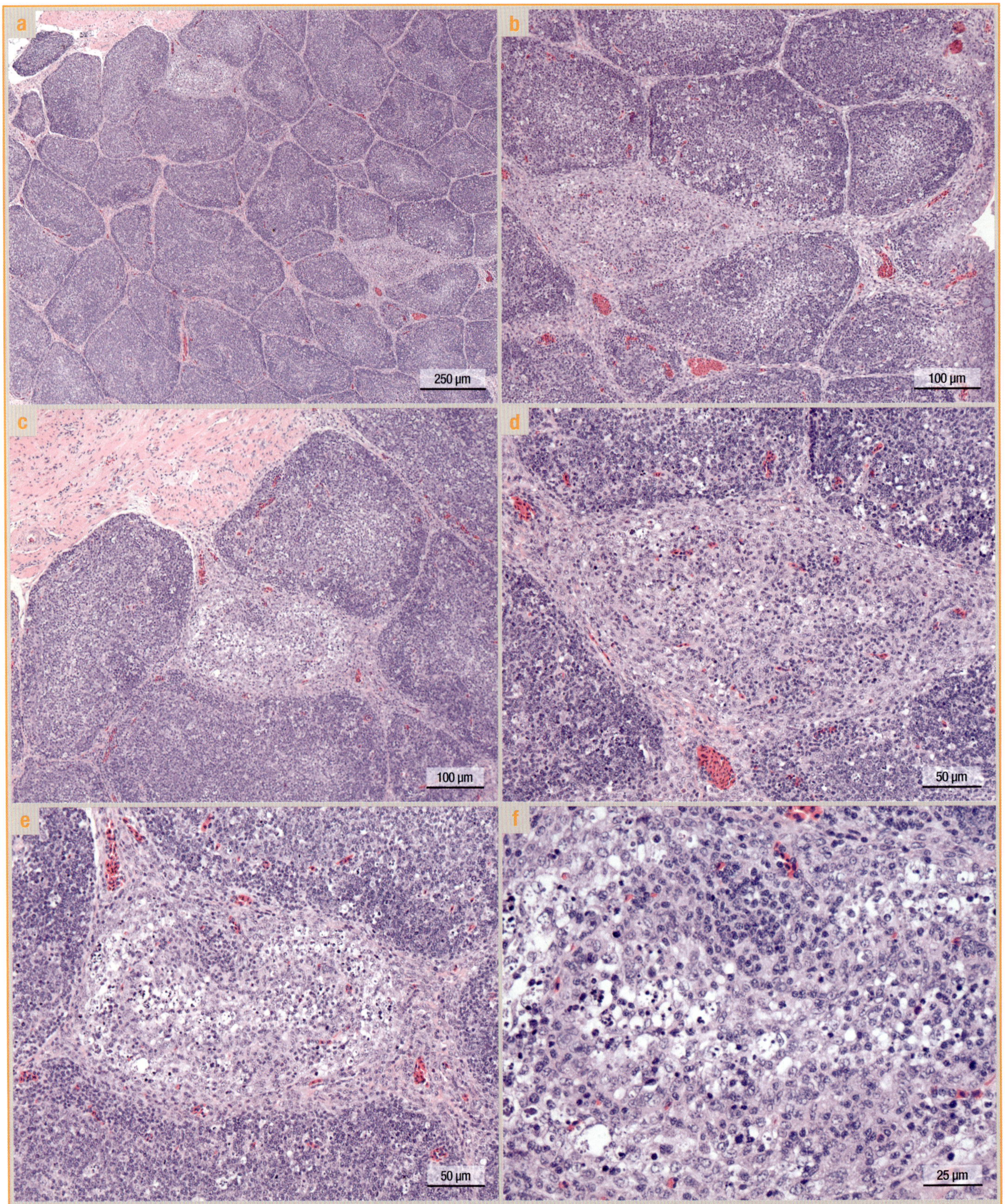

Fig. 8 Bursa of Fabricius from a 31 day-old broiler chicken shows focal lesions of lymphocyte necrosis resulting in atrophy of follicles. Lesion score is 2. These lesions are not disease specific, but MD is one differential. (a) Bar = 250 µm. (b) Bar = 100 µm. (c) Bar = 100 µm. (d) Bar = 50 µm. (e) Bar = 50 µm. (f) Bar = 25 µm.

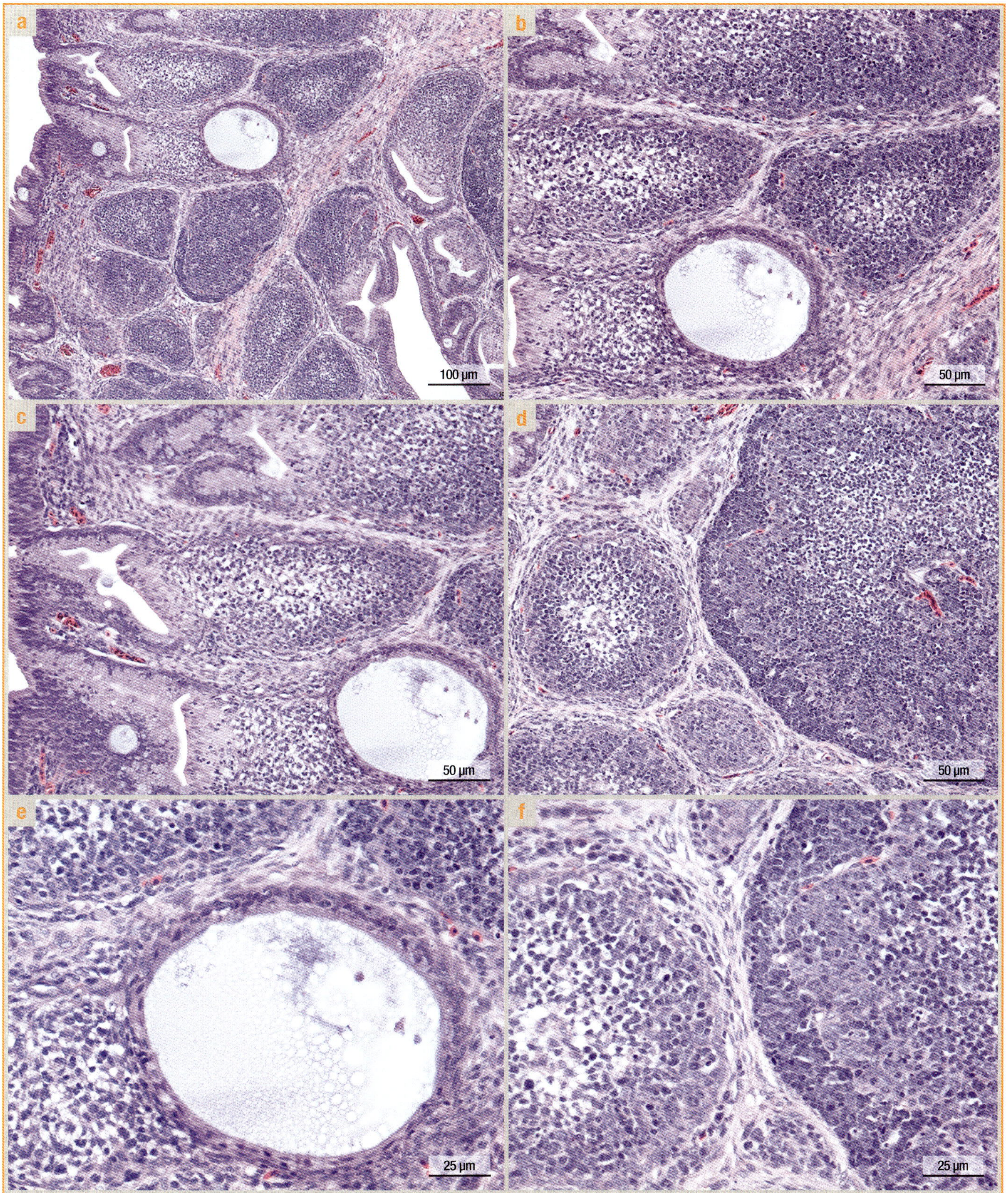

Fig. 9 Bursa of Fabricius from a 26 day-old broiler chicken shows a few follicles with relatively large populations of lymphocytes with distinct cortex and medulla. These may be regenerated follicles or follicles that had no or minimal damage. Some follicles are cystic, others are atrophic. Interfollicular region is expanded by fibrous tissue. Plical epithelium is hyperplastic. These are chronic lesions and not disease specific, but are consistent with IBD. The lesion score is 4. (a) Bar = 100 µm. (b) Bar = 50 µm. (c) Bar = 50 µm. (d) Bar = 50 µm. (e) Bar = 25 µm. (f) Bar = 25 µm.

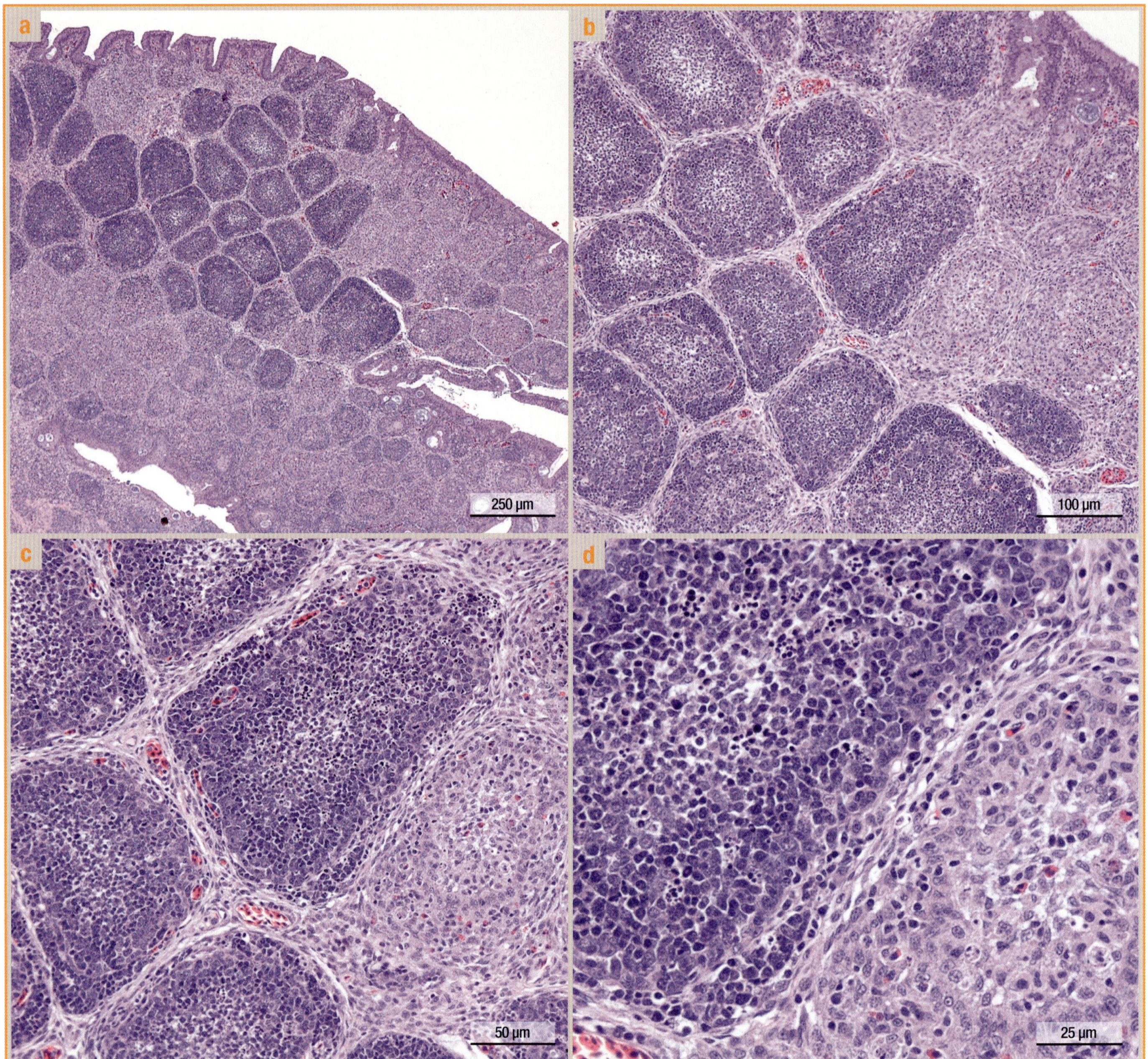

Fig. 10 Bursa of Fabricius from a 28 day-old broiler chicken shows the contrast between severe atrophy in most follicles with mild loss of lymphocytes in others. This lesion pattern is consistent with IBD. The larger, more normal follicles have regenerated. Lesion score is 4. (a) Bar = 250 µm. (b) Bar = 100 µm. (c) Bar = 50 µm. (d) Note the difference between the atrophic follicle (right) and the relatively normal follicle (left). Bar = 25 µm.

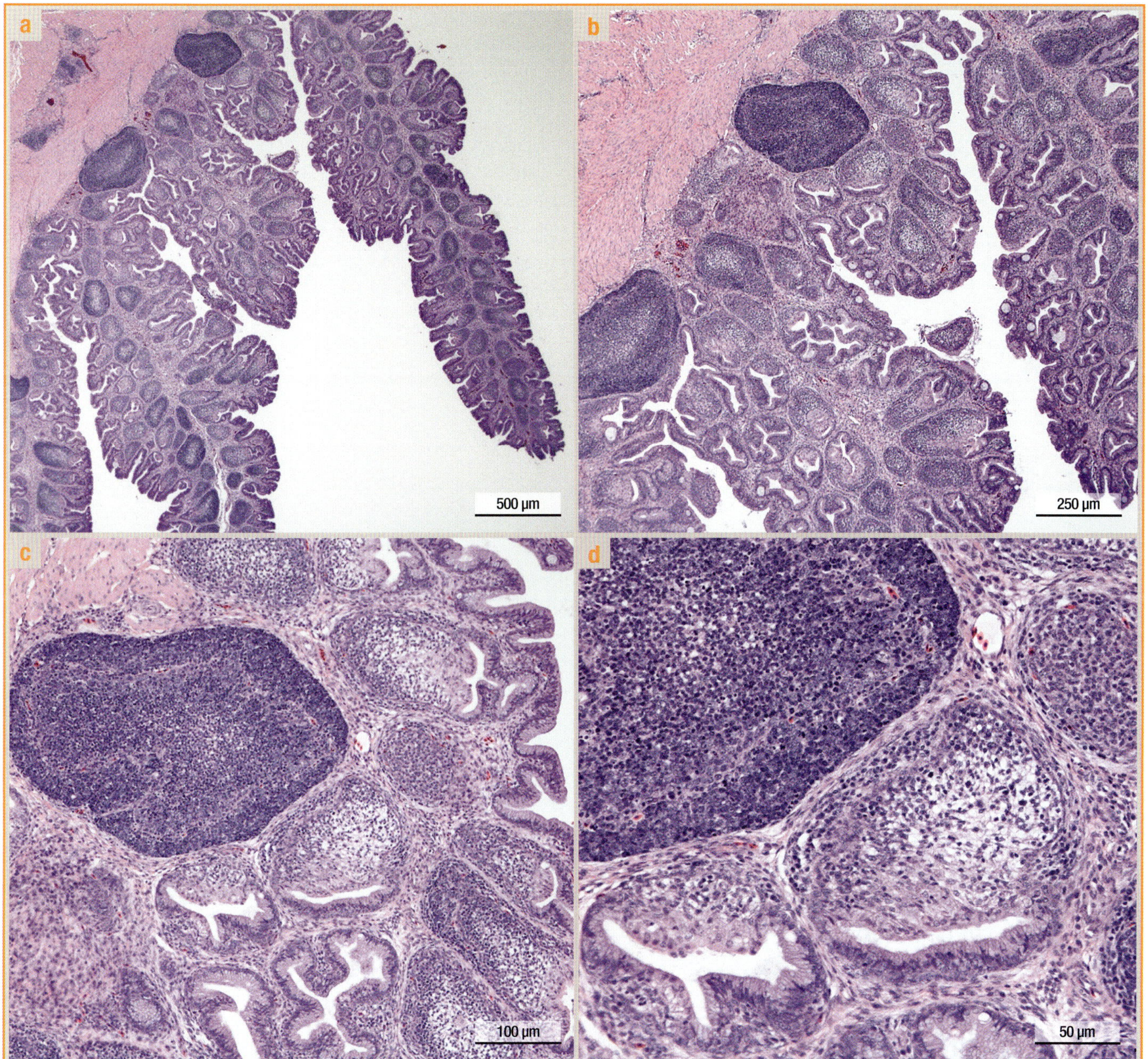

Fig. 11 Bursa of Fabricius from a 26 day-old broiler chicken shows diffuse atrophy with few relatively normal follicles. Lesion score is 4. This lesion is typical of post-IBD infection, but is not disease specific. Note the many folds in plical epithelium. (a) Bar = 500 µm. (b) Bar = 250 µm. (c) Isolated normal follicle is surrounded by atrophic follicles. Bar = 100 µm. (d) Bar = 50 µm.

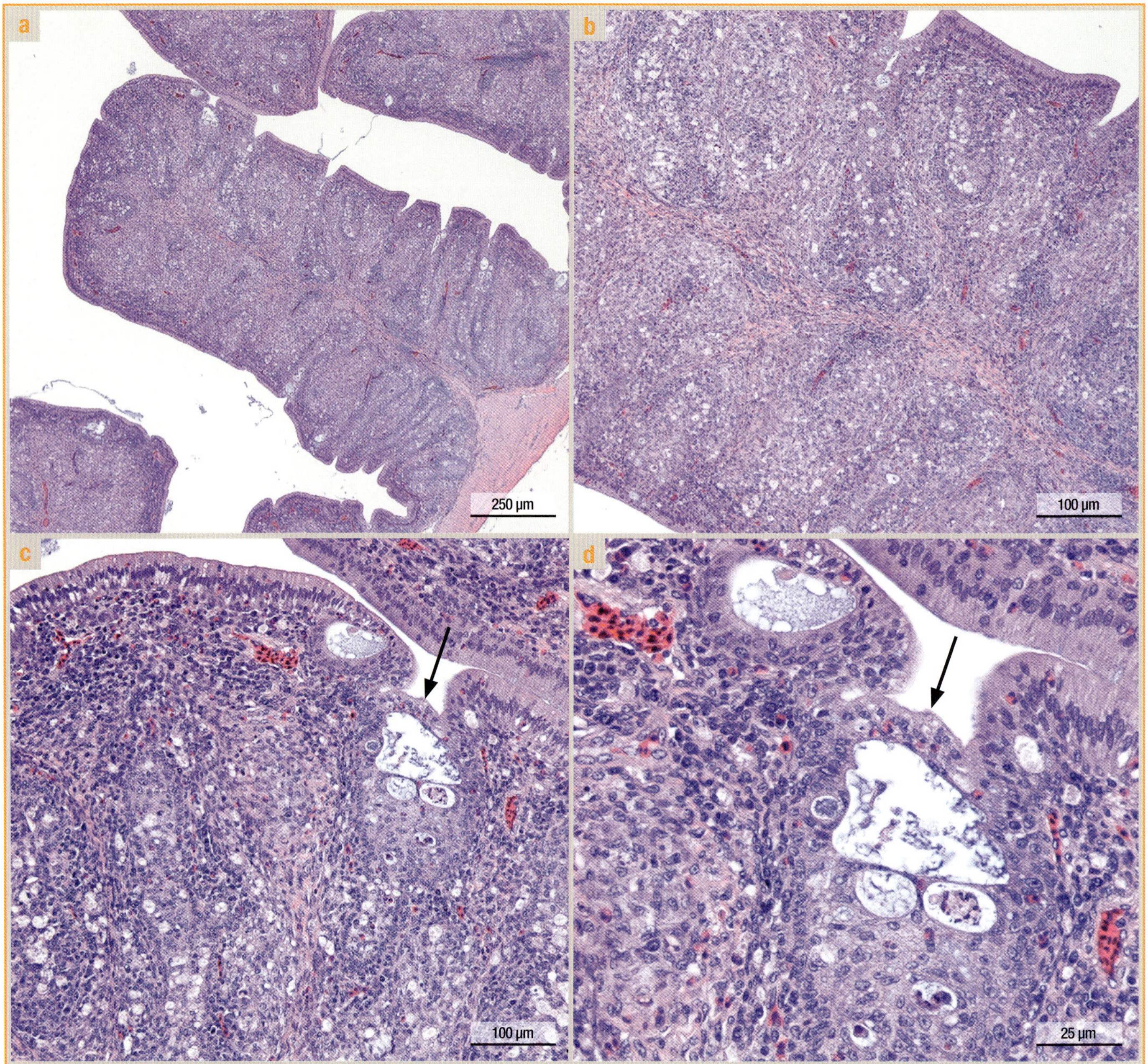

Fig. 12 Bursa of Fabricius from a 26 day-old broiler chicken shows diffuse atrophy. Lesions are typical of post-IBD. The lesion score is 4. (a) Bar = 250 µm. (b) Bar = 100 µm. (c) Bar = 100 µm. (d) Arrow shows specialized epithelium over a degenerating bursal follicle that has a small cyst within. Bar = 25 µm.

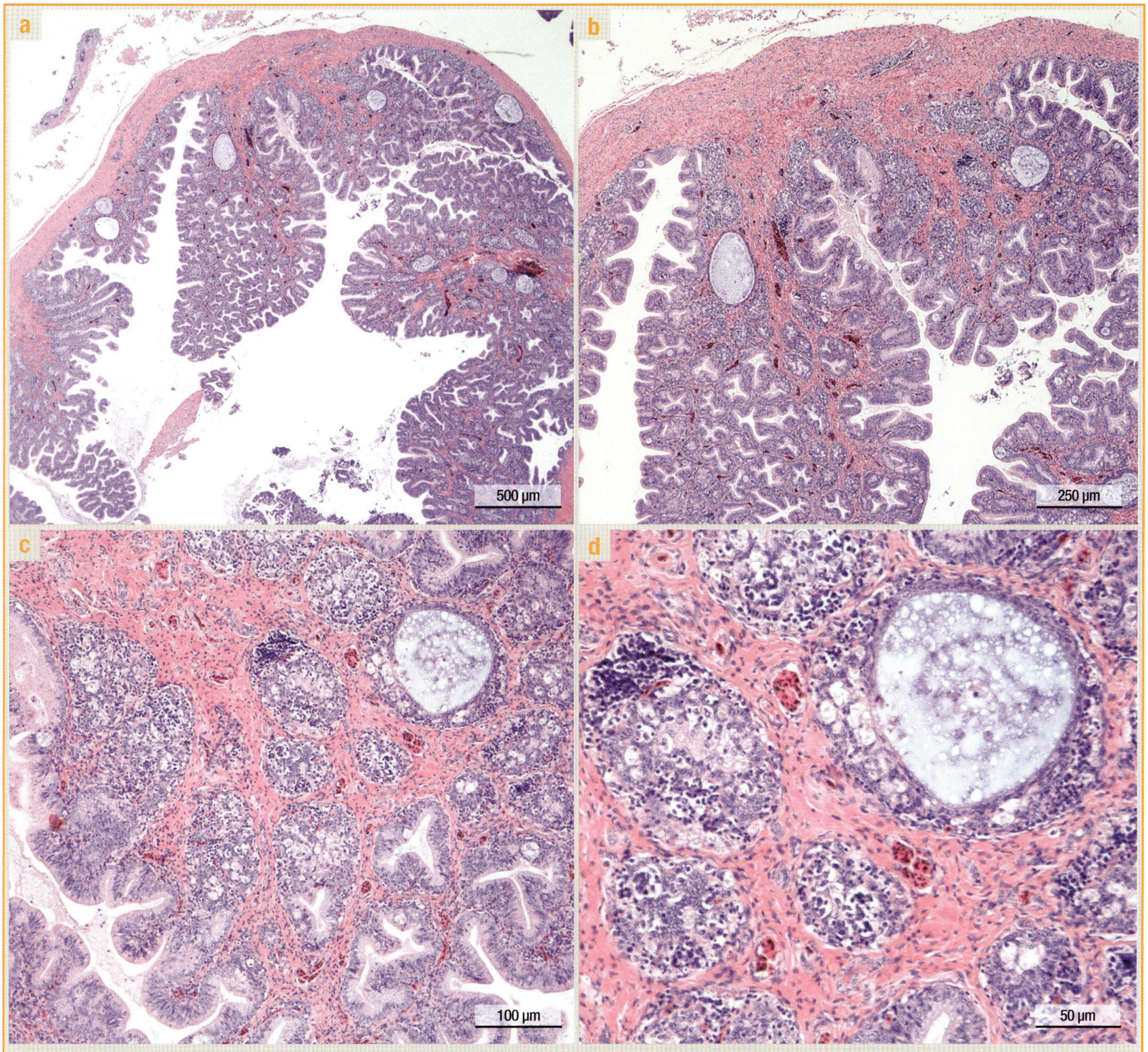

Fig. 13 Bursa of Fabricius from a 33 day-old broiler chicken shows diffuse atrophy, multiple cysts, expanded interfollicular region filled with collagen and pronounced plical epithelial hyperplasia. This is a typical, chronic, post-IBDV lesion. The lesion score is 4. (a) Bar = 500 µm. (b) Bar = 250 µm. (c) Bar = 100 µm. (d) Bar = 50 µm.

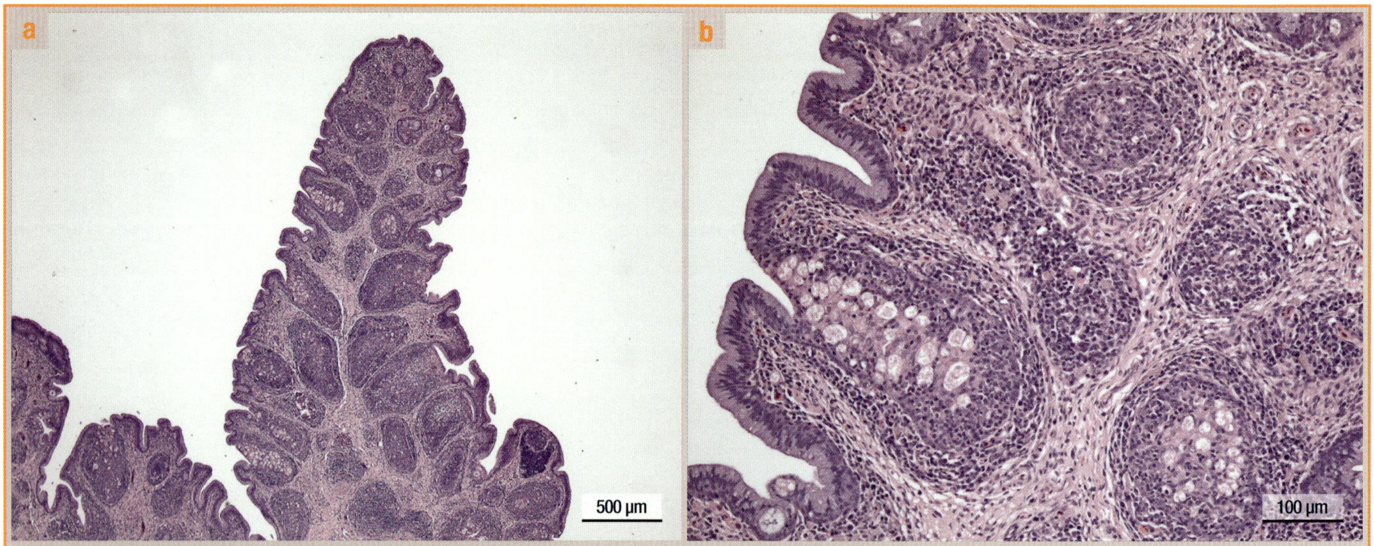

Fig. 14 | Bursa of Fabricius from a 42 day-old broiler chicken shows diffuse atrophy. Lesions are typical of post-IBDV infection. The lesion score is 4. (a) Bar = 500 µm. (b) Note the expansion of interfollicular space by dense fibrous tissue. Bar = 100 µm.

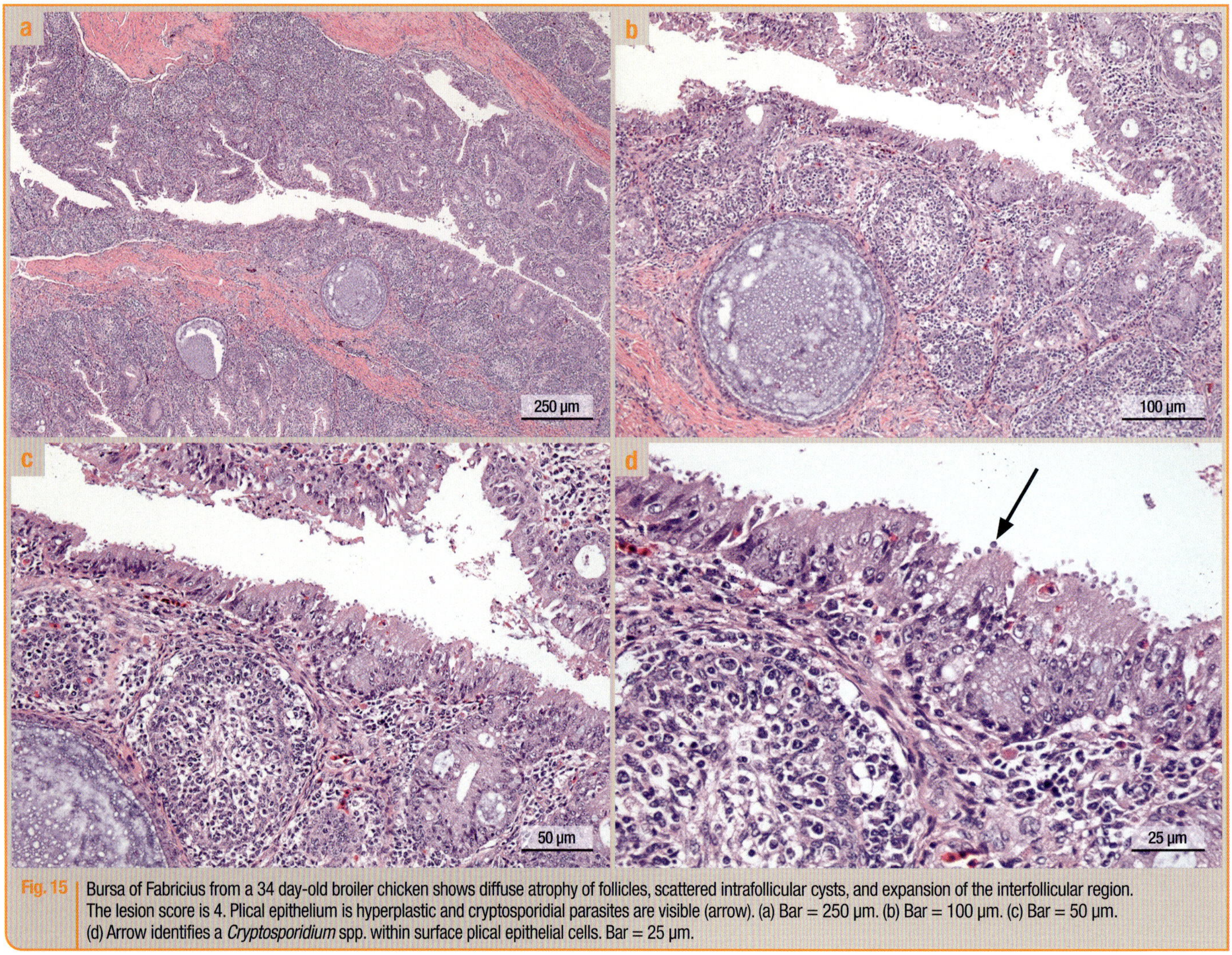

Fig. 15 | Bursa of Fabricius from a 34 day-old broiler chicken shows diffuse atrophy of follicles, scattered intrafollicular cysts, and expansion of the interfollicular region. The lesion score is 4. Plical epithelium is hyperplastic and cryptosporidial parasites are visible (arrow). (a) Bar = 250 µm. (b) Bar = 100 µm. (c) Bar = 50 µm. (d) Arrow identifies a *Cryptosporidium* spp. within surface plical epithelial cells. Bar = 25 µm.

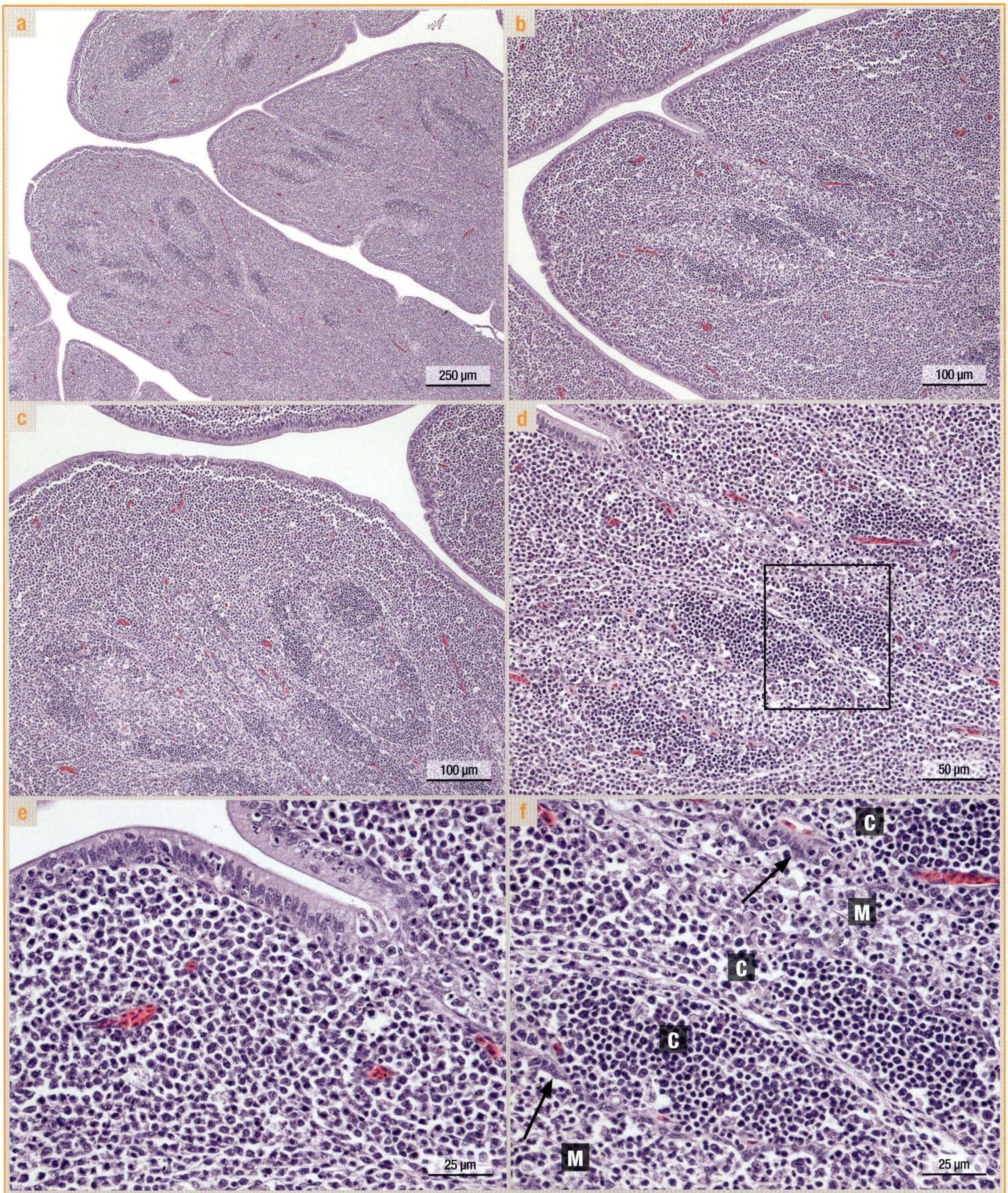

Fig. 16 Bursa of Fabricius from a 5 month-old pet/hobby chicken shows infiltration and expansion of the interfollicular region by neoplastic lymphocytes. Remnants of bursal follicles are visible. This pattern is characteristic of Marek's disease (MD). (a) Bar = 250 µm. (b) Bar = 100 µm. (c) Region in box is shown at higher magnification in (f). f) Bar = 100 µm. (d) Bar = 50 µm. (e) Bar = 25 µm. (f) Loss of lymphocytes from medulla (M) and cortex (C) are shown. Arrow shows epithelium between M and C. Bar = 25 µm.

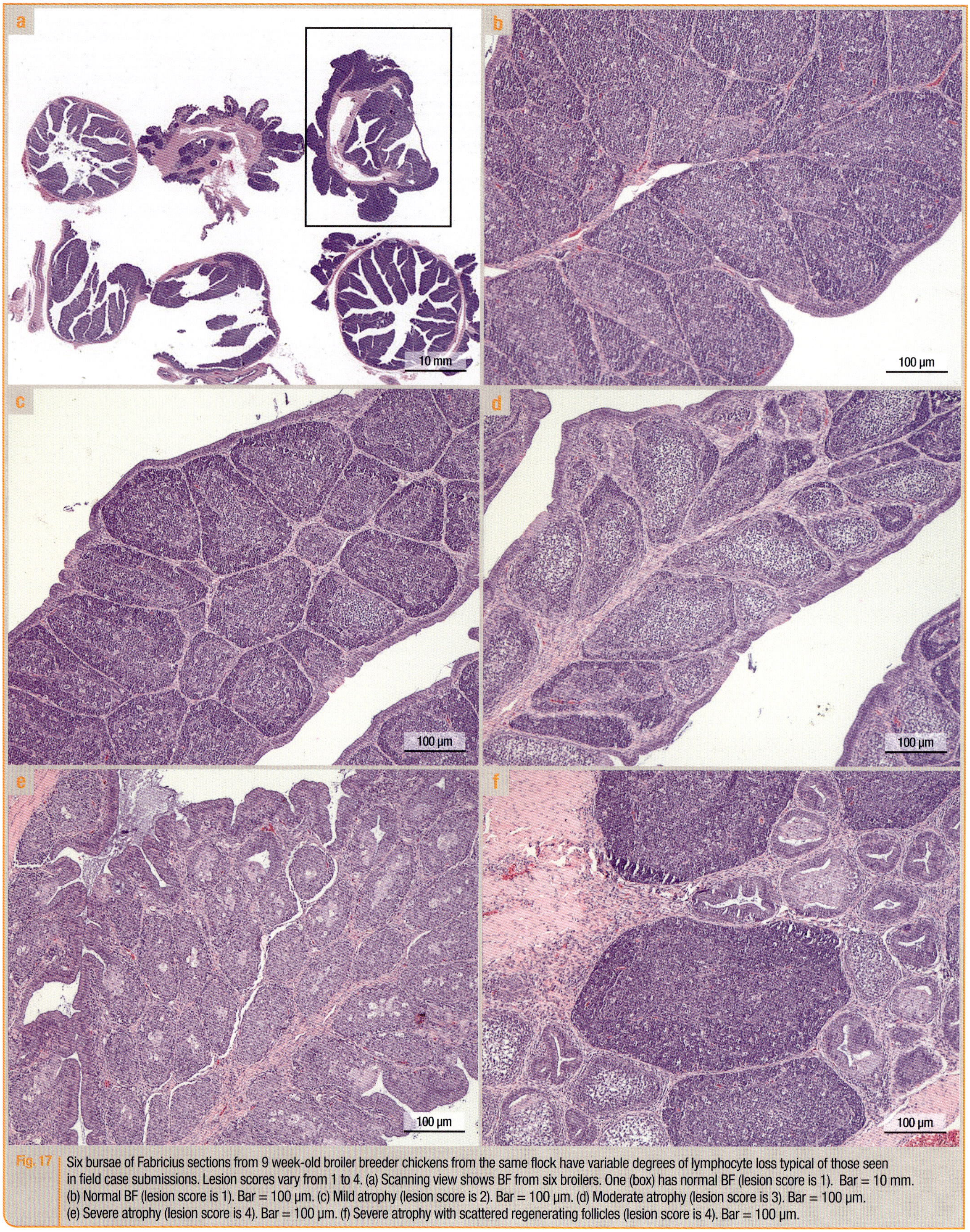

Fig. 17 Six bursae of Fabricius sections from 9 week-old broiler breeder chickens from the same flock have variable degrees of lymphocyte loss typical of those seen in field case submissions. Lesion scores vary from 1 to 4. (a) Scanning view shows BF from six broilers. One (box) has normal BF (lesion score is 1). Bar = 10 mm. (b) Normal BF (lesion score is 1). Bar = 100 µm. (c) Mild atrophy (lesion score is 2). Bar = 100 µm. (d) Moderate atrophy (lesion score is 3). Bar = 100 µm. (e) Severe atrophy (lesion score is 4). Bar = 100 µm. (f) Severe atrophy with scattered regenerating follicles (lesion score is 4). Bar = 100 µm.

Thymus

The thymus has multiple lobes each with a distinct cortex and medulla (Fig. 18) that provides the background for recognition of lesions and lesion patterns. Pyknotic nuclei scattered through the cortex create the appearance of a "starry sky". Some numbers of pyknotic nuclei are normal and this pattern is due to programmed cell death named apoptosis. It is difficult to determine the point at which the level of apoptosis becomes greater than normal. Equally impossible with standard H&E stains is the differentiation between apoptosis and necrosis. However, the net result is the same, reduction in the number of lymphocytes. The issue for the histopathologist is to determine whether lymphocyte loss is within expected or normal levels or excessive. Loss of cortical lymphocytes, when excessive, results in decrease in the width of the cortex. Decreased cortical width often is not uniform. Loss of lymphocytes in the medulla results in decreased medullary area, decreased basophilia of the region, increased space between cells, and increased numbers of pyknotic nuclei. Increased numbers of heterophils and macrophages may be found, but are not consistently present.

Transient depletion of cortical lymphocytes in the thymus is reported in Infectious Bursal Disease (IBD) and likely due to increased apoptosis.[30,55] This lesion is temporary and thus not likely to result in thymic atrophy.

The amount of blood in the thymus, typically within the medulla, is also difficult to gauge when borderline excessive. The blood illustrated in figure 19 is considered normal.

Chicken anemia virus (CAV) is documented as a major cause of immunosuppression and as a cause of thymic lesions.[1,13,24,27,29,33,36,40,41,58,59,64-66,68,69,74] CAV causes an abnormal increase in the rate of apoptosis resulting in loss of cortical and medullary lymphocytes. Lymphocyte loss may be accompanied by hemorrhage (Fig. 20). Lesions commonly are regional with adjacent lobes being unaffected. Not illustrated here is the significant loss of all cell types in the bone marrow.

Clinical case material often presents with normal sections of thymus (lesion score = 1) (Figs. 21a, c and e) adjacent to sections with diffuse atrophy (lesion score = 4) (Figs. 21b, d and f). Also common are sections with mild to moderate atrophy (lesion score = 3) (Figs. 22a, c and e) alongside sections with diffuse atrophy (lesion score = 4) (Figs. 22b, d and f). In some cases, severe atrophy is found in both cortex and medulla (Fig. 23). Each thymic section can be scored and a mean lesion score calculated for the submission. Examples of severe cortical atrophy with less atrophy in the medulla are common (Fig. 24). One can appreciate how easy it is to miss a section with diffuse atrophy and thus misinterpret the possible presence of immunosuppression.

The atrophic changes illustrated (Figs. 21-24) are not disease specific, but CAV is a major differential. Finding classic lesions (Fig. 20) of CAV is uncommon in field case submissions, but thymic atrophy typical of that described for post CAV infection is observed frequently. Finding evidence of thymic atrophy in the ranges illustrated here supports a prediction of immunosuppression. However, without measurement of immune function, histopathology is providing only a prediction. As restated from the BF section, increased incidence of diseases as the flock ages provides additional support for the theory of immunosuppression.

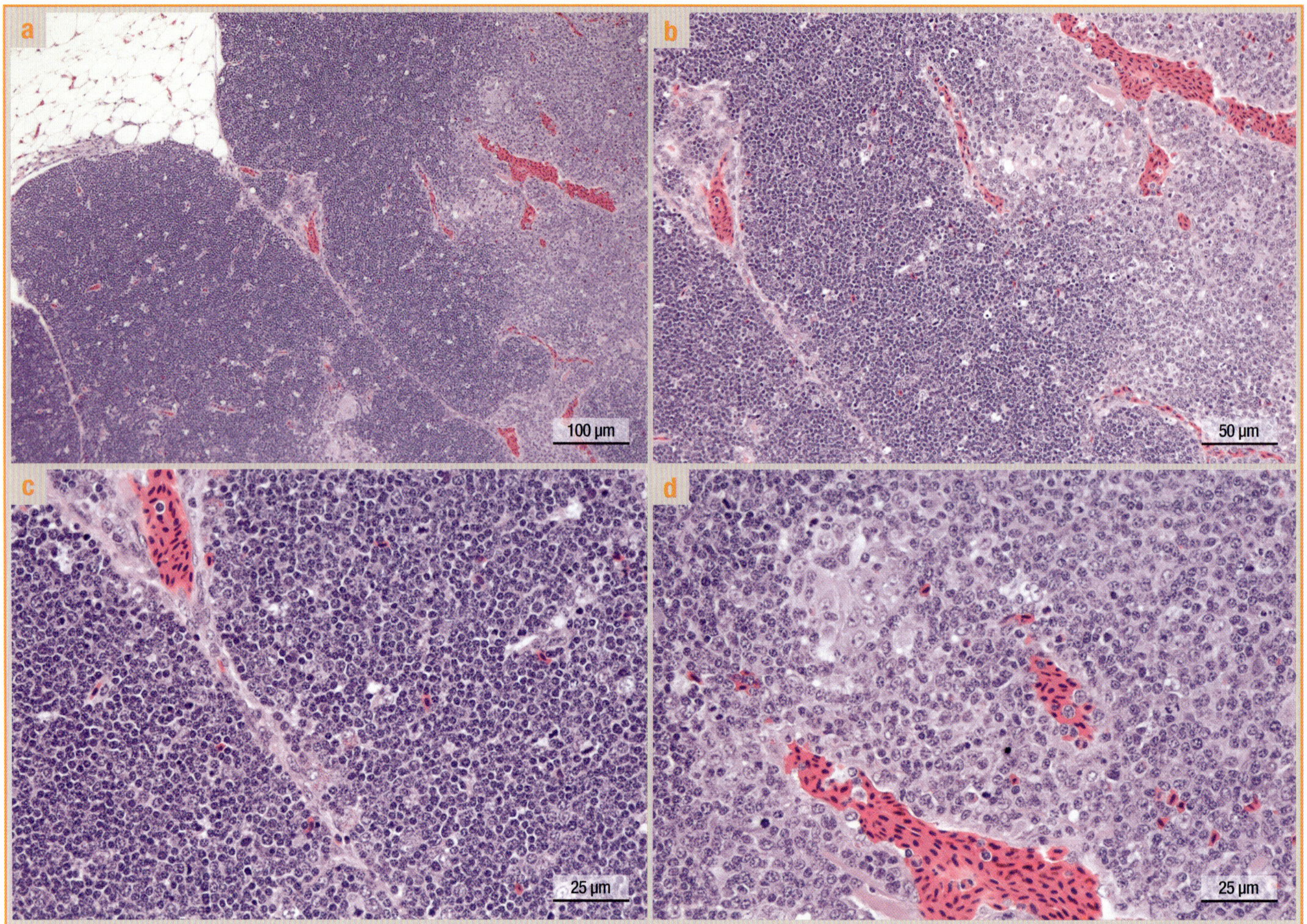

Fig. 18 Thymus from a 3.5 week-old broiler chicken is normal. (a) Wide cortex and portion of medulla are shown. Bar = 100 µm. (b) Bar = 50 µm. (c) Higher magnification of the cortex. Bar = 25 µm. (d) Higher magnification of the medulla. Bar = 25 µm.

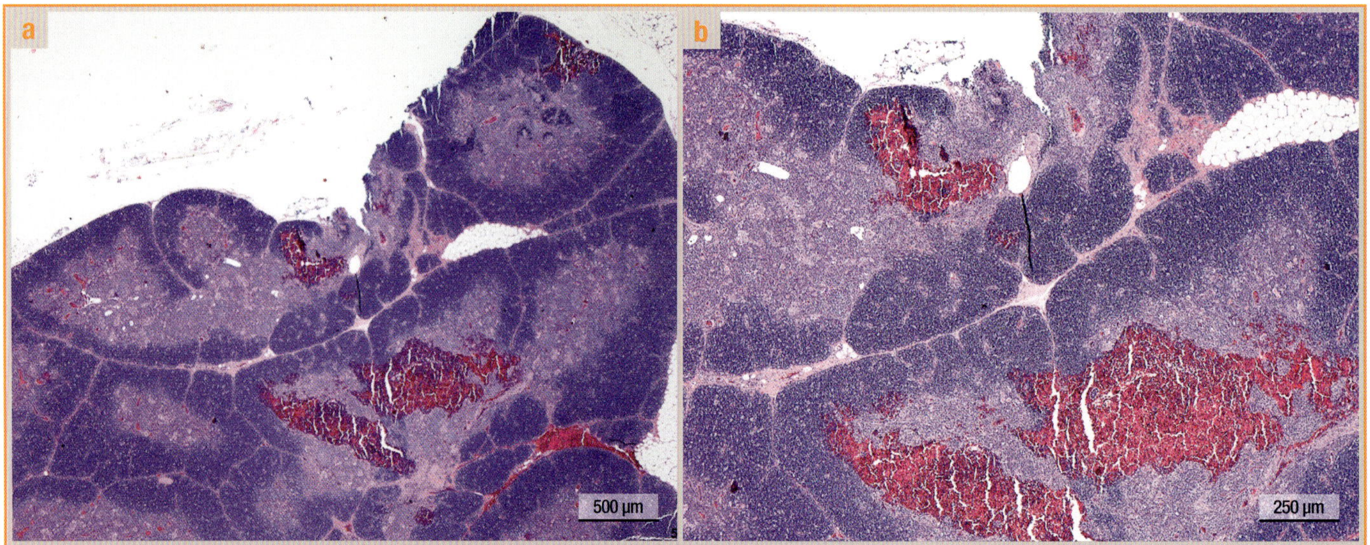

Fig. 19 Thymus from a 31 day-old broiler chicken is normal. Cortical width may be decreased, but this is a difficult assessment. Prominent blood vessels are in medulla and there may be some hemorrhage, but this is not considered a lesion. (a) Bar = 500 µm. (b) Bar = 250 µm.

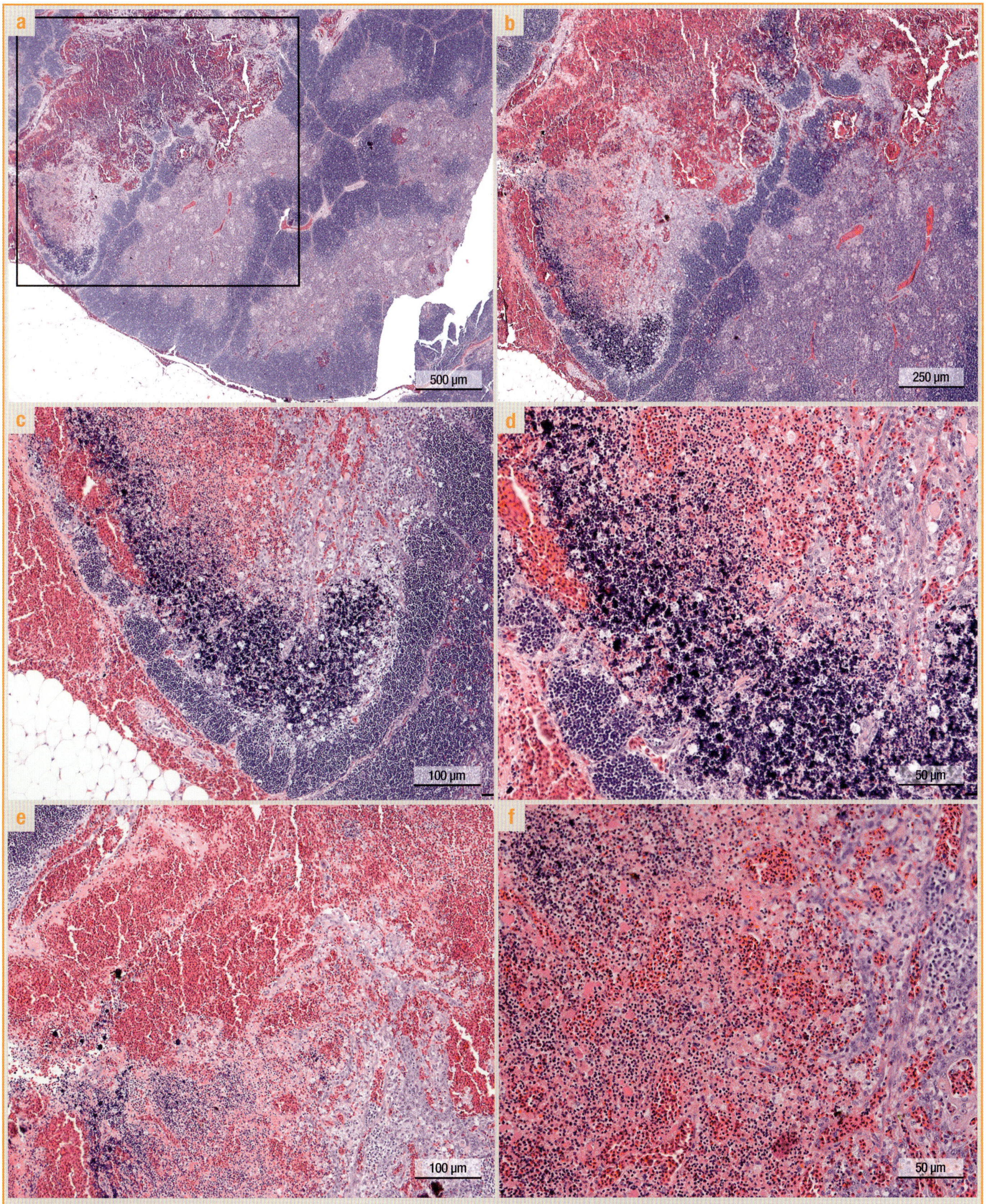

Fig. 20 Thymus from a 31 day-old broiler chicken shows lesions of regional acute hemorrhage and necrosis consistent with CAV. (a) Regional hemorrhage and necrosis (box). Bar = 500 µm. (b) Bar = 250 µm. (c) Bar = 100 µm. (d) Bar = 50 µm. (e) Bar = 100 µm. (f) Bar = 50 µm.

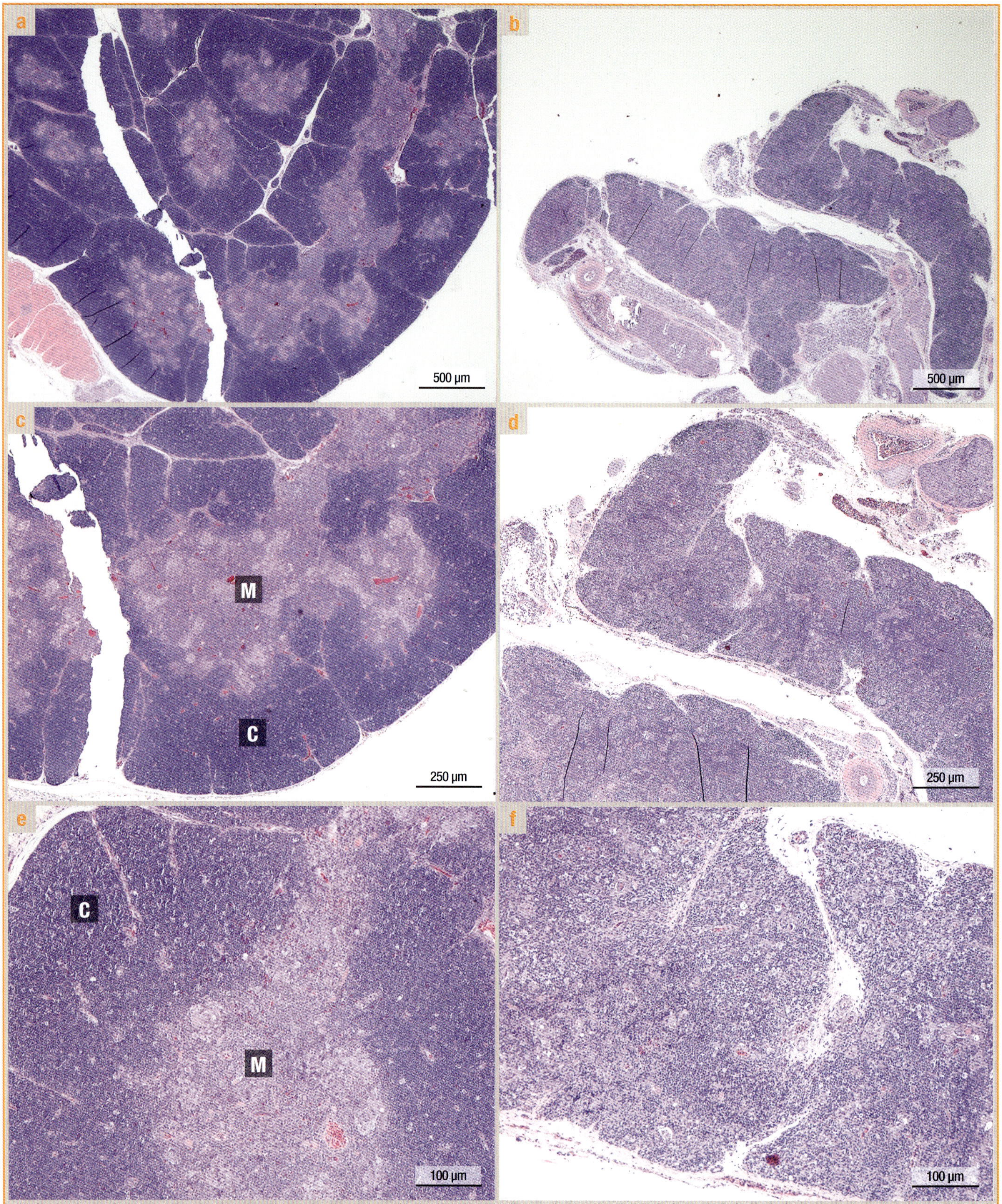

Fig. 21 Thymus from 2 week-old broiler breeder chickens from the same flock compares normal (a, c, e) with thymic atrophy (b, d, f). Cause of the atrophy was not determined but CAV is a differential. Cortex (C) and medulla (M) are visible in a, c and e, but not in b, d, or f. (a) Bar = 500 µm. (b) Bar = 500 µm. (c) Bar = 250 µm. (d) Bar = 250 µm. (e) Bar = 100 µm. (f) Bar = 100 µm.

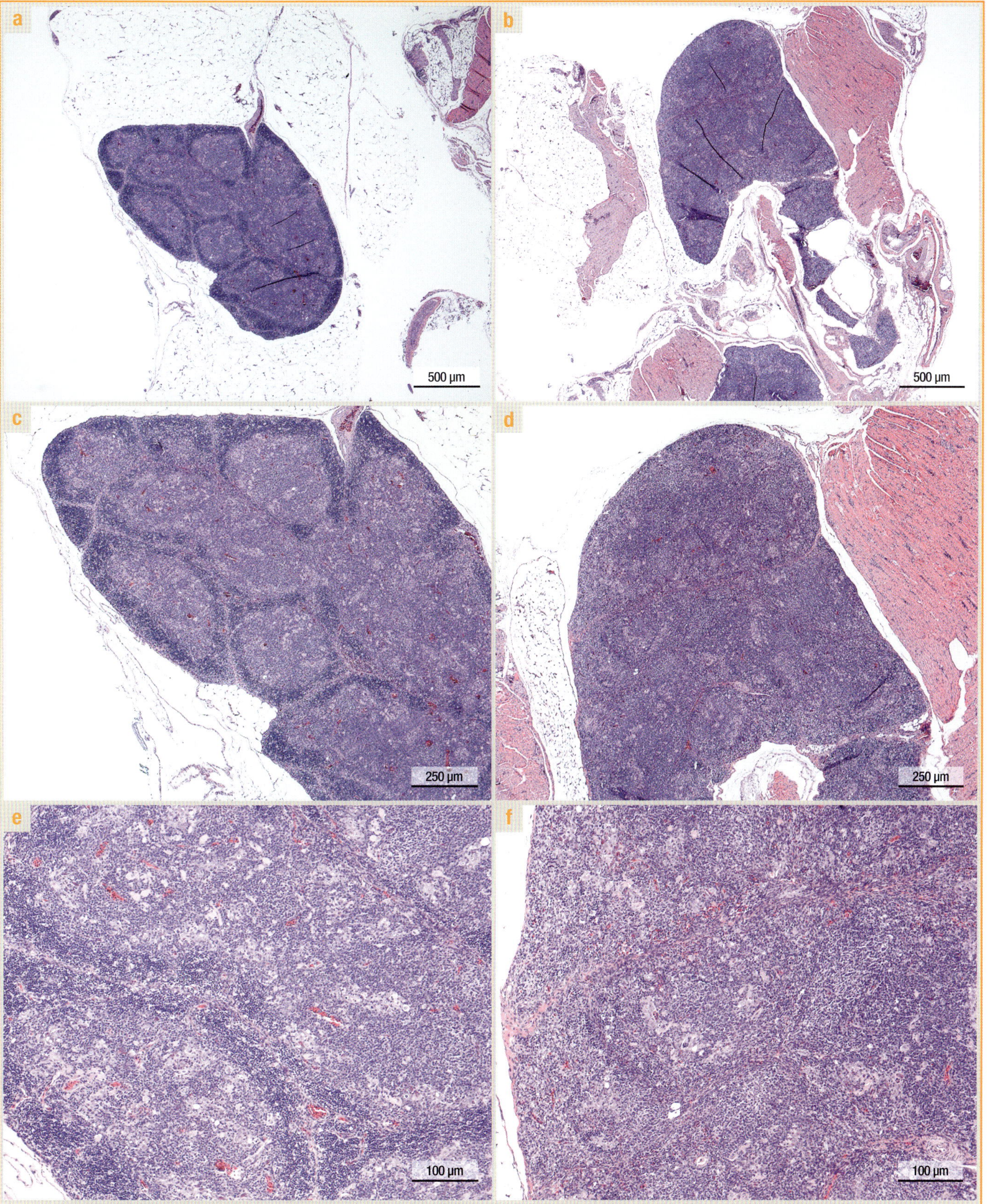

Fig. 22 Thymus from 3 week-old broiler breeder chickens from the same flock compares moderate atrophy (lesion score is 3 in a, c, e) with severe atrophy (lesion score is 4 in b, d, f). (a) Bar = 500 µm. (b) Bar = 500 µm. (c) Bar = 250 µm. (d) Bar = 250 µm. (e) Bar = 100 µm. (f) Bar = 100 µm.

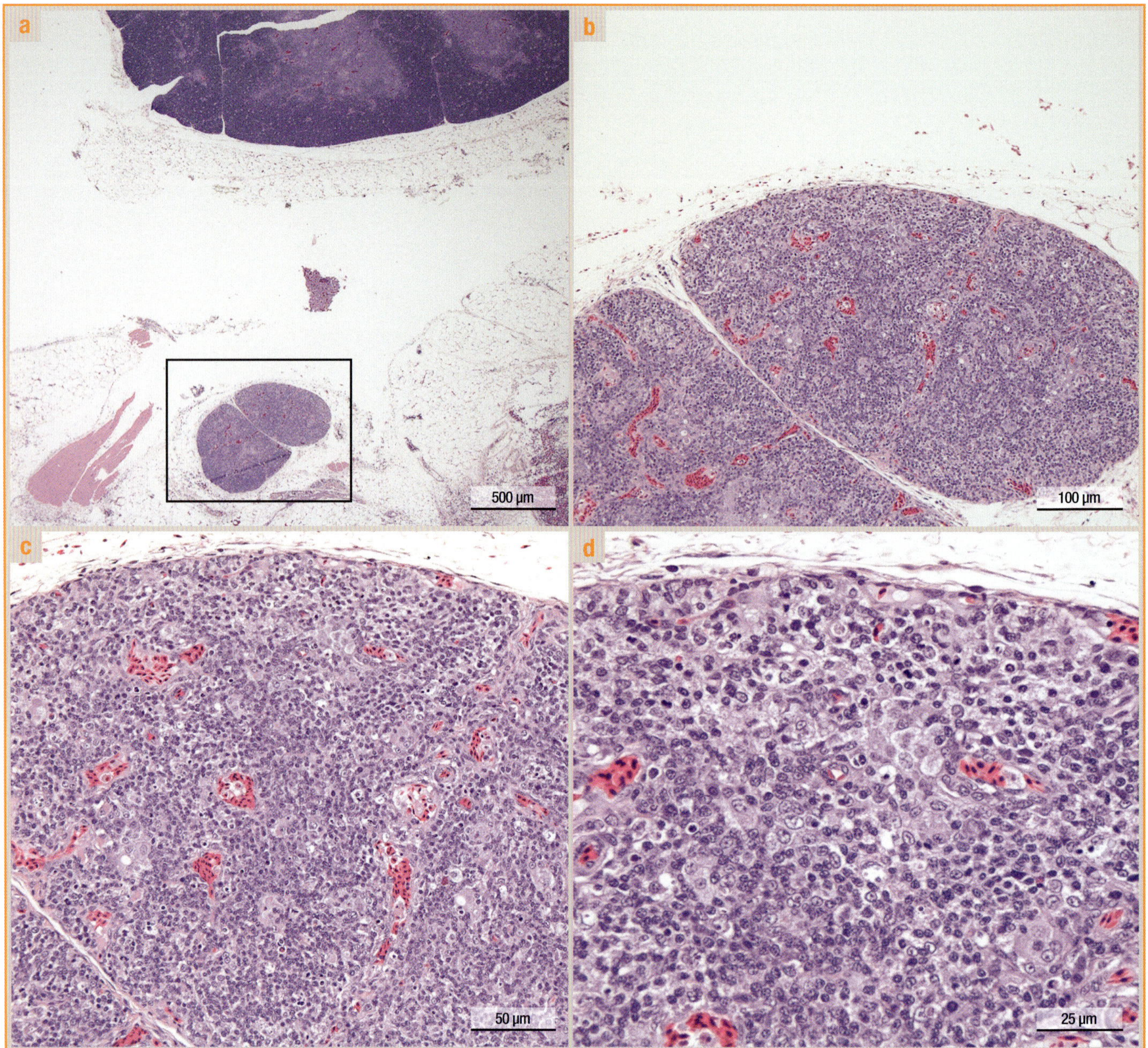

Fig. 23 Thymus lobes from a 3.5 week-old broiler chicken show the range of lesions that can be found in the same chicken.
(a) One lobe (top) is relatively normal and one lobe (box) is diffusely atrophic. Bar = 500 µm. (b) Higher magnification of atrophic lobe in box. Bar = 100 µm.
(c) Bar = 50 µm. (d) Bar = 25 µm.

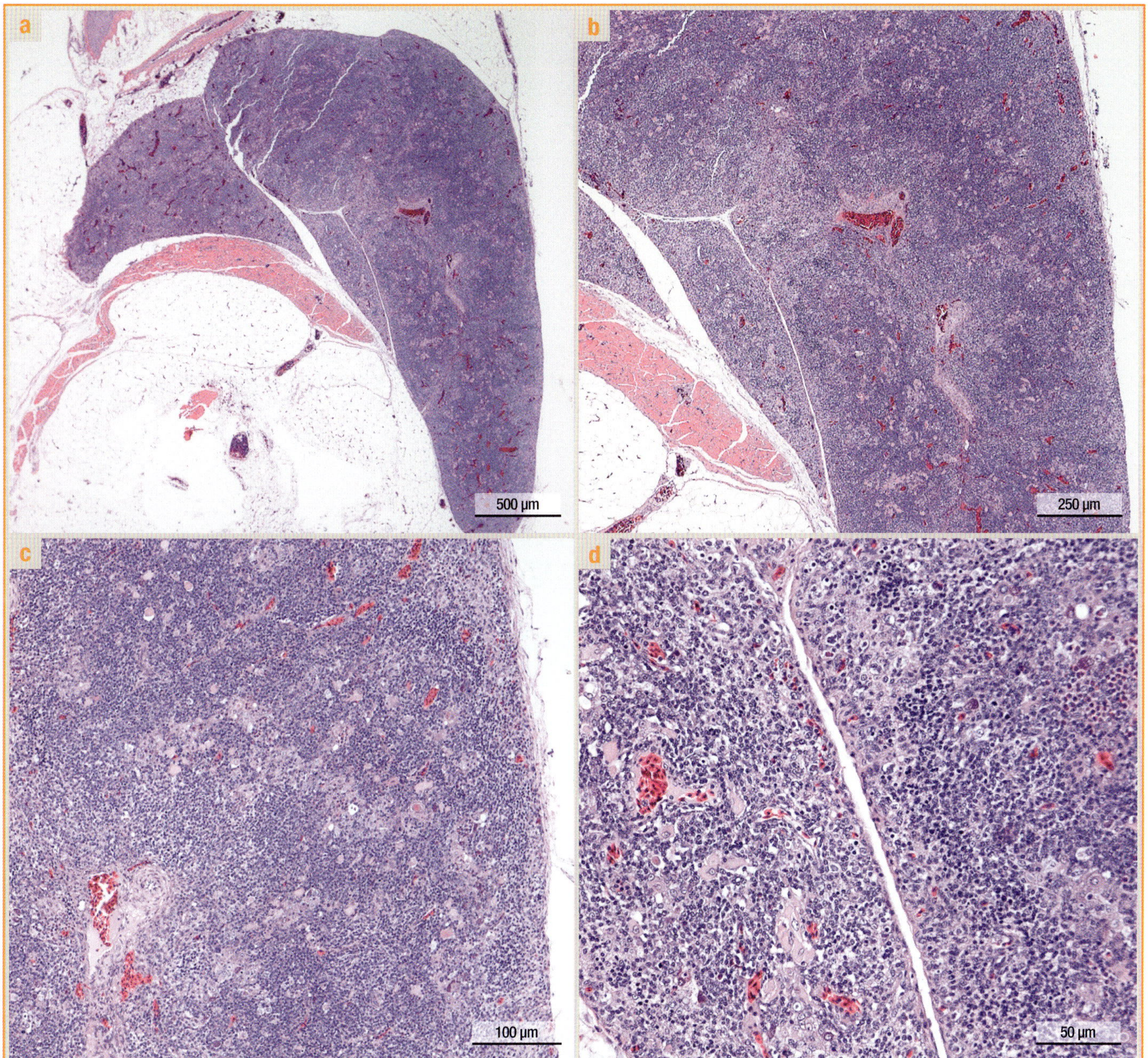

Fig. 24 Thymus from a 34 day-old broiler chicken shows diffuse atrophy with no distinct cortex or medulla and has a lesion score of 4. CAV is a possible cause. (a) Bar = 500 µm. (b) Bar = 250 µm. (c) Bar = 100 µm. (d) Bar = 50 µm.

Spleen

The spleen (Fig. 26) is organized into erythrocyte rich regions termed red pulp, and lymphocyte rich regions, termed white pulp. [31,32,34] White pulp regions are further compartmentalized. One compartment is composed of bursa-dependent lymphoid nodules (Figs. 26a, c and e) and T-dependent diffuse collections of lymphocytes located adjacent to arterioles –the periarteriolar lymphoid sheath or PALS (Figs. 26b, d and f). The second lymphoid cell compartment is composed of diffuse collections of B-dependent lymphocytes located around the sheathed venules –the periellipsoidal lymphoid sheath or PELS (Fig. 25). The sheathed venules have high and prominent endothelial cells and are surrounded by large, pale staining reticular cells. These two lymphoid cell compartments or regions are scattered throughout the spleen (Fig. 26). There is no regular, repeating pattern as seen in the BF; thus, the spleen is more difficult to evaluate. Loss of lymphocytes is seen as reduction in number and or size of bursa-dependent nodules, increase in pyknotic nuclei resulting in a "starry-sky" effect, loss of cells in diffuse collections in PALS and PELS, and increase in pale staining reticular cells. Decrease in lymphocytes can be relatively subtle (Figs. 27b, d and f) or striking (Fig. 28). Changes in other components of the spleen are difficult to assess with routine H&E staining methods. An example of such a difficult change to appreciate is the reduction in extracellular matrix associated with reduction in splenic reticular cells following IBDV infection. [6]

Increased numbers of lymphoid cells or hyperplasia may be observed when chickens are making an active immune response. This response is characterized by increase in number and size of bursa-dependent follicles and/or increase in cells in the PALS and PELS.

Increased numbers of reticular (histiocytic) cells is apparent when there is loss of lymphocytes (Figs. 29 and 30). Massive loss of lymphocytes and/or lymphoid cell hypoplasia in young broiler chickens results in the histologic pattern of generalized reticular cell hyperplasia and loss of splenic architecture (Fig. 29).

Significant increase in reticular cells in the PALS is a characteristic of multicentric histiocytosis (spindle cell proliferative disease) (Figs. 31 and 32). [3,23,60] The distinction between PALS and PELS is lost, bursa- dependent follicles are few or absent, and red pulp decreased in volume (Figs. 29 and 30). Subgroup J avian leukosis genes were detected in some of these lesions. [3,60]

Neoplastic lymphocytes proliferating in the spleen are features of MD, REV, and LL. The neoplastic lymphocytes in MD are pleomorphic, expand from the PALS and may invade blood vessels and the splenic capsule (Fig. 33). Neoplastic lymphocytes in LL are more uniform than in MD, but this can be difficult to determine, especially if post mortem autolysis is present. LL and REV tumors originate in one or more bursal follicles leading to proliferation of neoplastic lymphocytes within the bursa-dependent nodules followed by expansion resulting in a more diffuse, multinodular pattern (Fig. 34).

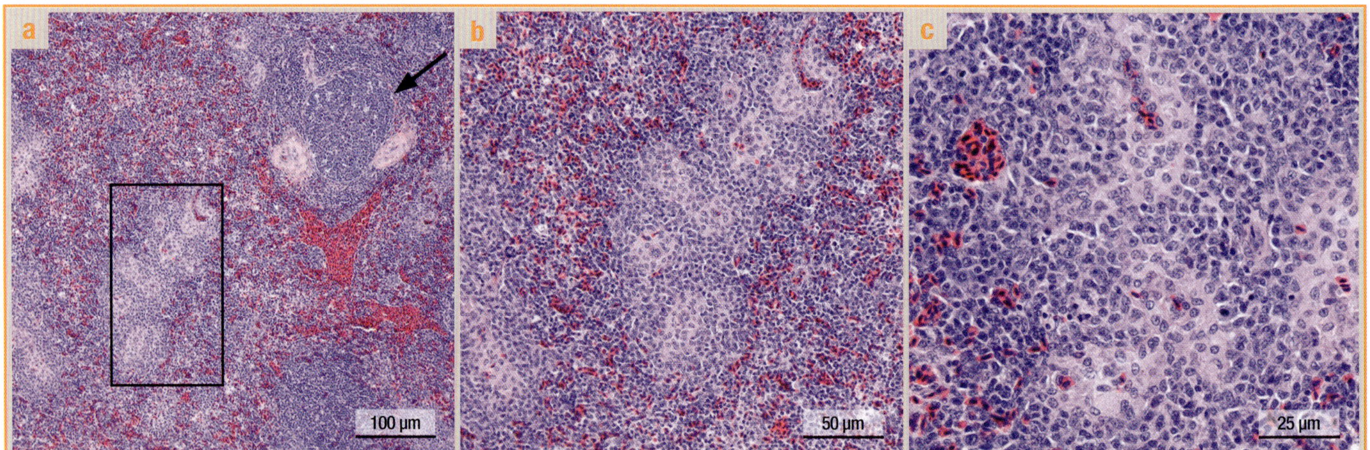

Fig. 25 Spleen from a pet/hobby chicken (age not reported). Normal periellipsoidal region (PELS in box) is shown at higher magnification in (b) and (c). (a) Shown are B-dependent lymphocytes in the PELS (box) and a diffuse collection of lymphocytes in the PALS with a bursa-dependent nodule (arrow). Bar = 100 µm. (b) Bar = 50 µm. (c) Note the pale stained reticular cells around the venules. Bar = 25 µm.

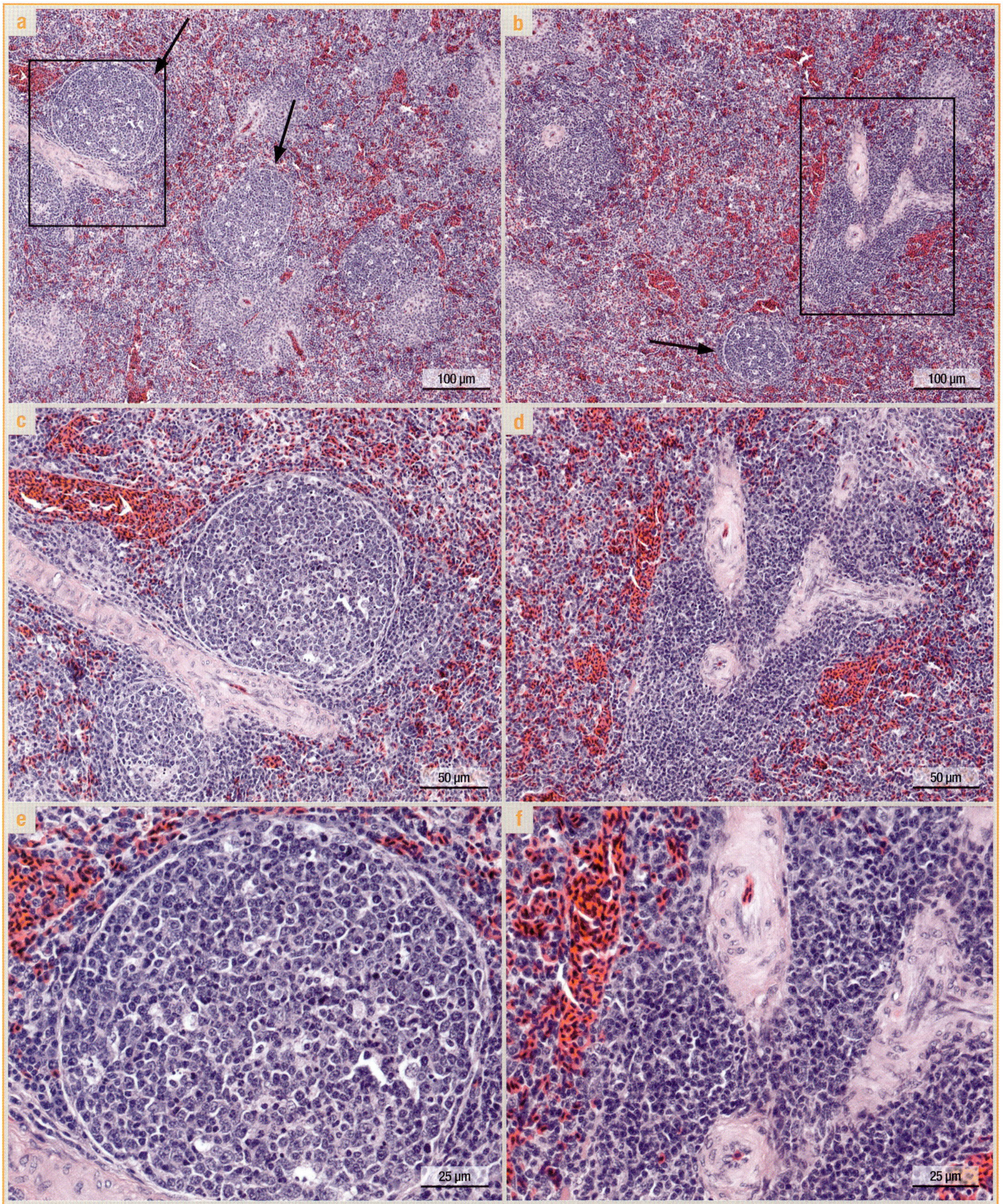

Fig. 26 Spleen from a pet/hobby chicken (age not reported) shows no lesions. (a) Shown are bursa-dependent lymphoid nodules (arrows) within the periarteriolar T-dependent lymphocyte (PALS) region. PALS (box) shown at higher magnifications in (c) and (e). Red pulp is also visible. Bar = 100 µm. (b) PALS (box) shown at higher magnification in (d) and (f). Arrow identifies a bursa-dependent nodule. Bar = 100 µm. (c) Bar = 50 µm. (d) Bar = 50 µm. (e) Bar = 25 µm. (f) Bar = 25 µm.

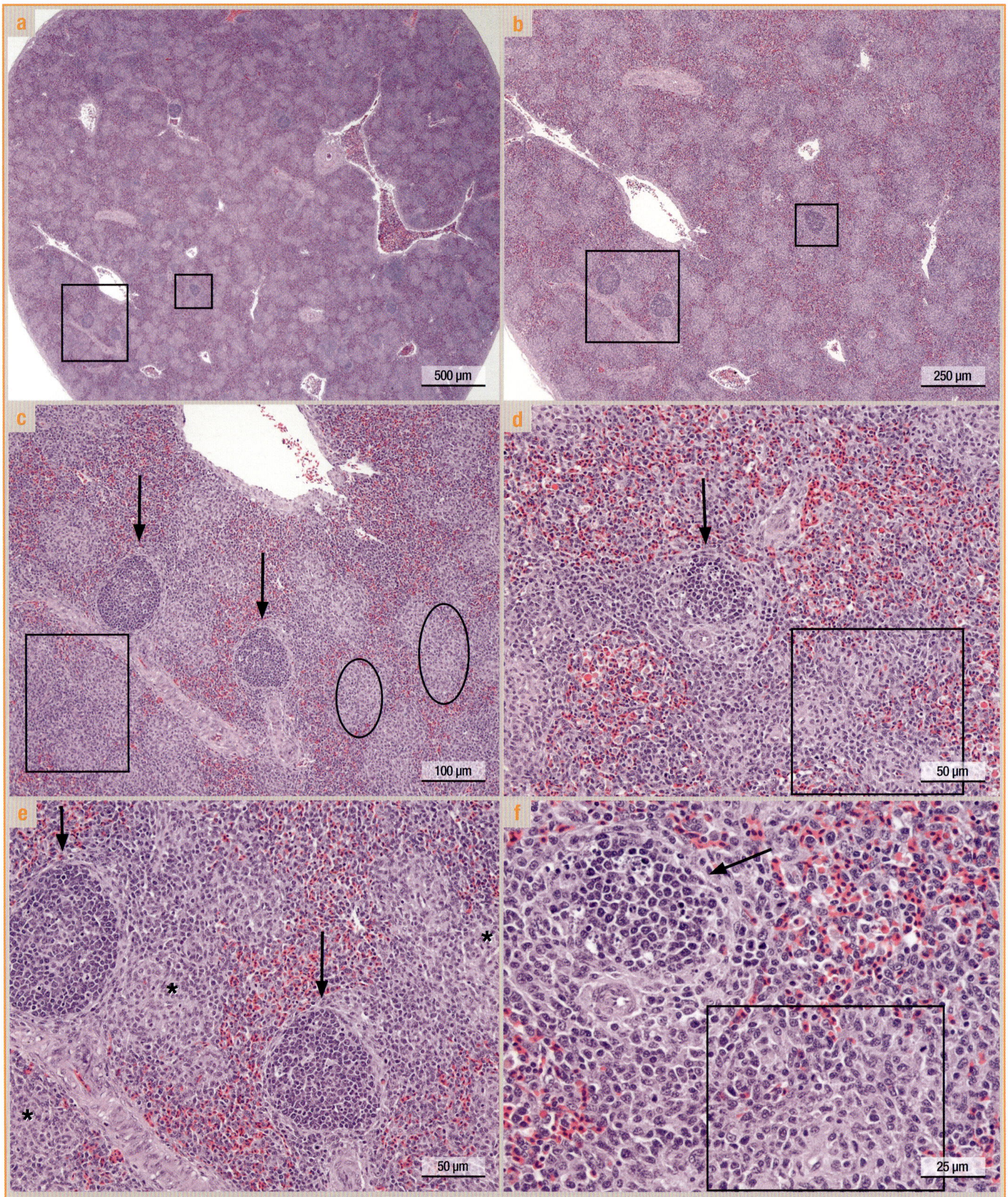

Fig. 27 Spleen from a 14 day-old broiler chicken with reticular hyperplasia and mild loss of lymphocytes. Lesions are not disease specific. (a) PALS (boxes) is shown at higher magnification in b-f. Bar = 500 µm. (b) Bar = 250 µm. (c) Increased reticular cells (ovals) are pale staining. Bar = 100 µm. (d) Loss of lymphocytes in bursa-dependent nodule (arrow). Region with reticular hyperplasia (box). Bar = 50 µm. (e) Reticular hyperplasia (*). Bar = 50 µm. (f) Bursa dependent nodule (arrow) has loss of lymphocytes. Note increased reticular cells (box). Bar = 25 µm.

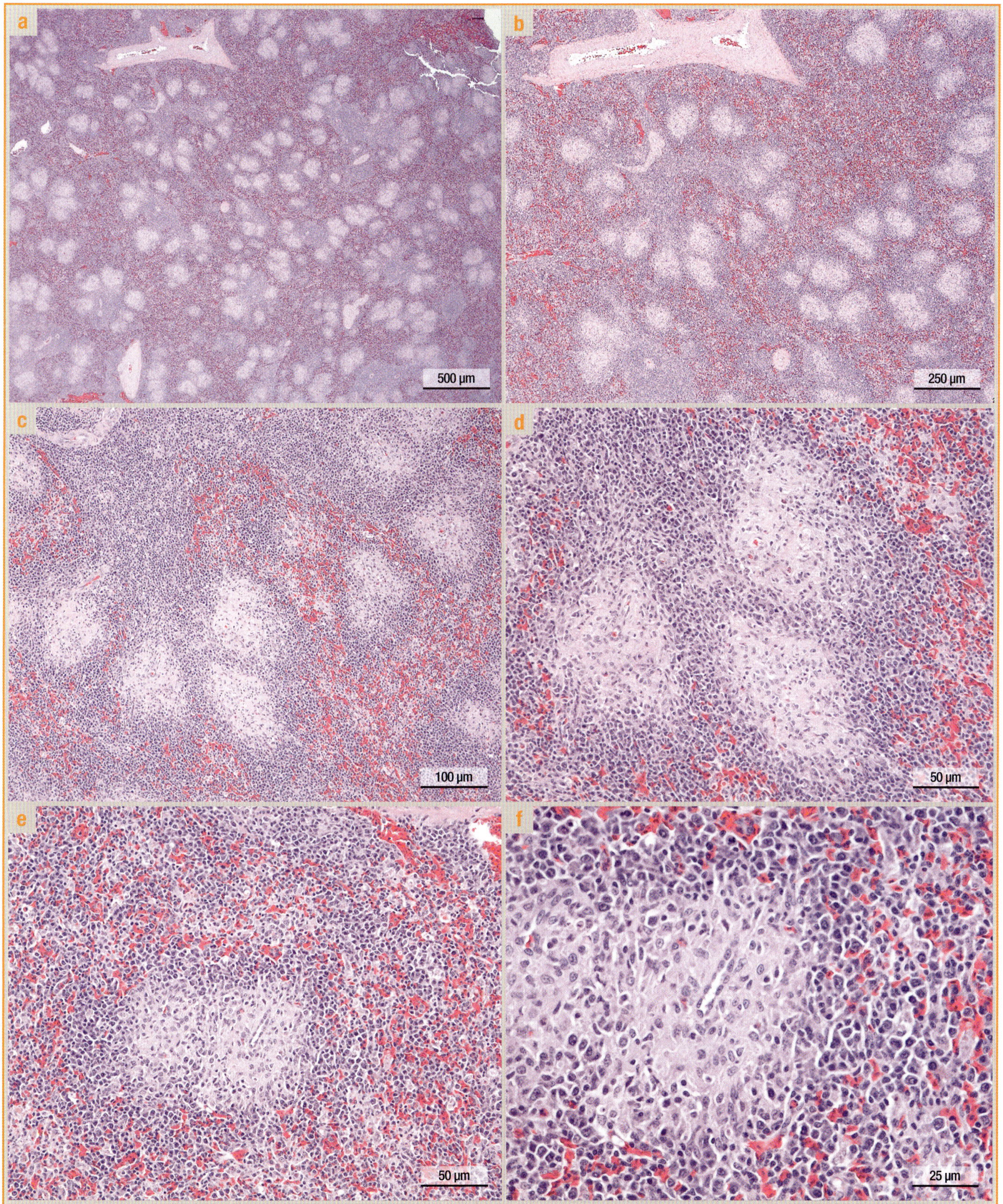

Fig. 28 Spleen from a 45 week-old broiler breeder chicken with pasteurellosis shows reticular hyperplasia. (a) Bar = 500 µm. (b) Bar = 250 µm. (c) Bar = 100 µm. (d) Bar = 50 µm. (e) Bar = 50 µm. (f) Bar = 25 µm. Note the loss of lymphocytes and increased reticular cells in this PELS region.

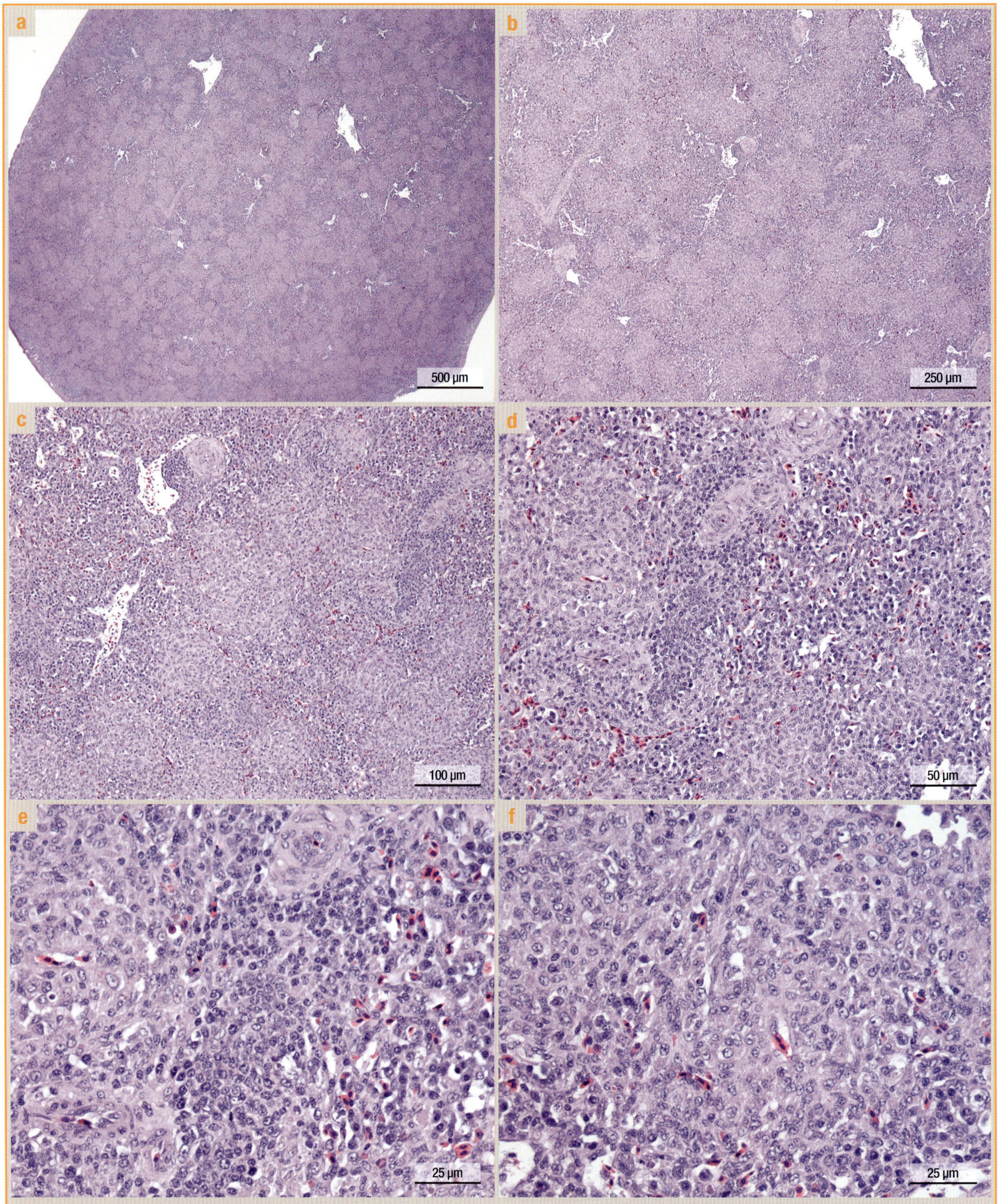

Fig. 29 Spleen from a 2 week-old broiler breeder chicken has severe reticular hyperplasia (lesion score is 4). Few lymphocytes remain. Cause was undetermined. (a) Bar = 500 µm. (b) Bar = 250 µm. (c) Bar = 100 µm. (d) Few lymphocytes remain in this PALS region. Bar = 50 µm. (e) Bar = 25 µm. (f) Bar = 25 µm.

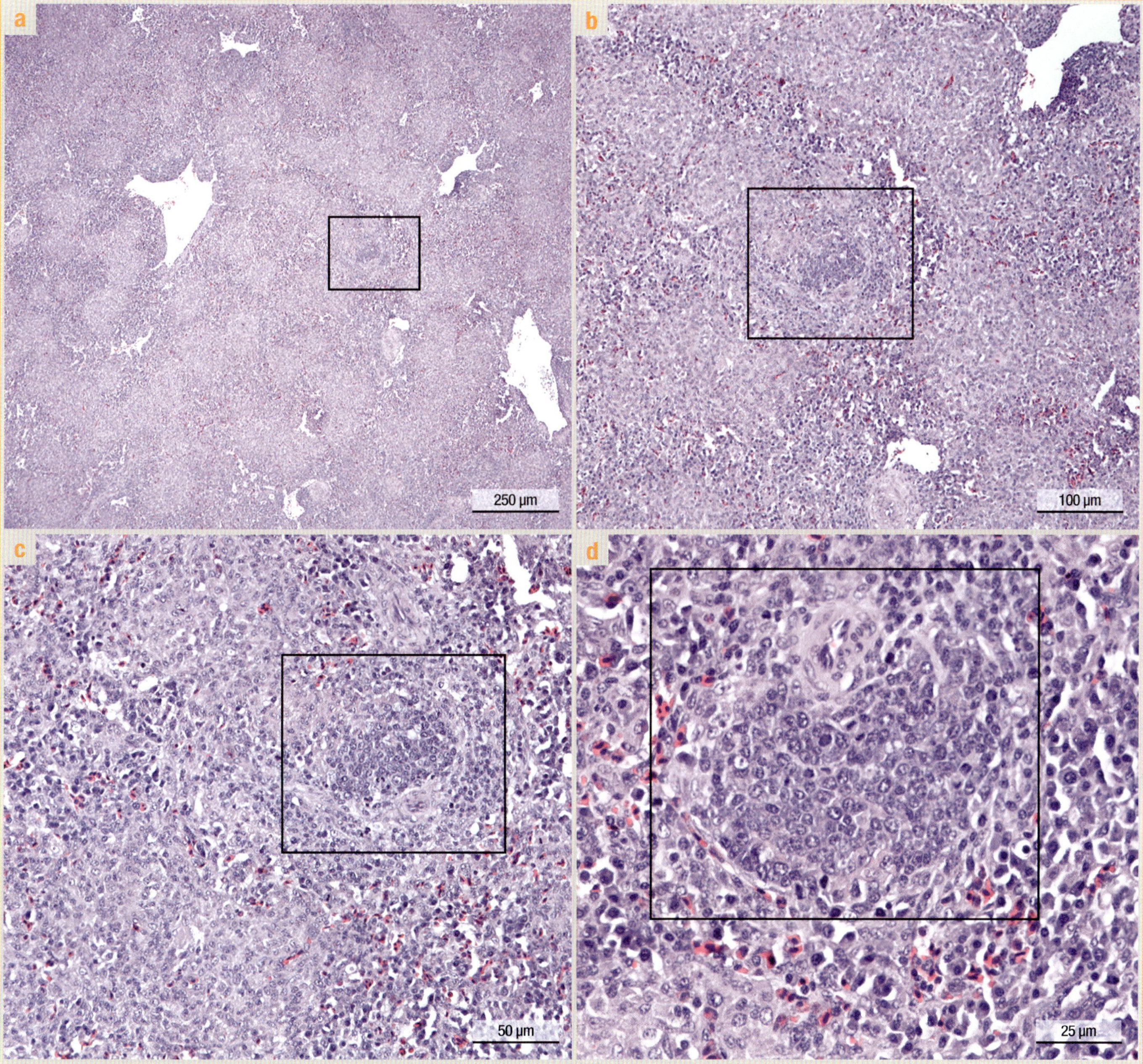

Fig. 30 Spleen from a 2 week-old broiler breeder chicken (see also Fig. 29). Reticular cells are replacing red pulp, PALS and PELS regions. Small bursa dependent nodule is shown (box), rest of PALS is region is filled with reticular cells. (a) Bar = 250 µm. (b) Bar = 100 µm. (c) Bar = 50 µm. (d) Bar = 25 µm.

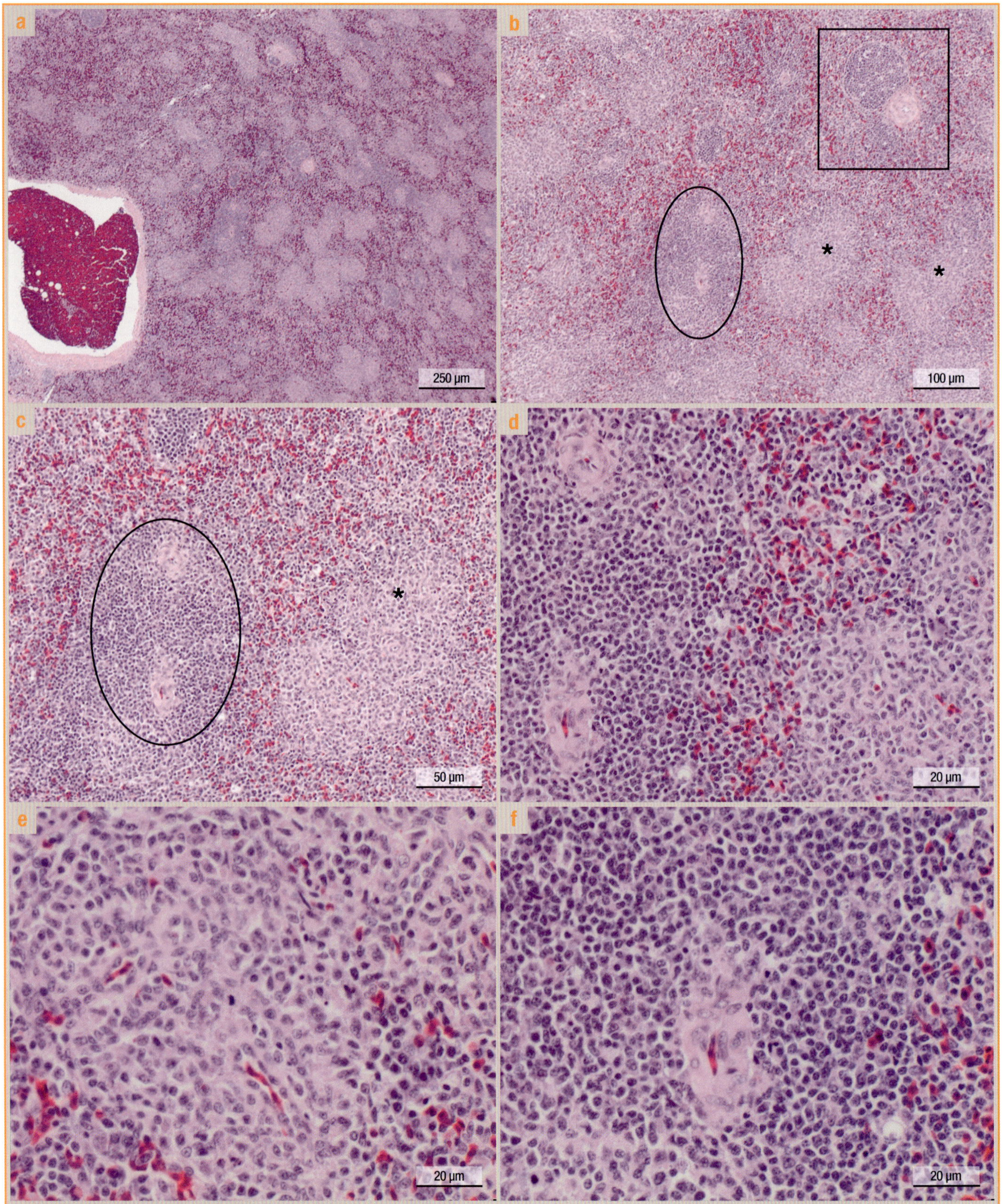

Fig. 31 Spleen form a 49 day-old broiler chicken has multicentric histiocytosis. (a) Bar = 250 µm. (b) Bursa dependent nodule (box) and T-dependent lymphocytes in PALS (oval). Proliferating reticular cells (*) are in the PELS. Bar = 100 µm. (c) PALS (oval) and reticular cells (*). Bar = 50 µm. (d) Bar = 20 µm. (e) Reticular cells in PELS. Bar = 20 µm. (f) Lymphocytes in PALS. Bar = 20 µm.

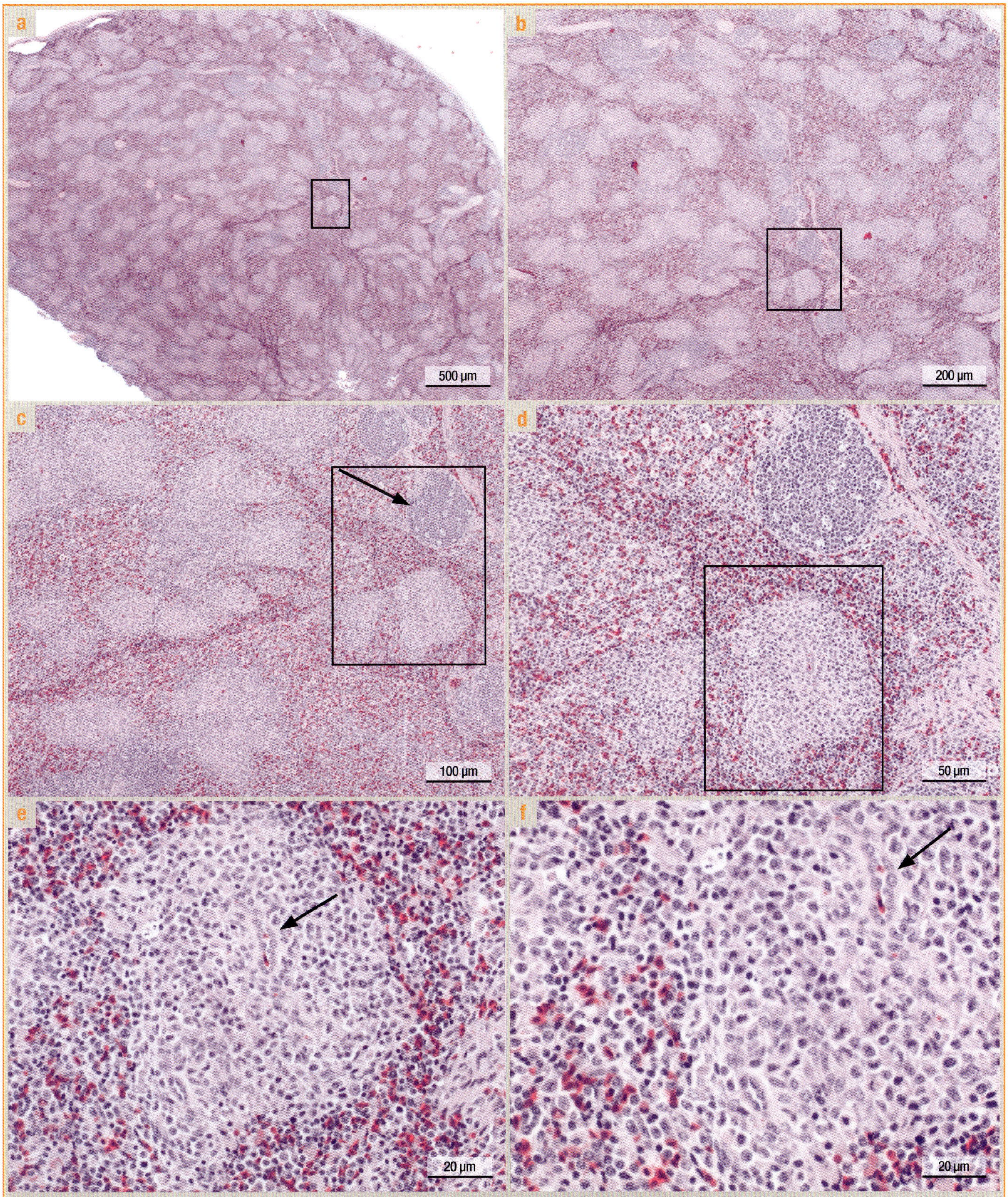

Fig. 32 Spleen from a 49 day-old broiler chicken with multicentric histiocytosis shows the nodular proliferation of reticular cells (histiocytes). Region in box is shown at progressively higher magnifications in b-f with bursa dependent nodule (arrow) and reticular hyperplasia in PELS (box). (a) Bar = 500 µm. (b) Bar = 200 µm. (c) Bar = 100 µm. (d) Bar = 50 µm. (e) Arrow identifies sheathed venule in PELS. Bar = 20 µm. (f) Arrow identifies sheathed venule in PELS. Bar = 20 µm.

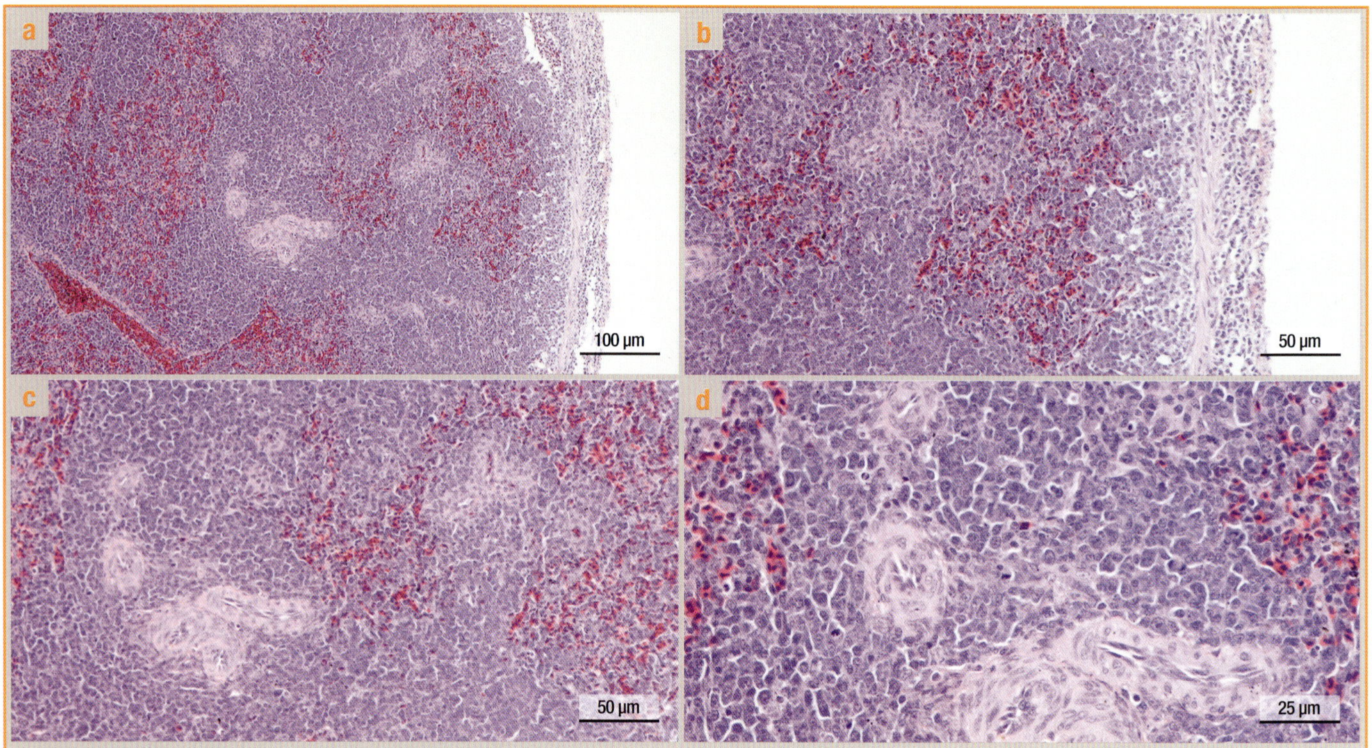

Fig. 33 Spleen from a 47 week old broiler breeder chicken shows proliferation of neoplastic lymphocytes that are expanding and replacing cells in the PALS, in the region just beneath the capsule and on the capsule. Diagnosis is MD. (a) Bar = 100 µm. (b) Bar = 50 µm. (c) Expansion of neoplastic lymphocytes in the PALS region. Bar = 50 µm. (d) PALS region. Bar = 25 µm.

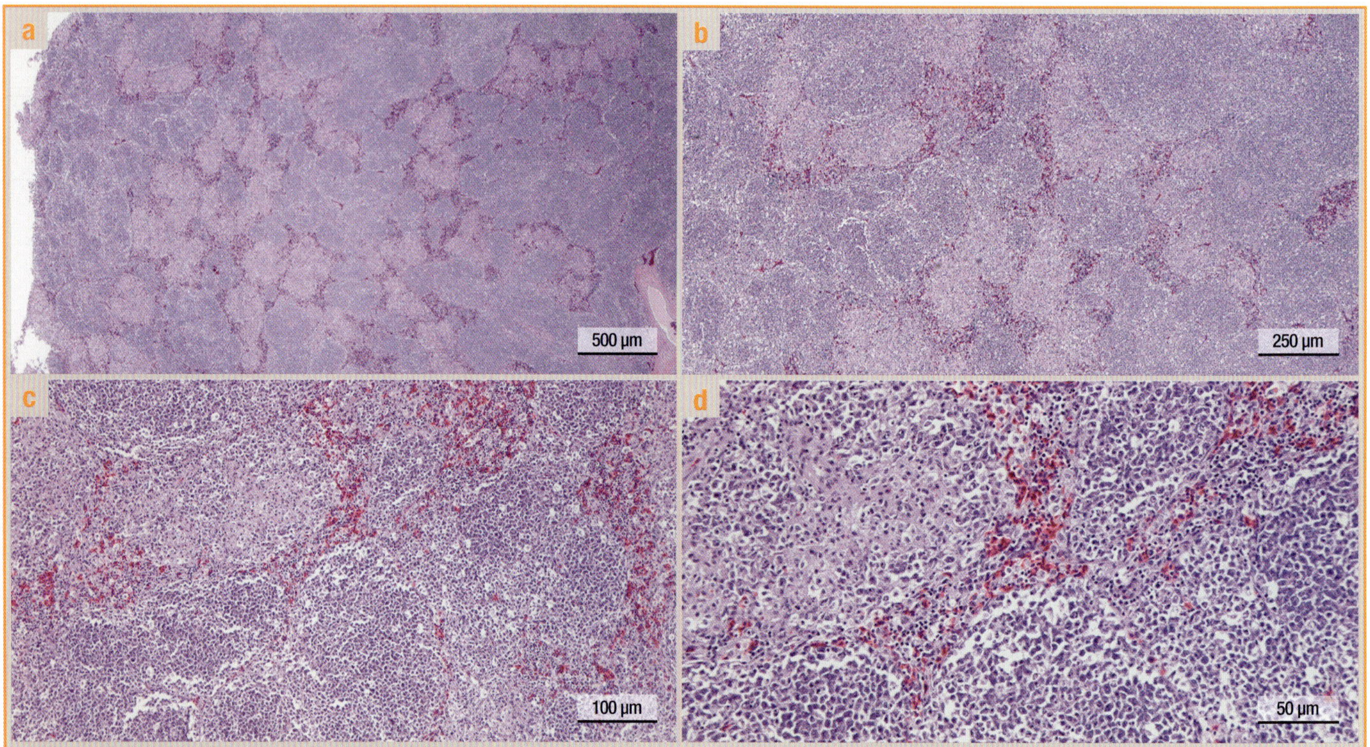

Fig. 34 Spleen from a 12 month-old pet/hobby chicken shows replacement of splenic tissue by neoplastic lymphocytes expanding in a nodular pattern. Diagnosis is lymphoid leukosis. Chicken had grossly enlarged liver and spleen. (a) Bar = 500 µm. (b) Bar = 250 µm. (c) Bar = 100 µm. (d) Nodular pattern is more apparent at this higher magnification. Bar = 50 µm.

Conclusions

Lymphocyte loss results from increased apoptosis or necrosis. Loss of lymphocytes is followed often by atrophy and, especially in the spleen, hyperplasia of reticular cells or histiocytes. These changes may be accompanied by inflammatory lesions including increased numbers of heterophils and macrophages and/or fibrosis and are consistent with a presumptive diagnosis of immunosuppression. Histopathology is one of the widely used, currently available tools that provide information upon which to base a presumptive diagnosis of immunosuppression. However, morphology alone is not a direct measurement of immune function. It would be better to measure immune system function directly, but current methods for measuring immune function are not cost effective or practical for application on farms (at "chicken-side").

It is possible for immunosuppression to be present in chickens having no or mild changes in BF, thymus, and/or spleen. It is also possible that chickens with lesions in these major lymphoid organs may lack detectable functional deficiencies of immune function. Thus, it is necessary to keep the limitations of our current methods of assessment in mind.

Post mortem changes make evaluation of these major lymphoid organs, or any tissues for that matter, difficult or impossible. Proper collection, handling and prompt fixation of organs are essential if good, useful information is to be obtained.

Lesions of lymphocyte depletion and atrophy in the major lymphoid organs of chickens examined as clinical case submissions are not likely to be disease specific. IBD, CAV, MD, and the mycotoxins should be considered in the differential diagnosis of such cases. Correlation of histopathology with lymphoid organ to body weight ratios and with functional evaluation of the immune system is recommended to maximize assessments of immunosuppression.

References

1. Adair, B.M. Immunopathogenesis of chicken anemia virus infection. Develop. Comp. Immun. 24:247-255. 2000.
2. Aly, M.M., R.L. Witter, and A.M. Fadly. Enhancement of reticuloendotheliosis virus-induced bursal lymphomas by serotype 2 Marek's disease virus. Avian Pathol. 25:81-94. 1996.
3. Arshad, S.S., A.P. Bland, S.M. Hacker, and L.N. Panyne. A low incidence of histiocytic sarcomatosis is associated with infection of chickens with the HPRS-103 strain of subgroup J avian leukosis virus. Avian Dis. 41:947-956. 1997.
4. Bang, B.G., M.A. Foard, and F.B. Bang. The effect of vitamin A deficiency and Newcastle disease on lymphoid cell systems in chickens. Proc. Soc. Exp. Biol. Med. 143:1140-1146. 1973.
5. Biggs, P.M., and V. Nair. The long view: 40 years of Marek's disease research and Avian Pathology. Avian Pathol. 41:3-9. 2012.
6. Biro, E., K. Kocsis, N. Nagy, D. Molnar, S. Kabell, V. Palya, and I. Olah. Origin of the chicken splenic reticular cells influences the effect of the infectious bursal disese virus on the extracellular matrix. Avian Pathol. 40:199-206. 2011.
7. Blagburn, B.L., D.S. Lindsay, F.J. Hoerr, J.F. Davis, and J.J. Giambrone. Pathobiology of cryptosporidiosis (*C. baileyi*) in broiler chickens. J. Protozool. 38:25. 1991.
8. Calnek, B.W., R.W. Harris, C. Buscaglia, K.A. Schat, and B. Lucio. Relationship between the immunosuppressive potential and the pathotype of Marek's disease virus isolates. Avian Dis. 42:124-132. 1998.
9. Cooper, M.D. A life of adventure in immunobiology. Ann. Rev. Immunol. 28:1-19. 2010.
10. Cooper, M.D., L.N. Payne, P.B. Dent, B.R. Burmester, and R.A. Good. Pathogenesis of avian lymphoid leukosis. I. Histogenesis. J. Natl. Cancer Inst. 41:373-378. 1968.
11. Cooper, M.D., R.D. Peterson, M.A. South, and R.A. Good. The functions of the thymus system and the bursa system in the chicken. J. Immunol. 176:75-110. 1996.
12. Cooper, M.D., H.G. Purchase, D.E. Bockman, and W.E. Gathings. Studies on the nature of the abnormality of B cell differentiation in avian lymphoid leukosis: Production of heterogeneous IgM by tumor cells. J. Immunol. 113:1210-1222. 1974.
13. Crowley, T.M., V.R. Haring, and R. Moore. Chicken Anemia Virus: An Understanding of the in-vitro host response over time. Viral Immunol. 24:3-9. 2011.
14. Dent, P.B., M.D. Cooper, L.N. Payne, J.J. Solomon, B.R. Burmester, and R.A. Good. Pathogenesis of avian lymphoid leukosis. II. Immunologic reactivity during lymphomagenesis. J. Natl. Cancer Inst. 41:391-401. 1968.
15. Dohms, J.E., and A. Metz. Stress-mechanisms of immunosuppression. Vet Immunol Immunopathol 30:89-109. 1991.
16. Ezeokoli, C.D., E.A. Ityondo, A.I. Nwannenna, and J.U. Umoh. Immunosuppression and histopathological changes in the bursa of Fabricius associated with infectious bursal disease vaccination in chicken. Comp. Immunol., Microbiol. Infect.Dis. 13:181-188. 1990.
17. Fletcher, O.J., C.S. Eidson, and S.E. Kleven. Bursal lesions in chickens inoculated with Marek's disease vaccines. Avian Dis. 16:153-162. 1972.
18. Fletcher, O.J., J.F. Munnell, and R.K. Page. Cryptosporidiosis of the bursa of Fabricius of chickens. Avian Dis. 19:630-639. 1975.
19. Gelb, J., Jr., D.J. Jackwood, E. Mundt, C.R. Pope, R. Hein, G. Slacum, J.M. Harris, B.S. Ladman, P. Lynch, D.A. Bautista, J.M. Ruano, and M.M. Troeber. Characterization of infectious bursal disease viruses isolated in 2007 from Delmarva commercial broiler chickens. Avian Dis. 56:82-89. 2012.
20. Glick, B. The bursa of Fabricius: The evolution of a discovery. Poult. Sci. 73:979-983. 1994.
21. Glick, B., T.S. Chang, and R.G. Jaap. The bursa of Fabricius and antibody production. Poult. Sci. 35:224-225. 1956.
22. Goodwin, M.A., J. Brown, and O.J. Fletcher. The relationship of Cryptosporidium sp. infection of the bursa of Fabricius, intestinal tract, and respiratory system of chickens in Georgia, 1974-1988. Avian Dis. 34:701-703. 1990.
23. Hafner, S., M.A. Goodwin, E.J. Smith, D.I. Bounous, M. Puette, L.C. Kelley, K.A. Langheinrich, and A.M. Fadly. Multicentric histiocytosis in young chickens. Gross and light microscopic pathology. Avian Dis. 40:202. 1996.
24. Haridy, M., J. Sasaki, M. Ikezawa, K. Okada, and M. Goryo. Pathological and immunohistochemical studies of subclinical infection of chicken anemia virus in 4-week-old chickens. J. Vet. Med. Sci. 74:757-764. 2012.
25. Henry, C.W., and R.N. Brewer. Scoring microscopic lesions in the bursa of Fabricius, thymus, spleen and kidney in chickens experimentally infected with infectious bursal disease virus. Poult. Sci. 58:1066-1067.1979.
26. Henry, C.W., R.N. Brewer, S.A. Edgar, and B.W. Gray. Studies on infectious bursal disease in chickens. II. Scoring microscopic lesions in the bursa of Fabricius, thymus, spleen, and kidney in gnotobiotic and battery reared White Leghorns experimentally infected with infectious bursal disease virus. Poult. Sci. 59:1006-1017. 1980.
27. Hoerr, F.J. Clinical aspects of immunosuppression in poultry. Avian Dis. 54:2-15. 2010.
28. Hoerr, F.J. Pathology of Multifactoral diseases in broiler chickens. In: 62nd Annual Meeting, The American College of Veterinary Pathologists. Nashville, TN. 2011.

29. Imai, K., M. Mase, K. Tsukamoto, H. Hihara, and N. Yuasa. Persistent infection with chicken anaemia virus and some effects of highly virulent infectious bursal disease virus infection on its persistency. Res. Vet. Sci. 67:233-238. 1999.
30. Inoue, M., M. Fukuda, and K. Miyano. Thymic lesions in chicken infected with infectious bursal disease virus. Avian Dis. 38:839-846. 1994.
31. Jeurissen, S.H.M. Structure and function in the chicken spleen. Res. in Immunol. 142:352-355. 1991.
32. Jeurissen, S.H.M., E. Claassen, and E.M. Janse. Histological and functional differentiation of non-lymphoid cells in the chicken spleen. Immunol. 77:75-80. 1992.
33. Jeurissen, S.H.M., F. Wagenaar, J.M.A. Pol, A.J. van der Eb, and M.H.M. Noteborn. Chicken anemia virus causes apoptosis of thymocytes after in vivo infection and of cell lines after in vitro infection. J. Virol. 66:7383-7388. 1992.
34. John, J.L. The avian spleen: A neglected organ. Quart. Rev. of Biol. 69:327-351. 1994.
35. Kim, I.J., M. Gagic, and J.M. Sharma. Recovery of antibody-producing ability and lymphocyte repopulation of bursal follicles in chickens exposed to infectious bursal disease virus. Avian Dis. 43:401-413. 1999.
36. Kuscu, B., and A. Gurel. Lesions in the thymus and bone marrow in chicks with experimentally induced chicken infectious anemia disease. J. Vet. Sci. 9:15-23. 2008.
37. Liu, H., M. Zhang, H. Han, J. Yuan, and Z. Li. Comparison of the expression of cytokine genes in the bursal tissues of the chickens following challenge with infectious bursal disease viruses of varying virulence. Virol. J. 7:364. 2010.
38. Mahgoub, H.A. An overview of infectious bursal disease. Arch. Virol. 157:2047-2057. 2012.
39. Mazariegos, L.A., P.D. Lukert, and J. Brown. Pathogenicity and immunosuppressive properties of infectious bursal disease "intermediate" strains. Avian Dis. 34:203-208. 1990.
40. McNeilly, F., J.A. Smyth, B.M. Adair, and M.S. McNulty. Synergism between chicken anemia virus (CAV) and avian reovirus following dual infection of 1-day-old chicks by a natural route. Avian Dis. 39: 532-537. 1995.
41. Miller, M.M., and K.A. Schat. Chicken infectious anemia virus: an example of the ultimate host-parasite relationship. Avian Dis 48:734-745. 2004.
42. Montgomery, R.D., P. Villegas, D.L. Dawe, and J. Brown. A comparison between the effect of an avian reovirus and infectious bursal disease virus on selected aspects of the immune system of the chicken. Avian Dis. 30:298-308. 1986.
43. Mundt, E. First ringtest on histopathological scoring of bursal section of IBDV infected chicken. In: Immunosuppressive Viral Diseases in Poultry. Proc. and Report 2002. European Communities, COST Action 839. T. van den Berg, ed. European Commission Directorate - General for Research, Brussels. pp 227-238. 2002.
44. Payne, L.N. Retrovirus-induced disease in poultry. Poult. Sci. 77:1204-1212. 1998.
45. Payne, L.N., and V. Nair. The long view: 40 years of avian leukosis research. Avian Pathol. 41:11-19. 2012.
46. Peterson, R.D., H.G. Purchase, B.R. Burmester, M.D. Cooper, and R.A. Good. Relationships among visceral lymphomatosis, bursa of Fabricius, and bursa-dependent lymphoid tissue of the chicken. J. Natl. Cancer Inst. 36:585-598. 1966.
47. Pope, C.R. Pathology of lymphoid organs with emphasis on immunosuppression. Vet. Immunol. Immunopathol. 30:31-44. 1991.
48. Pope, C.R. Lymphoid system. In: Avian Histopathology, 2nd ed. C. Riddell, ed. AAAP, New Bolton Center. pp 17-44. 1996.
49. Randall, C.J. Cryptosporidiosis of the Bursa of Fabricius and Trachea in Broilers. Avian Pathol. 11:95-102. 1982.
50. Rautenschlein, S., H.Y. Yeh, and J.M. Sharma. Comparative immunopathogenesis of mild, intermediate, and virulent strains of classic infectious bursal disease virus. Avian Dis. 47:66-78. 2003.
51. Rhee, J.K., H.C. Kim, and B.K. Park. Effects of Cryptosporidium baileyi infection on the bursa of Fabricius in chickens. Korean J. Parasitol. 35:181-187. 1997.
52. Rosales, A.G., P. Villegas, P.D. Lukert, O.J. Fletcher, and J. Brown. Immunosuppressive potential and pathogenicity of a recent isolate of infectious bursal disease virus in commercial broiler chickens. Avian Dis. 33:724-728. 1989.
53. Rosales, A.G., P. Villegas, P.D. Lukert, O.J. Fletcher, M.A. Mohamed, and J. Brown. Isolation, identification, and pathogenicity of two field strains of infectious bursal disease virus. Avian Dis. 33:35-41. 1989.
54. Ross, E.A., R.E. Coughlan, A. Flores-Langarica, S. Lax, J. Nicholson, G.E. Desanti, J.I. Marshall, S. Bobat, J. Hitchcock, A. White, W.E. Jenkinson, M. Khan, I.R. Henderson, G.G. Lavery, C.D. Buckley, G. Anderson, and A.F. Cunningham. Thymic function is maintained during *Salmonella*-induced atrophy and recovery. J. Immunol. 189:4266-4274. 2012.
55. Sharma, J.M., J. Dohms, M. Walser, and D.B. Snyder. Presence of lesions without virus replication in the thymus of chickens exposed to infectious bursal disease virus. Avian Dis. 37:741-748. 1993.
56. Sharma, J.M., I.J. Kim, S. Rautenschlein, and H.Y. Yeh. Infectious bursal disease virus of chickens: pathogenesis and immunosuppression. Dev. Comp. Immunol. 24:223-235. 2000.

57. Skeeles, J.K., P.D. Lukert, E.V. De Buysscher, O.J. Fletcher, and J. Brown. Infectious bursal disease viral infections. II. The relationship of age, complement levels, virus-neutralizing antibody, clotting, and lesions. Avian Dis. 23:107-117. 1979.
58. Smyth, J.A., D.A. Moffett, M.S. McNulty, D. Todd, and D.P. Mackie. A sequential histopathologic and immunocytochemical study of chicken anemia virus infection at one day of age. Avian Dis. 37:324-338. 1993.
59. Sommer, F., and C. Cardona. Chicken anemia virus in broilers: dynamics of the infection in two commercial broiler flocks. Avian Dis 47:1466-1473. 2003.
60. Takami, S., M. Goryo, T. Masegi, and K. Okada. Histopathological characteristics of spindle-cell proliferative disease in broiler chickens and its experimental reproduction in specific pathogen-free chickens. J. Vet. Med. Sci. 66:231-235. 2004.
61. Tanimura, N., and J.M. Sharma. In-situ apoptosis in chickens infected with infectious bursal disease virus. J. Comp. Pathol. 118:15-27. 1998.
62. Taylor, R.L., Jr., and F.M. McCorkle, Jr. A landmark contribution to poultry science--Immunological function of the bursa of Fabricius. Poult. Sci. 88:816-823. 2009.
63. Toro, H., J.C. Effler, F.J. Hoerr, and F.W. van Ginkel. Pathogenicity of infectious bursal disease virus variant AL2 in young chickens. Avian Dis. 53:78-82. 2009.
64. Toro, H., S. Ewald, and F.J. Hoerr. Serological evidence of chicken infectious anemia virus in the United States at least since 1959. Avian Dis. 50:124. 2006.
65. Toro, H., C. Gonzalez, L. Cerda, M. Hess, E. Reyes, and C. Geissea. Chicken anemia virus and fowl adenoviruses: association to induce the inclusion body hepatitis/ hydropericardium syndrome. Avian Dis 44:51-58. 2000.
66. Toro, H., V.L. van Santen, F.J. Hoerr, and C. Breedlove. Effects of chicken anemia virus and infectious bursal disease virus in commercial chickens. Avian Dis. 53:94-102. 2009.
67. Toro, H., V.L. van Santen, L. Li, S.B. Lockaby, E. van Santen, and F.J. Hoerr. Epidemiological and experimental evidence for immunodeficiency affecting avian infectious bronchitis. Avian Pathol. 35:455-464. 2006.
68. van Santen, V.L., K.S. Joiner, C. Murray, N. Petrenko, F.J. Hoerr, and H. Toro. Pathogenesis of chicken anemia virus: comparison of the oral and the intramuscular routes of infection. Avian Dis. 48:494-504. 2004.
69. Vaziry, A., A. Silim, C. Bleau, D. Frenette, and L. Lamontagne. Chicken infectious anaemia vaccinal strain persists in the spleen and thymus of young chicks and induces thymic lymphoid cell disorders. Avian Pathol. 40:377-385. 2011.
70. Wang, D., X. Jia, R. She, and Y. Liu. Acute hypersensitive-like injury in specific-pathogen-free chickens after infection with very virulent infectious bursal disease virus. Poult. Sci. 91:334-339. 2012.
71. Warner, N.L., and A. Szenberg. Effect of neonatal thymectomy on the immune response in the chicken. Nature 196:784-785. 1962.
72. Warner, N.L., A. Szenberg, and F.M. Burnet. The immunological role of different lymphoid organs in the chicken. I. Dissociation of immunological responsiveness. Aust. J. Exp. Biol. Med. Sci. 40:373-388. 1962.
73. Williams, A.E., and T.F. Davison. Enhanced immunopathology induced by very virulent infectious bursal disease virus. Avian Pathol. 34:4-14. 2005.
74. Yuasa, N., T. Taniguchi, and I. Yoshida. Isolation and some characteristics of an agent inducing anemia in chicks. Avian Dis. 23:366-385. 1979.

CHAPTER 2

NON-INFECTIOUS CAUSES OF IMMUNOSUPPRESSION: MYCOTOXINS AND STRESS

MYCOTOXINS AND IMMUNOSUPPRESSION

Orlando Osuna

STRESS AND IMMUNOSUPPRESSION

Enrique Montiel

MYCOTOXINS AND IMMUNOSUPPRESSION

Orlando Osuna

Introduction

All animals require an effective immune system that protects them from invasion by microorganisms, parasites, fungi, viruses and any foreign molecules. In commercial animal production systems, it is very difficult to completely avoid nutritional or environmental stressors, which are responsible for immunosuppression and increased susceptibility to various diseases and consequently decrease the productive and reproductive performance of farm animals. In this respect, from a nutritional perspective, mycotoxins are one of the most immunosuppressive factors in animal diets. [49,57,68]

A properly functioning immune system is of special importance to poultry because most commercial flocks are raised under intensive rearing conditions. Under such conditions, the flocks are vulnerable to rapid spread of infectious agents and disease outbreaks. [54] Both natural and acquired immunity could be severely affected by mycotoxins. [12,15,22-25,37,50,56,60]

Lymphoid organs constitute the main structural category of the avian immune system. Among the lymphoid components, the bursa of Fabricius (a site of B-lymphocyte development and differentiation) and the thymus (a site of T-lymphocyte development and differentiation) are considered to be the primary lymphoid organs. [49,50] The secondary lymphoid organs, characterized by aggregates of lymphocytes and antigen-presenting cells, are scattered throughout the body. Spleen, bone marrow, Harderian gland, bronchial-associated (BALT) and gut-associated (GALT) lymphoid tissues are the examples of secondary lymphoid organs. [54] In chickens, GALT includes the bursa of Fabricius, cecal tonsils, Peyer's patches, and lymphoid aggregates in the urodeum and protodeum. [54] Mycotoxins can affect the embryonic development and functionality of the lymphoid organs. [49,56]

The clinical toxicological syndromes caused by the ingestion of mycotoxins have been characterized in domestic animals, poultry and laboratory animals. They range from acute mortality to decreased performance and immunosuppression. In fact, consumption of certain mycotoxins, at far lower concentrations than those that produce clinical micotoxicosis, suppresses immune functions and decrease resistance to infectious diseases. [13,15,43,47,48,60]

Mycotoxin-induced immunosuppression in poultry may be manifested as:

- Decreased antibody production to antigens and impaired delayed hypersensitivity response.
- Reduction in bacterial clearance (e.g. *Salmonella*, *Brucella*, *Listeria* and *Escherichia*).
- Decreased lymphocyte proliferation (response to mitogens).
- Alterations in macrophage phagocytic ability.
- Alteration in $CD4^+/CD8^+$ ratio.
- Alteration in immune organ weights (spleen, thymus, bursa of Fabricius).
- Histological changes (lymphocyte depletion, degeneration and necrosis).

Mycotoxins can adversely affect intestinal barrier functions by reducing the intestinal epithelial integrity and removing tight junction proteins. [6,35,68] These affect, directly or indirectly, the host immune response. Such immunotoxic effects of mycotoxins render poultry susceptible to many infectious diseases. Both cell-mediated and humoral immunity may be adversely affected after feeding mycotoxins to poultry. [25]

Field diagnosis of these mycotoxins is, at times, very difficult and this emphasizes the importance of fully characterizing them so that they can be recognized as they occur in the animal industry. It appears that the level of a particular mycotoxin in the field that produces a certain effect can be much lower than the level that produces the same effect under laboratory conditions. Obviously, this difference can be explained by the complexity of environmental, social and other stressors that exist in the field compared to those in a carefully controlled laboratory experiment. Also, in the field, it is common for certain animals in a flock or herd to have subclinical disease, which would make mycotoxin interactions in the diet more severe for these animals. This difference in minimal effective dosage may be due, to some extent, to the complexity of the total and multiple mycotoxin exposure of the animal versus any single mycotoxin. [3,17,25,32,67]

The goal of this chapter is to aid in the understanding of the most toxic mycotoxins affecting the immune system of poultry at very low level of concentration in the feed such as aflatoxin, ochratoxin and the trichothecenes. In addition, other mycotoxins such as citrinin, fumonisin and ooporein can induce clinical signs and lesions very similar to those observed in infectious diseases and they are briefly described in this chapter. Nevertheless, more detail information could be found in the cited references.

Etiology

Mycotoxins are a group of structurally diverse secondary metabolites of fungi that occur as contaminants of grains worldwide. *Aspergillus*, *Alternaria*, *Claviceps*, *Fusarium* and *Penicillium* species of fungi are ubiquitous in nature and, under ideal conditions, often infect economically important crops and forages in the field, as well as during their storage, shipment and processing. Many of the secondary metabolites produced by these fungi can cause serious health problems in animals and their presence in agricultural commodities may result in serious economic losses. [36,37,41]

According to the United Nation's Food and Agricultural Organization (FAO), approximately 25 % of the world's grain supply is contaminated with mycotoxins. Worldwide, the economic losses due to mycotoxins in poultry feeds can be as much as several hundred million dollars (USD) annually. [11]

Several hundred mycotoxins have been reported in the literature, with their target sites and different mechanisms of toxicity, as their chemical structures vary for each one. More than a single mycotoxin may simultaneously contaminate feed ingredients and finished feed. When more than one mycotoxin is present in feed, the toxicity and clinical signs observed in the animals are complex and diverse. When mycotoxins are present simultaneously, interactive effects can be classified as additive, antagonistic or synergistic. [32-34] The interaction of mycotoxins in animal feeds can help to determine the levels of mycotoxins which do not cause any problems. Those levels could be lower due to the synergistic or additive effect when multiple mycotoxins interact simultaneously compared with those levels that may be required to induce problems when a single mycotoxin is found in the contaminated animal feed.

EFFECTS OF CLIMATE ON MYCOTOXIN PRODUCTION

- Aflatoxin predominates in grain in warm climates.
- Fumonisin, deoxynivalenol and zearalenone predominate in cool climates.

Mycotoxins can also interact with other factors including feed ingredients, infectious diseases, environmental conditions, heat or cold stress, ammonia, heavy metals, etc., just to mention few of the many possibilities that could interact under field conditions. [18,32]

Epidemiology

Mycotoxicosis is a general term that applies to a broad range of clinical syndromes caused by the ingestion of feed contaminated with one or more mycotoxins. The severity of the disease condition varies with the concentration of toxin ingested and the duration of toxin exposure. There are many types of mycotoxins recognized. However, the ones most commonly associated with disease in poultry include aflatoxins, ochratoxins, fusarium toxins, trichothecene, fumonisin, moniliformin, zearalenone, and fusarochromanone. [9,17,43,67]

No practical way has been found to completely prevent the formation of mycotoxins in grains prior to harvest. Since their discovery, mycotoxins have been a thorn in the side of feed mills and poultry production facilities. They will continue to be unavoidable contaminants in animal feed due to the ubiquitous nature of molds. Virtually all-animal feed grains contain molds and viable mold spores. These molds are capable of producing mycotoxins when the environmental conditions are correct. Infections of the grain usually occur in the field during the pre-harvest stage and contamination levels vary from year to year. High contamination levels are frequently associated with pre-harvest physiological stressors such as drought or insect damage. In addition, aflatoxin tends to predominate in grain that is produced in warmer climates. Grain that is produced in cooler climates is likely to contain the Fusarium toxins such as fumonisin, deoxynivalenol and zearalenone. [44]

Aflatoxins

Aflatoxin production occurs when *Aspergillus flavus* and *Aspergillus parasiticus* attack peanuts, cottonseed, white and yellow corn, certain nuts and wheat. Chemically, they are polycyclic furan compounds possessing intense blue or green fluorescence under long wave UV light. There are four frequently reported aflatoxin contaminants in grain identified as aflatoxin B1, B2, G1 and G2. Aflatoxin B1 is the most toxic, and hepatotoxicity and immunotoxicity are the primary effects in nearly all animals. Drought, extreme heat and corn ear injury from insect feeding stress the corn and create an environment favorable to these molds and to eventual aflatoxin production. It is now known that aflatoxin can be produced in standing grain before harvest and can continue to be produced during storage, especially when moisture content is above 12 % and temperature is greater than 21 °C (70 °F). Aflatoxin, once produced, is quite stable to heat, milling, pelleting and many chemicals. [35,52,53]

Clinical signs of aflatoxicosis

Clinical signs of mycotoxicosis vary significantly with avian species, type of mycotoxin, dose ingested, and the duration of the toxin exposure to poultry. [18,19,43] Aflatoxins are primarily associated with liver disease and immunotoxicity. Aflatoxins, such as AFB1, are known hepatocarcinogens and causes liver lesions in both mammalian and avian species. [49]

Clinical signs associated with aflatoxin exposure in broilers include:

- Anorexia.
- Poor growth (Fig. 1).
- Impaired feed utilization.
- Passage of undigested feed particles.
- Increased feed conversion.
- Increased morbidity and mortality.
- Increased leg problems.
- Increased carcass condemnations.

In addition, in broilers clinical signs include:

- Poor feather growth.
- Loss of pigmentation on the feet and legs.
- Bruising and changes in relative organ weights. [27,36,37]

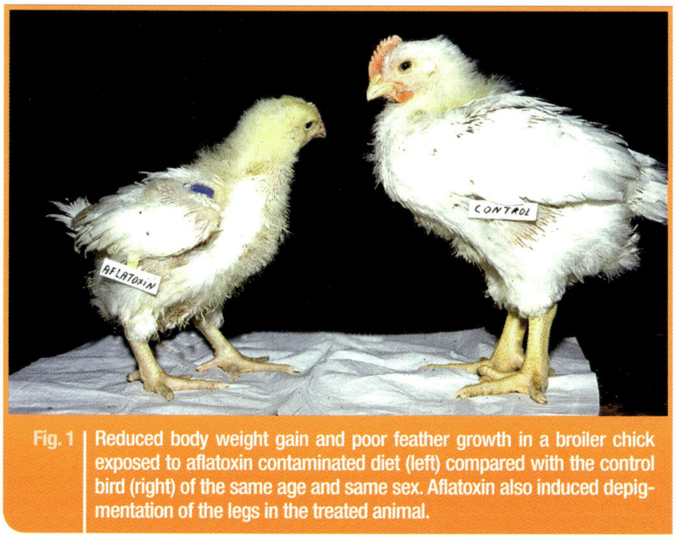

Fig. 1 Reduced body weight gain and poor feather growth in a broiler chick exposed to aflatoxin contaminated diet (left) compared with the control bird (right) of the same age and same sex. Aflatoxin also induced depigmentation of the legs in the treated animal.

EFFECTS OF MYCOTOXINS ON IMMUNITY OF POULTRY

- Involution of the bursa of Fabricius.
- Involution of the thymus.
- Decrease immunoglobulin production.
- Decrease mucosal immunity.
- Decrease complement and interferon production.
- Decrease phagocytosis of neutrophils, monocytes, thrombocytes, and macrophages.
- Humoral immunity affected.
- Cell mediated immunity affected.
- Skin of legs, feathers, oral cavity, and gastrointestinal mucosa affected.

In all cases, aflatoxicosis may also be associated with an increase susceptibility to infectious diseases and failure of vaccination programs. [22,37] Without doubt, one of the major manifestations of mycotoxicosis is the loss of the flock's body weight uniformity.

Feeding aflatoxin to laying hens has been shown to:

- Increase relative liver weights.
- Reduce relative ovary weights.

This decrease of relative ovary weight adversely affects the size and number of the ova, a phenomenon detrimental to future egg production. [59]

Outbreaks of aflatoxicosis in laying hens have been documented with:

- A marked decrease in egg production.
- A reduced egg size.
- A decreased pigmentation of the egg yolk.
- Feather picking.
- Characteristically enlarged fatty livers. [65]

Chronic ingestion of aflatoxin affects renal function of laying hens and induces calcium, phosphorus and sodium losses. [40] Aflatoxin could also induce nutrient loss in laying hens due to a direct or indirect effect, or both, on functionality and characteristics of the gastrointestinal tract. [4]

In mature broiler breeders aflatoxins are reported to:

- Decrease fertility and hatchability.
- Increase embryo mortality mainly increasing the percentage of early-dead and late-dead embryos. [49]

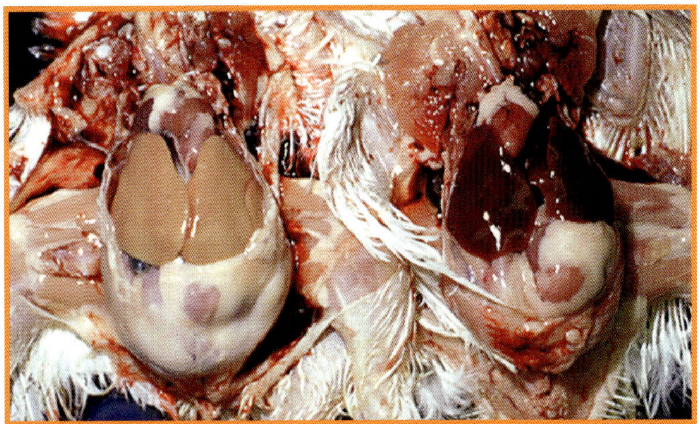

Fig. 2 | Friable, pale and enlarged liver in a broiler chicken fed aflatoxin-contaminated diet (left) and compared to the liver of the control group (right). Image kindly provided by Dr. David Ledoux.

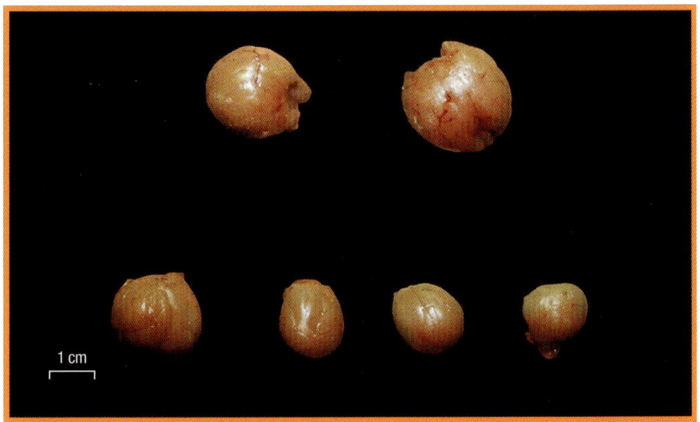

Fig. 3 | Reduced size of the bursa of Fabricius of chicken exposed to dietary aflatoxin (below) and compared with the normal size of the bursa of Fabricius of the control diet group (above).

The cause of the increase in embryo mortality is most likely due to the transfer of toxic metabolites from the diet of the hen to the egg.[65] This hypothesis agrees with the findings of residues of aflatoxicol and aflatoxin B1 in eggs of both egg-type laying hens as well as broiler breeder hens within 24 hours after initiation of aflatoxin being incorporated into the diet.[49,58] This would also permit the developing embryo contact with these toxicants, both prior to and during the incubation process. Poor progeny performance has been reported in chicks from eggs laid by dams exposed previously to dietary aflatoxins.[49]

SENSITIVITY OF THE AVIAN SPECIES TO MYCOTOXINS

Among poultry, ducks are the most susceptible to aflatoxins, followed by turkeys, broilers, laying hens and quail.

It was recently demonstrated that broilers fed diets containing 50 % or more corn naturally contaminated with aflatoxin continuously for 21 or 42 days, decreased body weight gain and decreased liver protein with concentrations of aflatoxin as low as:[67]

36.9 ng/g AFB1 + 6.4 ng/g AFB2

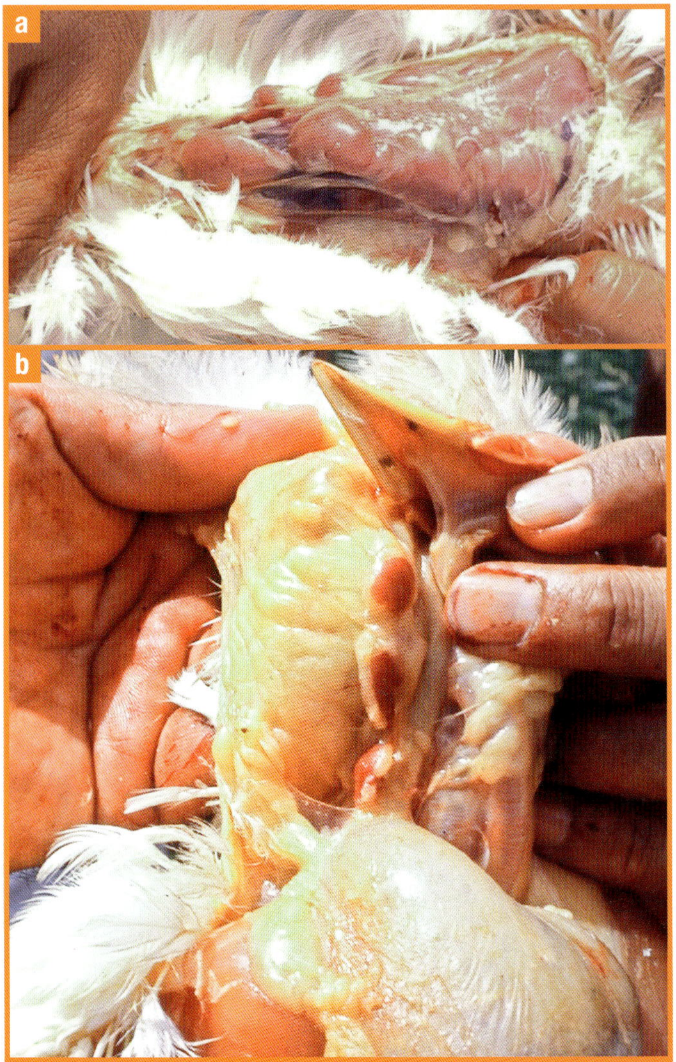

Fig. 4 | (a) Normal size and structure of the thymus gland of a broiler chicken. (b) Decreased size of the thymus gland of a broiler chicken of the same age and sex. Aflatoxin can decrease the cell-mediated immunity, as measured by graft-versus-host reactions.

Gross lesions of aflatoxin

Changes associated with the visceral organs in response to aflatoxin can assist in the initial recognition of aflatoxicosis in poultry. For example, the livers of birds with aflatoxicosis will be

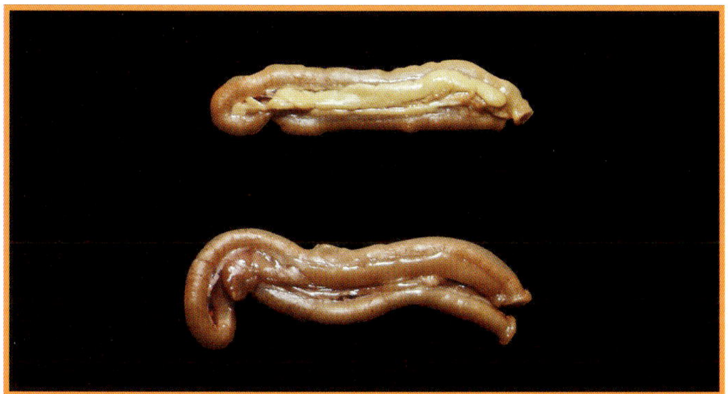

Fig. 5 | Depigmentation of the pancreas in broiler chicks exposed to aflatoxin contaminated diets (2.5 µg/g) (above) compared with the pancreas of the control group (below). A severe reduction in plasma carotenoids of broiler chicks was also observed in the same aflatoxin treated group.

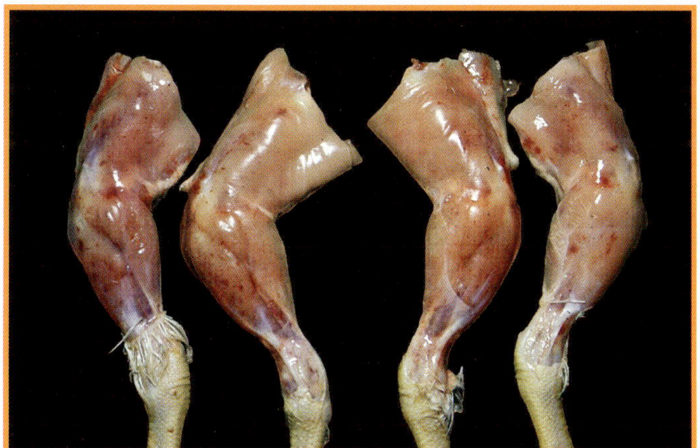

Fig. 6 | Bruising in broiler chicks exposed to diets experimentally contaminated with aflatoxin. This increased susceptibility to bruising could be due to the increased capillary fragility, decrease integrity of tissue and inadequate synthesis of blood clotting factors by the liver.

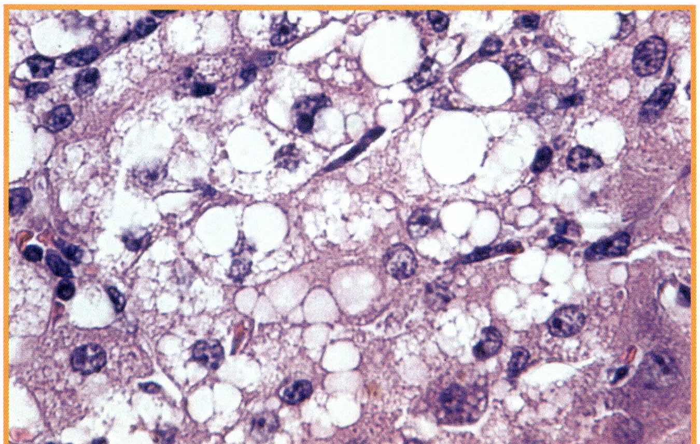

Fig. 7 | Histopathology of a liver section obtained from a broiler chick fed aflatoxin contaminated diets. This acute poisoning include disorganization of the hepatocytes with vacuolation in cytoplasm, swelling of cells, necrosis and leukocyte infiltration.

characteristically yellow, pale, friable and enlarged (Fig. 2), with microscopic changes including fatty infiltration, hepatic necrosis, and biliary hyperplasia. The gall bladder is usually enlarged and filled with bile. Kidneys of affected birds appear enlarged, congested and pale. [31,36,65]

In addition, liver, spleen, proventriculus, pancreas and kidneys are increased in size, whereas the bursa of Fabricius (Fig. 3) and thymus gland are decreased (Fig. 4). [12,23,24,36,65] The excretory potential of the kidney is reduced by aflatoxin, which could be associated with the marked thickening of the glomerular capillary membrane. [36,65] Detection of these changes is not sufficient evidence upon which to make a complete diagnosis; however, knowledge of these responses can be used as an aid in the diagnosis of aflatoxicosis and can assist in the differential diagnosis with other mycotoxins or with any other diseases. [18,25,53,65,68]

Broilers exposed to dietary aflatoxin may result in depigmentation of the pancreas (Fig. 5) as well as depigmentation of the blood serum samples. Most important, aflatoxin decreases in serum albumin, globulin, and total protein, which are indicators of impaired protein synthesis. [36,67]

An increased susceptibility to bruising (Fig. 6), resulting from increased capillary fragility, is often observed. This effect is manifested by an increased incidence of petechial hemorrhages of the musculature of young animals. This increased susceptibility to bruising occurs quite rapidly once aflatoxin is introduced into the diet of chickens. [65]

Histopathology of aflatoxin

Microscopically, liver changes following acute poisoning include disorganization of hepatocytes with vacuolation in the cytoplasm (Fig. 7), swelling of cells, centrilobular congestion, necrosis and leukocyte infiltration. Swelling and necrosis of the renal tubules epithelium have also been reported. In case of chronic exposure to toxic levels, there is a diffuse fatty change of the liver, and proliferation of the bile ducts. Mitotic figures might be seen in biliary cells. [1,31,43]

Effect of aflatoxin on the immune system of poultry

The relative sizes of the bursa of Fabricius and the thymus, primary initiators of immunity in the chickens, were reduced by aflatoxin in a dose-related fashion. The regression of these two organs by aflatoxin would be expected to result in impaired immunological performance.[22,60] It should be noted that the regression of the bursa and the suppression of antigen responses occurred with concentrations of aflatoxin that do not inhibit growth.[55]

A major concern of poultry producers is the immunosuppression caused by aflatoxin and the increase in susceptibility to a wide variety of infectious diseases along with accompanying vaccine failure and therapeutic drug failures. Aflatoxin-induced immunosuppression produces a cascading effect starting with depressed protein synthesis, lowered serum albumin and globulin levels, reduction in circulating antibody levels, impairment of the reticulo-endothelial system, reduced cell-mediated immunity, and abnormal development of the thymus and bursa of Fabricius.[17]

Aflatoxin is an immunotoxic agent that acts primary on both humoral immunity as well as on cell-mediated immunity and phagocytic cell functions.[13,23,25,49,50,56,60] In addition, aflatoxin exposure has been shown to reduce resistance to various bacterial, viral and protozoan diseases in poultry.[18,19,25,47,48]

Aflatoxin has been reported to increase the susceptibility to some infectious diseases and severity of avian infectious diseases such as salmonellosis, crop mycosis, aspergillosis, coccidiosis, infectious bursal disease (IBD), and Marek's disease (MD).[9,12,18,19,23,28,49,66] Aflatoxin caused failure of vaccine against fowl cholera in turkeys and chickens[13,15,22], Newcastle Disease (ND) and IBD in chickens.[22,24,37]

The results demonstrate that aflatoxin in feed can increase chicken susceptibility to IBDV infection.[12,24] Chickens having simultaneous aflatoxicosis and IBD had higher mortality, more severely depressed body weight, and more extensive gross and microscopic lesions associated with IBD than did chickens having IBDV alone. Thus, subclinical IBD might be accentuated by dietary aflatoxin.[24] It was also reported that IBD during aflatoxicosis could in many regards appear to be a different disease with high mortality and with major kidney involvement, coagulopathy, hypocalcemia, hypoproteinemia and enhanced enlargement of the spleen. Certainly, the changes were enough to offer difficulties for any diagnostician, and the fate of the birds could be markedly different.[12]

The combination of aflatoxin and *Eimeria tenella* has been reported to result in a synergistic effect on mortality.[64] In addition with *E. acervulina* and *E. tenella*, weight gain and body weights are reduced significantly more when coccidia and dietary aflatoxin were present together. Even mortality, which is rare with *E. acervulina,* was markedly increased by dietary aflatoxin. Either aflatoxin or *E. acervulina* alone reduced the concentration of plasma pigments. When both were present, depigmentation was greater than with each alone.[52]

Broiler breeder hens fed a diet containing aflatoxin have been shown to transfer active aflatoxin metabolites into their eggs resulting in a significant immune dysfunction in progeny chicks. In other words, the progeny of hens consuming an AFB1-contaminated diet may be increasingly susceptible to disease owing to suppression of humoral and cellular immunity.[49,56,57]

Diagnosis of aflatoxin

When aflatoxicosis is suspected, a complete diagnostic evaluation should be performed, including:

- Thorough feeding history.
- Observation of clinical signs.
- Necropsy exam.
- Tissue collection for histopathology.
- Bacterial and virus cultures.
- Serology.

These tests will help to rule out other diseases.

Analytic confirmation of aflatoxin in the material ingested is necessary to aid in the diagnosis. Feed and grain can be analyzed by several methods including the use of thin layer chromatography (TLC), high performance liquid chromatography (HPLC) and the monoclonal antibody detection (ELISA) kits. Toxin detection in tissues, particularly liver, is possible.[41]

Differential diagnosis

In general, aflatoxicosis must be differentiated from:[10,12,19,23,24,26,66]

- Poor nutrition.
- Poor management.
- Infectious diseases that could induce immunosuppression (IBD, inclusion body hepatitis, malabsorption syndrome, MD).
- Fatty liver syndrome.
- Coccidiosis.
- Selenium poisoning.
- Deficiency of linoleic acid.
- *Crotalaria* seed poisoning.

Ochratoxin A (OTA)

Ochratoxins are isocoumarin metabolites produced by certain species of *Aspergillus* and *Penicillium* fungi. Four ochratoxins –designated as A, B, C, and D– have been identified. Of these, ochratoxin A (OTA) appears as the most common in nature and has been considered to be the most potent ochratoxin that adversely affects production parameters and the health of poultry. [29,33,34] Ochratoxin is known as a nephrotoxin as it damages predominantly kidney tissue (Fig. 8). [1]

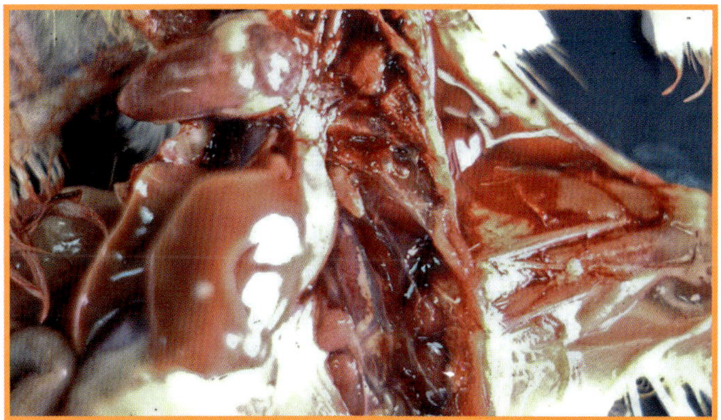

Fig. 8 | Nephrotoxic effect in broiler chicks experimentally induced with diets contaminated with ochratoxin. Note the anticoagulant effect induced by ochratoxin as an isocoumarin mycotoxin.

Clinical signs of ochratoxicosis

Typical signs of ochratoxicosis include: [20,29]

- Severe stunting.
- Suppressed feed intake.
- Poor feathering.
- Dehydration.
- Increased feed conversion.

Independent outbreaks of ochratoxicosis involving turkeys, laying hens, and broilers have previously been documented in the U. S. [20,29] Field outbreaks of ochratoxicosis in broilers were characterized by rupture of the large intestine during processing. The fragile large intestine was characterized as enlarged, with increased fat content, decreased collagen content, and decreased radial length of the collagenous longitudinal folds. [63]

Ochratoxicosis in laying hens is characterized by.

- Severe nephropathy.
- Body weight loss.
- Decreased feed intake with impaired feed efficiency.
- Delay in sexual maturity.
- Decreased egg production.
- Depressed hatchability of fertile eggs.
- Poor progeny performance in chicks from eggs laid by hens with ochratoxicosis.

Also, it has been reported that a yellow staining of eggshells is associated with ochratoxicosis. [17,65]

Gross lesions of ochratoxin A (OTA)

The nephrotoxicity of ochratoxin is easily observed upon necropsy of affected birds. The kidneys appear extremely swollen and pale in color. The ureters will often be very distinct due to the accumulation of urates. However, visceral and articular gout have not been reported in field outbreaks of ochratoxicosis. [29,32-34,65]

Perhaps the most distinctive change associated with the liver during ochratoxicosis in several species of poultry is an accumulation of glycogen. Detection of glycogen granules by microscopic examination or analysis of liver for total glycogen can be useful in the documentation of ochratoxicosis in poultry. [65]

When broiler chicks were fed simultaneously ochratoxin A and aflatoxin, synergistic toxicity resulted. The effects observed in the combination treatment were greater than could have been produced by individual mycotoxins. The kidneys appeared to be the target organ of this mycotoxin combination. Ochratoxin A's lesions persisted longer than the aflatoxin effect. [32-34]

Histopathology of ochratoxin A (OTA)

In the kidneys, OTA causes:

- Necrosis of tubular epithelial cells, glomerular infiltration and distended glomerular spaces. [1,35]
- Degeneration of the epithelium of convoluted tubules and Malpighi corpuscles, increase in the size of epithelial cells, distended and degenerated epithelium of proximal convoluted tubules and pyknotic nuclei in the cytoplasm of epithelial cells. [1,20]

Effect of OTA on the poultry immune system

Feeding OTA-contaminated diets may increase the severity of secondary infections in poultry and hence poses a threat to poultry production. [35] OTA causes reduction in the size of lymphatic organs such as spleen and bursa of Fabricius. [35]

In the bursa, OTA causes atrophy of follicles and reduction in the lymphocytic mass present in the medulla. Follicles of cortex and medulla also show vacuolar degeneration. Within the thymus, OTA exposure reduced lymphocytic mass in the parenchyma and localized congested areas were observed. [1,35] It could be hypothesized that reduced thymus weight and/or bursa of Fabricius weight, as well as reduced leucocyte counts, indicate alterations in the functioning of the immune system. [1,14,20,29]

Diagnosis of ochratoxicosis

Ochratoxin can be found in grains, feed and often in tissues such as liver and kidney. The mycotoxin can also be found in muscle and fat tissue. Residues in eggs are possible following consumption of a diet containing 1 μg/g dietary level for several weeks. Chemical analytic and immunoassay methods are available. [1,41,65]

Differential diagnosis

Ochratoxicosis must be differentiated from: [38,39,46,53]

- Aflatoxicosis.
- Visceral gout.
- Nephrotropic strains of infectious bronchitis.
- Infectious bursal disease.
- Mycotoxicosis (citrinin, oosporein, fumonisin).
- Sodium toxicosis or "salt poisoning".
- Water deprivation.
- Calcium nephropathy.
- Sesquicarbonate poisoning.
- Bicarbonate poisoning.
- Organophosphorus insecticide poisoning.
- Carbamate insecticide poisoning.
- Vitamin A deficiency.
- Malabsorption syndrome.
- Heat stress and cold stress.

Citrinin

Citrinin, like ochratoxin A, is a nephrotoxin mycotoxin in poultry. [38] Citrinin can be produced by a number of *Penicillium* and *Aspergillus* spp., usually in concert with ochratoxins. [65] The most constant clinical sign of citrinin toxicosis is the rapid increase in water consumption and the severe watery diarrhea in both laying hens and young broiler chicks (Fig. 9). Field observations indicate that most frequent clinical signs are increase in water consumption and water excretion. [38,41,42,65]

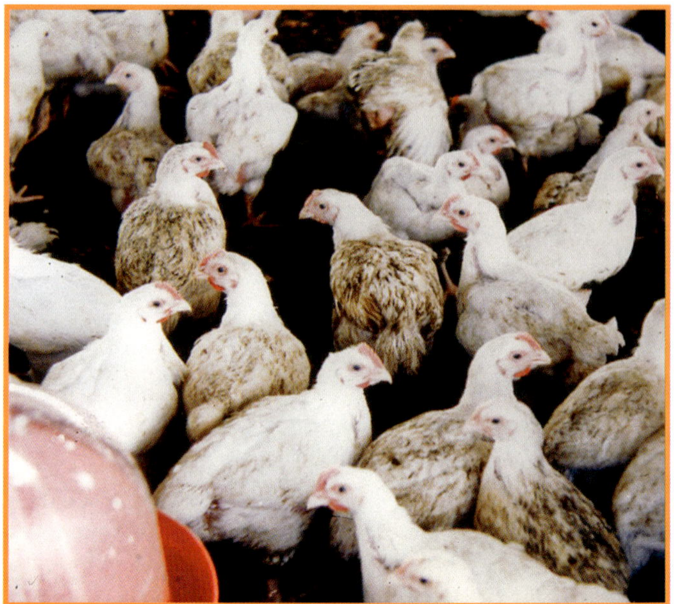

Fig. 9 Dirty feathers and wet litter resulting from an increase in water consumption induced by citrinin in broiler chickens few hours after initial exposure. Similar clinical signs and lesions can be seen with infectious enteritis, fumonisin toxicosis, ochratoxicosis, insecticide poisoning, sodium bicarbonate poisoning, and nephrotoxic strain of infectious bronchitis.

For diagnostic purposes, of citrinin toxicosis, feed analysis is recommended. [38,42] The lack of an effect on the bursa of Fabricius and spleen by citrinin should aid diagnosticians in differentiating it from ochratoxin. [42,65]

Oosporein

Oosporein has been identified as a nephrotoxin produced by the fungi *Oospora colorans*, *Chaetomium trilaterale*, *C. aureum* and numerous other filamentous. Finished poultry feeds, cereal grains, peanuts, and other feedstuffs have been identified as favorable substrates. [39,46]

Birds fed the diets with 200 μg oosporein/g of feed or more were observed to have both visceral and articular gout. Turkeys are more resistant to oosporein than chickens. [39,41,46,65]

Birds that die acutely of oosporein toxicosis have visceral gout especially of the pericardium (Fig. 10). If the exposure to oosporein is of an extended period of time, it is possible to observe both visceral and articular urate deposits (Fig. 11). [39,46]

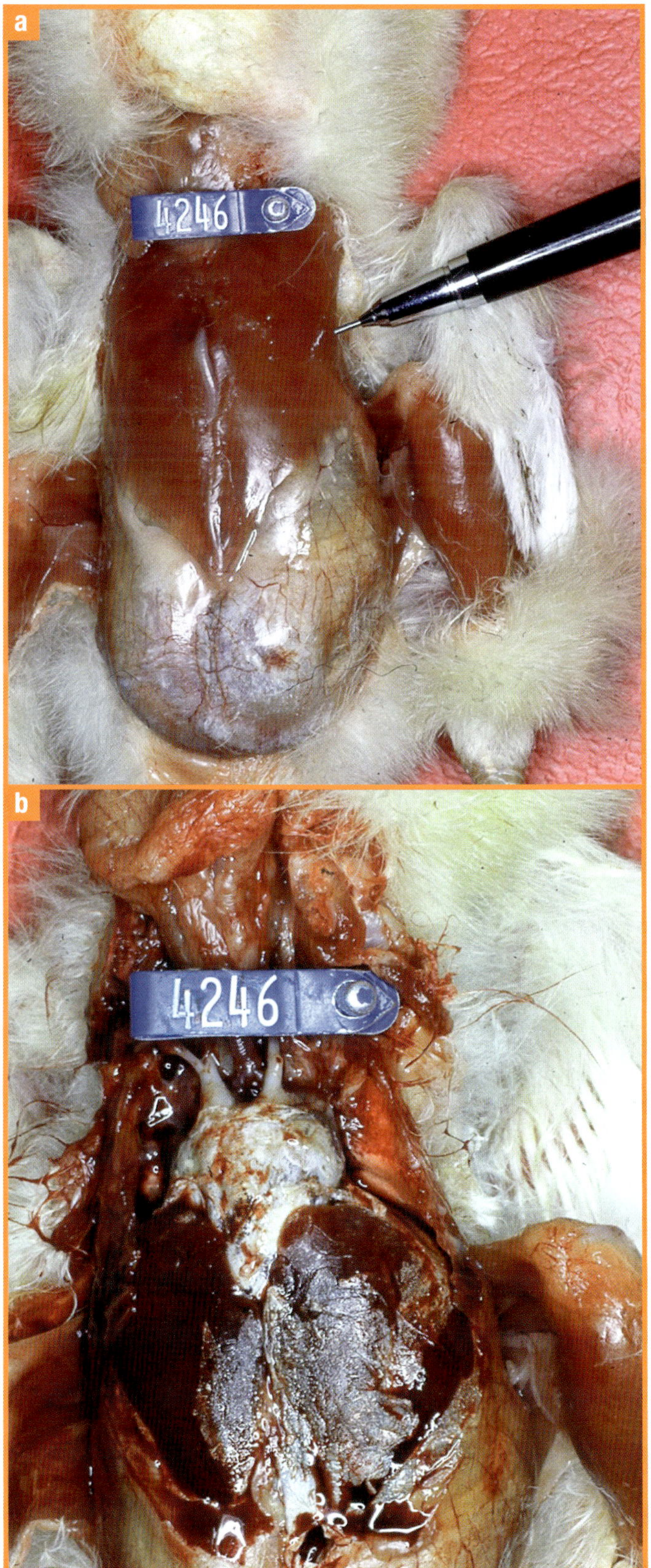

Fig. 10 | Severe visceral gout in a broiler chicken exposed to dietary oosporein. (a) Urate deposits in the abdominal cavity and breast muscle. (b) Urate deposits in the pericardium.

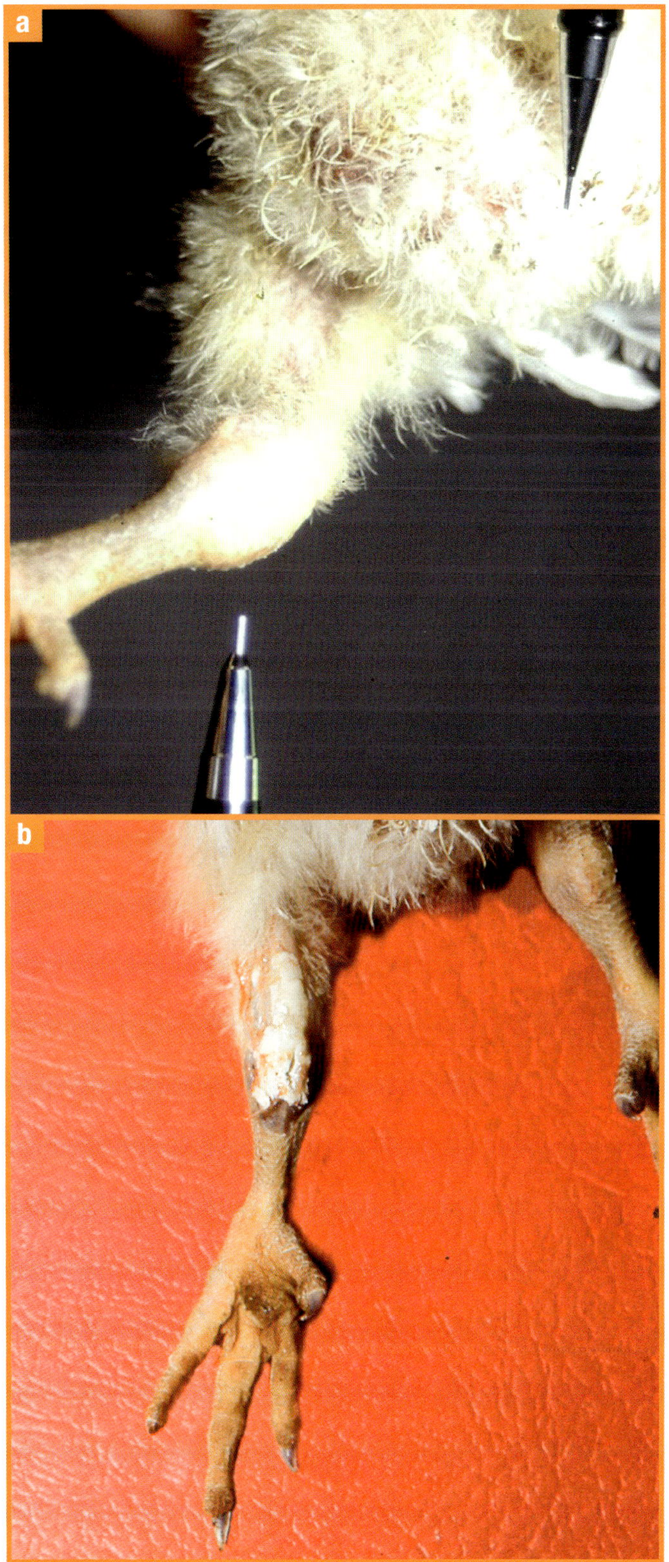

Fig. 11 | Severe articular gout in a broiler chicken fed diets contaminated with oosporein. (a) Note the urate deposits around the cloaca area and the severe swelling of the distal tibiotarsal joint. (b) An incision was made to expose the massive urate accumulation in that distal tibiotarsal joint. The kidneys of those chickens were very pale and enlarged with detectable urate deposits in the renal tubules.

Upon necropsy, the prominent lesions observed were:

- Massive urate deposits in various tissues.
- Swollen and pale kidneys.
- Dehydration.
- Proventricular enlargement with mucosal necrosis.
- Green discoloration of the gizzard lining.

In the acute phase of the toxicosis, macroscopic lesions included: enlarged pale kidneys, and white granular urate crystals in the pericardium and peritoneal surfaces.[39,41,46,65]

Fusarium toxins

Fusarium toxins are produced by certain species of *Fusarium* toxigenic molds including *F. tricinctum, F. roseum, F. verticillioides* (*F. moniliforme*). *Fusarium* spp. toxins, such as trichothecenes, fumonisins, moniliformin, fusaric acid, fusarochromanone and zearalenone can be associated with a wide range of clinical signs in poultry. Early signs may include feed refusal, depression, and necrosis of any epithelium that comes into contact with the toxin. Most commonly the oral mucosa, but sometimes the feet and legs that come in contact with *Fusarium* toxins, are affected. In case of long-term ingestion, reduced growth rate, decreased egg production, thin-shelled eggs, as well as abnormal feathering are common signs. Other possible signs include diarrhea, loss of motor control, abnormalities of the legs, rickets, dyspnea, cyanosis of the comb and wattles, edema of head and neck, hydropericardium, enlargement of the heart and sudden death within a poultry flock.[2,7,21,30,45,51,58,61,62]

Poultry are relatively resistant to zearalenone in comparison to pigs. Zearalenone in pigs is responsible for reproductive disorders due to its estrogenic effects. However, at high dietary concentrations vent enlargement and enhanced secondary sex characteristics have been reported in turkeys and chickens.[17,65]

Fumonisins

It is already well known that fumonisins induce equine leukoencephalomalacia and porcine pulmonary edema. Hepatic and renal toxicity can be observed in several animal species, including broilers, turkeys and ducks.[6,62] Although fumonisin B1 (FB1) is the most abundant fumonisin, however FB2 and FB3 closely mimic the toxicological and cancer-initiating activity of FB1.[6,21]

Chickens, turkeys and ducks are relatively resistant to fumonisin due to poor absorption and rapid excretion following metabolism, while horses, rabbits and pigs are very susceptible to this mycotoxin.[6,30,62] Dietary FB1, at concentrations of 80 mg/kg or less, did not adversely affect body weight, feed efficiency, or water consumption of broiler chicks.[30] The relative weights of the liver, spleen, kidney, proventriculus, and bursa of Fabricius, were also unaffected ($P > 0.05$) by any dietary concentration of 80 mg FB1/kg or less compared with the control (0 mg/kg) group.[30] Since FB1 induces disruption of the sphingolipids biosynthesis, the sphinganine:sphingosine ratios (Sa:So ratio) were increased significantly at concentrations of 20, 40 and 80 mg FB1/kg.[30] The increase Sa:So ratio in the serum and tissue of poultry, pigs and horses may be used to diagnose fumonisin toxicosis.[30,41]

Diarrhea has been described in chicks fed *Fusarium*-contaminated feeds. These lesions and clinical signs are not specific and have been described in chicks and poults with enteritis due to rotaviruses, parvoviruses, reoviruses, enteroviruses and coronaviruses.[6,15,21,30,31]

Trichothecenes

Trichothecenes belong to a class of chemicals called sesquiterpene lactones. More than 50 different compounds belong to this group and are characterized by similar chemical structures and similar biological activities.[65] Many of the trichothecenes are produced in nature by *Fusarium* fungi, which infect corn, wheat, barley, and other cereals in the field. The compounds of greatest concern in domestic animals include T-2 toxin, diacetoxyscirpenol (DAS), nivalenol (NIV), and deoxynivalenol (vomitoxin or DON). Most of these mycotoxins are potent tissue irritants and inflammatory agents. As a group, but within individual variations, trichothecenes are potent inhibitors of protein synthesis, and some inhibit DNA synthesis.[31,61]

Clinical signs of trichothecenes

Manifestations of trichothecene toxicosis such as T-2 toxicosis in broiler chicks include growth depression accompanied by decreased feed intake, poor or abnormal feathering, neurological disturbances and oral lesions (Fig. 12). Development of oral lesions associated with trichothecenes has been reported in broilers, laying hens and turkey poults.[2,31,41,51,61,65]

Feed refusal can be caused by several mycotoxins, particularly the trichothecene toxins that include T-2 toxin, diacetoxyscirpenol (DAS) and deoxynivalenol (vomitoxin, DON). There is some specificity in feed refusal caused by these various toxins. DON does not appear to cause much feed refusal in chickens, whereas it is extremely potent in swine. Ochratoxin causes feed refusal in turkeys, but not in chickens.[2,27,34,65]

In a field case of T-2 toxicosis in laying hens, egg production dropped from 72 % to 50 %. Of the eggs that were produced, the percentage of cracked eggs increased from 3 % to 15 %. Of the eggs that were packed and shipped, an additional 18 % were cracked by the time they arrived in the hands of consumers. The incidence of blood spots in the eggs went from essentially zero to 3 %. Eighty five percent of the birds displayed oral lesions. A consequence of this outbreak was that this flock of about 150,000 laying hens had to be terminated before their normal scheduled laying cycle ended.[27]

Diacetoxyscirpenol (DAS) exhibited a more pronounced effect on body weight compared to T-2 toxin.[2,7] The consumption of DAS by broiler breeders produced oral lesions. The location of the oral lesions corresponded to the location of the glandular taste buds and the corresponding salivary glands of the upper beak, lower beak and tongue. The tongue tip possesses taste buds and was very sensitive to the effects of DAS.[2,7]

Abnormal feathering of chicks by scirpenol mycotoxins depends on the degree of acetylation of each mycotoxin.[45] The most severe feather abnormalities were induced by 15-MAS at the lowest concentration of 0.5 μg/g feed ($P < 0.05$). The T-2 toxin was thought to cause abnormal feathering by interference with protein synthesis or by a more direct effect on the follicular tissue where feathers are formed.[45,65]

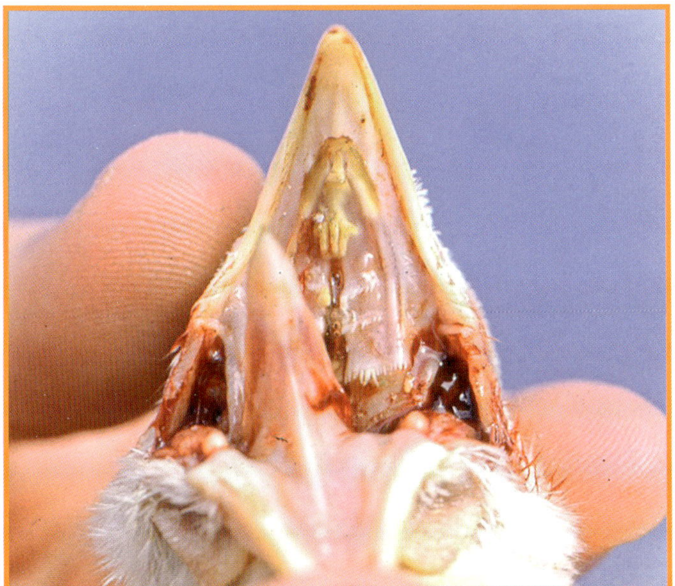

Fig. 12 | Typical oral lesions in broilers resulting from the ingestion of experimentally contaminated diet with T-2 toxin. This type of lesion can assist in early recognition of trichothecene intoxication.

Gross lesions of trichothecenes

The gross pathology of trichothecenes is mainly associated with:[7,27,31,41,65]

- Oral lesions.
- Feathering alterations.
- Dermal necrosis.
- Liver lesions.
- Gastroenteric effects.
- Coagulopathies.
- Immunologic dysfunctions.

Contamination of the feed and litter with trichothecene mycotoxins caused vesicular lesions on the feet and legs of poultry. At necropsy, lymphoid tissues are atrophied, and bone marrow is pale yellow in broilers.[31]

At necropsy of laying hens exposed to trichothecenes, atrophy of the ovary and oviduct will often be observed. T-2 toxin and HT-2 toxin were identified in the feed. A decrease in egg production was accompanied by reductions in feed consumption and thin-shelled eggs. Oral and feather lesions were neither uniform throughout the layer facility, nor were lesions uniform within a cage of hens.[31]

Histopathology of trichothecenes

The histopathology confirms mucosal necrosis and ulcerations of the oral lesions, submucosal granulation tissue and inflammatory cells, and crusts composed of exudate, bacterial colonies, and feed components.[31,41]

Histopathologic changes include necrosis with cell depletion of lymphoid and hematopoietic tissues and necrosis of hepatocytes, bile ducts, and enteric mucosa. Hepatocytes have vacuolar change due to lipid accumulation, accompanied by hyperplasia of bile ducts. Thyroid gland follicles are small, contain pale colloid, and have tall epithelial cells.[35] Chickens exposed to dietary trichothecene mycotoxins, exhibited microscopic lesions in the integument, including necrosis of feather epidermis and of follicular epidermis at the neck of the feather follicle.[31,45]

Effects of trichothecenes on the poultry immune system

Trichothecen toxins (T-2, DAS) may depress bone marrow and cause lymphopenia and thymic involution. Parameters of humoral immunity (globulin, complement) and cell-mediated immunity are altered. Decreased leukocyte count and regression of the bursa of Fabricius are common immunosuppressive effects associated with T-2 toxicosis. Increasing the concentration of T-2 toxin derivatives reduces macrophage viability.[9] It was demonstrated that an increased susceptibility of chicks to *Salmonella* spp. occurred when chicks were fed a diet containing 16 ppm T-2 toxin.[9]

Diagnosis of trichothecenes

The recommended method of establishing a diagnosis is by representative sampling and analysis of feed and grains for T-2 toxin, DAS, DON or any other trichothecenes. Feed and grain can now be rapidly screened for several mycotoxins including T-2 toxin, vomitoxin (DON), fumonisin B1, zearalenone, using monoclonal antibody detection (ELISA) kits. The use of thin layer chromatography (TLC) and high performance liquid chromatography (HPLC) is also recommended for the identification and quantification of mycotoxins in grains and feeds.

Differential diagnosis

Oral lesions in poultry are commonly attributed to trichothecene mycotoxins. However, other agents associated with oral lesions include:

- Excess of copper in the diet.
- Quaternary ammonium disinfectant toxicity.
- Deficiency of pantothenic acid, biotin, and vitamin A
- Infectious diseases (such as avian pox, trichomoniasis, candidiasis).
- Trauma.

It was demonstrated that fine particles that could be found in certain mash feed could induce bilateral oral lesions in laying hens under the stress of egg production.[16] It has been also been reported severe beak damage in poultry induced by ergot alkaloid poisoning.[5,16,31]

It is clear that trichothecene mycotoxins should be suspected when feather abnormalities occur and particularly when *Fusarium* is associated with the mixed feed or its ingredients. However, feather abnormalities can also be caused by:

- Low-protein diets.
- Deficiencies of arginine, leucine, and glycine.
- Deficiencies of vitamin E and selenium, pyridoxine, biotin and zinc.[2,45]
- Reticuloendotheliosis for the feather lesions.

Regarding the reduction in egg production, changes in the egg characteristics (egg-shell quality and internal egg quality) a differential diagnosis should be made between fusarium toxins and other etiologies such as:

- Heat stress.
- Excess of sulphonamides, nicarbazin, arasan (thiram) fungicide, organochlorine insecticides (DDT, chlordane).
- Infectious diseases (avian influenza, infectious bronchitis, Newcastle disease, EDS76, TRT).
- Ammonia, gossypol, sterculic acid (cottonseed oil) and vanadium.[8]

References

1. Abidin, Z., A. Khatoon, and M. Numan. Mycotoxins in broilers: Pathological alterations induced by aflatoxins and ochratoxins, diagnosis and determination, treatment and control of mycotoxicosis. World Poultry Science, 67 (September): 485-496, 2011.
2. Ademoyero, A. A. and P.B. Hamilton. Mouth lesions in broiler chickens caused by scirpenol mycotoxins. Poultry Science, 70: 2082- 2089, 1991.
3. Andretta, I, M. Kipper, C.R. Lehnen, L. Hauschild, M.M. Vale, and P.A. Lovatto. Meta-analytical study of productive and nutritional interactions of mycotoxins in broilers. Poultry Science, 90: 1934-1940, 2011.
4. Applegate, T.J., G. Schatzmayr, K. Pricket, C. Troche, and Z. Jiang. Effect of aflatoxin culture on intestinal function and nutrient loss in laying hens. Poultry Science, 88: 1235-1241, 2009.
5. Bailey, C.A., Fanzzino, Jr., J. J., Ziehr, M. S., Sattar, M., Haq, A., U., Odvody, G., and Porter, J. K.: Evaluation of sorghum ergot toxicity in broilers. Poultry Science, 78: 1391-1397, 1999.
6. Benlashehr, I., C. Repussard, J.Y. Jouglar, D. Tardieu, and P. Guerre. Toxicokinetics of fumonisin B2 in ducks and turkeys. Poultry Science, 90: 1671-1675, 2011.
7. Brake, J., P.B. Hamilton, and R.S. Kitrell. Effects of the trichothecene mycotoxin diacetoxyscirpenol on feed consumption, body weight, and oral lesions of broiler breeders. Poultry Science, 79: 856-863, 2000.
8. Bressman, R.B., R.D. Miles, C.W. Comer, H.R. Wilson, and G.D. Butcher. Effect of dietary supplementation of vanadium in commercial egg-type laying hens. Journal of Applied Poultry Research, 11: 46-53, 2002.
9. Boonchuvit, B, and P.B. Hamilton. Interaction of T-2 toxin with Salmonella infections of chickens. Poultry Science, 54: 1693-1696, 1975.
10. Burguera, J.A., G.T. Edds, and O. Osuna. Influence of selenium on aflatoxin B1 or crotalaria toxicity in turkey poults. American Journal of Veterinary Research, 44: 1714-1717. 1983.
11. CAST, Council for Agricultural Science and Technology. Mycotoxins: Risk in plant, animal, and human systems. Ames, Iowa, USA, 2003.
12. Chang, C.F. and P.B. Hamilton. Increased severity and new symptoms of infectious bursal disease during aflatoxicosis in broiler chickens. Poultry Science, 61: 1061-1068. 1982.
13. Chang, C.F. and P.B. Hamilton. Impaired phagocytosis by heterophils from chickens during aflatoxicosis. Toxicology and Applied Pharmacology, 48: 459-466, 1979.
14. Chang, C.F., W.E. Huff, and P.B. Hamilton. A leucocytopenia induced in chickens by dietary ochratoxin A. Poultry Science, 58: 555-558, 1979.
15. Corrier, D. E. Mycotoxicosis: mechanism of immunosuppression. Veterinary Immunology and Immunopathology, 30: 73-87. 1991.
16. Daft, B., Read, D., Manzer, M., Bickford, A. and Kinde, H.: The influence of crumble and mash feed on oral lesions of White Leghorn laying hens. Avian Diseases, 45: 349 –354, 2001.
17. Devegowda, G and T.N.K. Murthy. Mycotoxins: Their effects in poultry and some pratical solutions. In: The Mycotoxin Blue Book. Diaz, D., eds Nottingham University Press, Nottingham, NG11 OAX, United Kingdom, pp. 25-56, 2005
18. Edds, G.T., and C. F. Simpson. Cecal coccidiosis in poultry as affected by prior exposure to aflatoxin B1. American Journal of Veterinary Research, 37(1): 65-68. 1976.
19. Edds, G.T., K.P. C. Nair, and C. F. Simpson, C.F. Effect of aflatoxin B1 on resistance in poultry against cecal coccidiosis and Marek's disease. American Journal of Veterinary Research, 34 (6): 819-826.1973.
20. Elaroussi, M.A., E.R. Mohamed, E.M. El Barkouky, A. M. Atta, A.M. Abdou, and M.H. Hatab. Experimental ochratoxicosis in broiler chickens. Avian Pathology, 35: 263-269, 2006.
21. Gelderbrom, W.C., W.F. Marasas, R. Vleggaar, P. G. Thiel, and M. E. Cawood. Fumonisins: Isolation, chemical characterization and biological effects. Mycopathologia, 117: 11-16, 1992.
22. Ghesquiere, L. H. The impact of mycotoxins on the vaccination of poultry. International Poultry Production, 21 (1): 7 – 11, 2013.
23. Giambrone, J.J., D.L. Ewert, R.D. Wyatt, R.D., and C.S. Eidson. Effect of aflatoxin on the humoral and cell-mediated immune systems of the chicken. American Journal of Veterinary Research, 39 (2): 305 – 307, 1978.
24. Giambrone, J.J., M. Partadivedja, C.S. Edison, and S.H. Klevan. Interaction of aflatoxin with infectious bursal disease virus infection in young chickens. Avian Diseases, 22: 431-439, 1978.
25. Girish, C. K., and T.K. Smith. Impact of feed-borne mycotoxins on avian cell-mediated and humoral immune system. World Mycotoxin Journal, 1 (2): 105-121, 2008.
26. Gregory III, J.F., and G.T. Edds. Effect of dietary selenium on the metabolism of aflatoxin B1 in turkeys. Food and Chemical Toxicology, 22 (8): 637-642, 1984.
27. Hamilton, P.B. Determining safe levels of mycotoxins. J. Food. Prot. 47: 570-575, 1984.
28. Hamilton, P.B. and J. R. Harris. Interactions of aflatoxicosis with Candida albicans infections and other stresses in chickens. Poultry Science, 50: 906-912, 1971.

29. Hamilton, P.B., W.E. Huff, J.R. Harris, and R.D. Wyatt. Natural occurrences of ochratoxicosis in poultry. Poultry Science, 61: 1832-1834, 1982.
30. Henry, M. H., Wyatt, R. D., and Fletcher, O. J.: The toxicity of purified fumonisin B1 in broiler chicks. Poultry Science, 79: 1378-1384, 2000.
31. Hoerr, F.J. Mycotoxicosis. In: Diseases of Poultry. 10th ed. B. W. Calnek, H.J. Barnes, C. W. Beard, L. R. McDougald and Y. M. Safi, ed. Iowa State University Press, Ames, IA, pp. 958-962, 1997.
32. Huff, W. E., L.F. Kubena, R. B. Harvey, and J.A. Doerr. Mycotoxin interactions in poultry and swine. Journal of Animal Science, 66: 2351-2355, 1988.
33. Huff, W.E. and J.A. Doerr. Synergism between aflatoxin and ochratoxin A in broiler chickens. Poultry Science, 60: 550- 555, 1981.
34. Huff, W.E., J. A. Doerr, C.J. Wabeck. G. W. Chaloupka, J. D. May, and J. W. Merkley. Individual and combined effects of aflatoxin and ochratoxin A on bruising in broilers chickens. Poultry Science, 62: 1764 -1771, 1983.
35. Kumar, A., N. Jindal, C.I. Shukla, R.K. Asrani, D.R. Ledoux, and G. T. Rottinghaus. Pathological changes in broiler chickens fed ochratoxin A and inoculated with Escherichia coli. Avian Pathology, 33:413-417, 2004.
36. Ledoux, D. R., Rottinghaus, G. E., Bermudez, A. J., and Alonso- Debolt, M.: Efficacy of a hydrated sodium calcium aluminosilicate to ameliorate the toxic effects of aflatoxin in broiler chicks. Poultry Science, 78: 204 – 210, 1999.
37. Manegar, G.A., B. E. Shambulingappa and K.J. Ananda. Studies on tolerance limit of aflatoxin in commercial broilers. Lybian Agriculture Research Center Journal International, 1(3): 177-181, 2010.
38. Manning, R. O., T. P. Brown, R. D. Wyatt and O. J. Fletcher. The individual and combined effects of citrinin and ochratoxin A in broiler chicks. Avian Diseases, 29: 986-988, 1985.
39. Manning, R.O. and R.D. Wyatt. Comparative toxicity of Chaetomium trilaterale contaminated corn and various chemical forms of oosporein in broiler chicks. Poultry Science, 63: 251-259, 1984.
40. Martinez-de-Anda, A., A.G. Valdivia, F. Jaramillo-Juarez, J.L. Reyes, R. Ortiz, T. Quezada M.C. de Luna, and M.L. Rodriguez. Effects of aflatoxin chronic intoxication in renal function of laying hens. Poultry Science, 89:1622-1628, 2010.
41. Meerdink, G.L. Mycotoxins. In: Clinical Veterinary Toxicology (K. H. Plumlee ed.). Mosby, St. Louis, Missouri, pp. 231-281, 2004.
42. Mehdi, N.A.Q., W.W. Carlton, G.D. Boon, and J. Tuite. Studies on the sequential development and pathogenesis of citrinin micotoxicosis in turkeys and ducklings. Veterinary Pathology, 21: 216-223, 1984.
43. Osuna, O: Micotoxinas e Micotoxicosis: Chapt 36. In Revolledo, L. e Piantino-Ferreira, A. J. (orgz): Patologia Aviária. Editorial Manole Ltda, Barueri, SP – Brasil, 2009, pp. 348-362, 2009 (In Portuguese).
44. Osuna, O. and R. Miles. Strategies Exist for Coping with Poor Quality Grain. Feedstuffs, 69 (3): 1 - 34, 1997.
45. Parkhurst, C.R., P.B. Hamilton, and A.A. Ademoyero. Abnormal feathering of chicks caused by Scirpenol mycotoxins differing in degree of acetylation. Poultry Science, 71: 833-837, 1992.
46. Pegram, R.A. and R. D. Wyatt. Avian gout caused by oosporein, a mycotoxin produced by Chaetomium triaterale. Poultry Science, 60: 2429-2440, 1981.
47. Pier, A.C. Effects of aflatoxin on immunity. JAVMAK, 163 (1): 1267-1269, 1973.
48. Pier, A.C., R.E. Fitchtner, R.E., and S.J. Cysewski. Effects of aflatoxin on the cellular immune system. Ann. Nutr. Alim., 31: 781 – 788, 1977.
49. Qureshi, M.A., J. Brake, P.B. Halminton, W.M. Hagler, and S. Nesheim. Dietary exposure of broiler breeders to aflatoxin results in immune dysfunction in progeny chicks. Poultry Science, 77: 812- 819, 1998.
50. Qureshi, M.A., I. Hussain, and C.L. Heggen. Understanding Immunology in disease development and control. Poultry Science, 77: 1126-1129, 1998.
51. Richardson, K. E. and P.B. Hamilton. Comparative toxicity of scirpentriol and its acetylated derivatives. Poultry Science, 69: 397 – 402, 1990.
52. Ruff, M.D., and R.D. Wyatt. Influence of dietary aflatoxin on the severity of Eimeria acervulina infection in broiler chickens. Avian Diseases, 22: 471-480, 1978.
53. Sander, J. E., Savage, S. I. and Rowland G. E.: Sodium sesquicarbonate toxicity in broiler chickens. Avian Diseases, 42: 215 – 218, 1998.
54. Sharma, J.M. The avian immune system. In: Diseases of Poultry. Y. M. Saif, ed. Iowa State University Press, Ames, pp. 5 – 16, 2003.
55. Smith, J.W., and P.B. Hamilton. Aflatoxicosis in the broiler chickens. Poultry Science, 49: 207-215, 1970.
56. Sur, E., I. Celik, Y. Oznurlu, M.F. Aydin, H. Oguz, V. Kurtoglu, and T. Ozaydin. Enzyme histochemical and serological investigations on the immune system from chickens treated in ovo with aflatoxin B1 (AFB1). Revue Med Vet., 162 (10): 443-448, 2011.
57. Surai, P. F. and J.E. Dvorska. Effects of mycotoxins on antioxidant status and immunity. In: The Mycotoxin Blue Book. Diaz, D. eds Nottingham University Press, Nottingham, NG11 OAX, United Kingdom, pp. 93-137, 2005
58. Tardieu, D., J.D. Baily, F. Skiba, J.P. Métayer, F. Grosjean, F., and P. Guerre. Chronic toxicity of fumonisins in turkeys. Poultry Science, 86: 1887-1893, 2007.

59. Trucksess, M. W., Staloff, L., Young, K., Wyatt, R. D., and Miller, B. L. Aflatoxicol and aflatoxin B1 and M1 in eggs and tissues of laying hens consuming aflatoxin-contaminated feed. Poultry Science, 62: 2176 – 2182, 1983.
60. Thaxton, J.P., H.T. Tung, and P.B. Hamilton. Immunosuppression in Chickens by aflatoxin. Poultry Science, 53: 721-725, 1974.
61. Ueno, Y.: Toxicological features of T-2 toxin and related trichothecenes. Fundam. Appl. Toxicol., 4: s124 – s132, 1984.
62. Vudathala, D.K., D.B. Prelusky, M. Ayroud, H.L. Trenholm, and J.D. Miller. Pharmacokinetic fate and pathological effects of ^{14}C- fumonisin B1 in laying hens. Natural Toxins 2: 81-88, 1994.
63. Warren, M. F. and P. B. Hamilton. Intestinal fragility during ochratoxicosis and aflatoxicosis in broiler chickens. Applied and Environmental Microbiology, 40 (3): 641-645, 1980.
64. Witlock, D.R. and R. D. Wyatt. Effects of Eimeria tenella infection and dietary aflatoxin on blood coagulation of young broiler chicks. Avian Diseases, 22 (3): 481- 486, 1978.
65. Wyatt, R.D. Poultry, Chapter 24. In: Mycotoxins and Animal Foods (John E. Smith and Rachel S. Henderson, ed). CRC Press, Boca Raton, pp. 553-605, 1991.
66. Wyatt, R.D., Ruff, M.D., and Page, R.K. Interactions of aflatoxin with Eimeria tenella infection and monensin in young broiler chickens. Avian Diseases, 19: 730-740, 1975.
67. Yang, J., F. Bai, K. Zhang, S. Bai, X. Peng, X. Ding, Y. Li, J. Zhang, and L. Zhao. Effects of feeding corn naturally contaminated with aflatoxin B1 and B2 on hepatic functions of broilers. Poultry Science, 91: 2792 2801, 2012.
68. Yegani, M. and D.R. Korver. Factors affecting intestinal health in poultry. Poultry Science, 87: 2052-2063, 2008.

STRESS AND IMMUNOSUPPRESSION

Enrique Montiel

Introduction

A good functioning immune system is the cornerstone of protection against disease. This fact is crucial to obtain good economic results in commercial poultry. The avian immune system involves a multiplicity of tissues, cells, and mediators that allow birds to recognize foreign antigens, mount a response, and eliminate them. Various stress factors can affect the proper development of immune organs or specific functions. Direct environmental changes, mostly management-related such as temperature, density, nutrition and housing conditions [1,7,8,10,21,27] are capable of affecting immune responses and therefore disease susceptibility. [3,16,17,28,37-40,45,50] The impact of stress on the immune system has a tremendous importance for the poultry industry. There are some specific stress agents that may impact performance, affect the immune system, compromise flock health, and limit the efficiency of modern poultry production. This chapter will review relevant findings on stress-related immunosuppression and present a practical approach to understand and manage stress within a cost-effective poultry industry.

The connection between stress, immunosuppression and decreased performance

Among the various causes of immunosuppression, stress is perhaps one of the most complex and least understood. In poultry, the negative effect of stress caused by infectious and environmental factors on decreased performance has been greatly studied. It is widely understood that certain management conditions such as temperature, humidity, and space need to be met to achieve meat or egg production goals. Failing to comply with good poultry production practices leads to negative economic consequences. However, the impact of a stressor on the physiology of the bird leading to a dysfunctional immune system is less understood. For example, it is widely known that subjecting the birds to extreme temperatures may increase mortality and decrease growth, thus affecting the overall performance of the flock. However, temperature is not perceived as a potential immunosuppressor capable of impairing innate immune responses and transiently suppressing immunity against *Escherichia coli*. [28,39,40] In fact, birds exposed to low temperatures after the administration of respiratory vaccines may experience rolling reactions, develop secondary *E. coli* infections [48], and suffer increased condemnations due to airsacculitis at processing. Recent findings also suggest that birds raised in slats versus litter had decreased cellular and humoral immune responses and increased heteterophil/lymphocyte ratios. The detrimental effect of stress on antibody production was not the same for all the antigens tested. [11]

STRESS AT EARLY AGES

Stress during incubation or at an early age has an important effect on the whole life of chickens.

The exposure to stressful situations at the parental level, during incubation or at the early age may have a long lasting effect in the bird's life. [18,24,42,47] Stress at an early age and even during incubation may impair immune responses to coccidia and infectious bronchitis in commercial layers up to 106 days of age. The early stress has been also proven to cause long lasting consequences on the hypothalamic-pituitary-adrenal axis (HPA) in wild birds and commercial poultry. [24,42] More recently, studies in broiler breeder pullets to compare skip-a-day feeding *vs.* daily programs used during rearing until 18 weeks of age showed that innate responses to *E. coli* and *Salmonella* spp. where lower in the skip-a-day feeding groups up to 60 weeks of age (Montiel et al., unpublished).

Understanding stress

The mechanisms of stress-induced immunosuppression are not well understood. One of the best studied mechanisms is interaction between the neuroendocrine and immune systems, usually involving the HPA. The impact of stress on birds usually results in the release of glucocorticoids (e.g. corticosterone) that affect metabolism, may negatively affect performance, and cause immunosuppression. Administration of adrenocorticotropin (ACTH) and corticosterone have been shown to decrease performance in broilers [46] and cause lymphoid depletion in the bursa, spleen and thymus. [9] Moreover, increased glucocorticoids levels after stress situations have been associated with a decrease on innate or induced immunity. [2,11,26,30,34,36,39,41] Administration of corticosterone and ACTH can reactivate viremia and cloacal shedding in birds infected with avian leukosis virus that had seroconverted and cleared viremia for long periods of time. [12,32] Development of Marek's disease in chickens that had been properly vaccinated and protected for months was also observed when administered corticosterone or dexamethasone. [35] Protection against Marek's disease was also higher in birds selected for low concentrations of blood corticosterone. [43] Because of the clear detrimental effect on the avian immune system, corticosterone administration is perhaps the most widely used model to reproduce stress-derived immunosuppression in birds. However, in addition to corticosterone, there are a number of other mediators such as epinephrine, norepinephrine and dopamine that can work as immunomodulators. [9] The cytokines derived from the immune responses have in turn an effect on the endocrine system. [5] Immune response has been also suggested to produce oxidative stress in birds. [4] Lymphocytes seem to have endocrine functions and hormone release from lymphocytes may have an important role in the initiation of antibody production in commercial birds. [29] Therefore, stress establishes a bidirectional interaction between the immune and the endocrine systems. This interaction is usually the ultimate physiological consequence of stress induced by the various agents. [6,11,16,17,20,22,38,39]

Measuring stress or immunosuppression?

Immunosuppression induced by a stressor can be assessed by evaluating immune system tissues or by functional tests. Evaluation of corticosterone in circulating blood has been used to assess the level of stress. [16,41] In fact, administration of corticosterone by feed, injection or other methods has been used to reproduce stress-effect under laboratory conditions. [9,11,12,14,22,26,28,33,41,45] However, although levels of corticosterone in circulating blood are typically associated with stress and immunosuppression, recent studies have shown that stress-derived immunosuppression can occur without high levels of blood corticosterone. [11] In these studies the lack of foraging materials was compared to the injection of corticosteroids. The results showed that the lack of foraging materials did not cause a significant elevation of the blood levels of corticosterone in spite of the fact that the antibody response to sheep red blood cells (SRBC) and tetanus toxoid (TT) were decreased. Additionally, in studies to investigate the effect of corticosterone levels on populations of the northern fowl mite in cockerels, the highest mite populations were found in birds with low blood corticosterone concentrations. [16] Therefore, to determine if any given stressor is causing immunosuppression in birds, one or more immune assays to measure immune responses need to be in place.

The following are some of the methods commonly used to determine if a given stressor has the potential to cause immunosuppression:

1. The heterophil/lymphocyte ratio in circulating blood is commonly used to measure stress in birds. [3,15,19,30] This test determines changes in blood cell populations. Decrease in lymphocyte numbers indicates lymphoid depletion. The severity of the immunosuppression induced by the tested agent is assessed by determining differences between the challenged birds and the unchallenged controls. Higher ratios indicate stronger immunosuppressive effect.
2. Humoral immunity can be evaluated by measuring seroconversion against SRBC [11,14], TT, and other antigens. [11] Production of circulating or local antibodies to a foreign antigen is the primary consequence of humoral immune responses. Decreased antibody titers of treated vs. untreated birds is a sign of immunosuppression. Other antigens such as TT can be used for the same purpose. The detrimental effect of stress on antibody levels depends on the antigen used and the responses to some of them, such as human serum albumin (HSA) may not be affected. [11]
3. Cell-mediated immunity can be measured using lymphocyte transformation assays. These tests detect the response of lymphocytes to mitogens like concanavalin-A (Con-A) or phytohemagglutinin (PHA) from spleen lymphocytes. [31,44] The test is commonly conducted using Con-A, and evaluates the activation potential of lymphocytes under antigen stimulation.
4. The time of clearance of *E. coli* after intravenous inoculation is another test used to quantify cellular immune responses. This method consists of the inoculation

of a known amount of *E. coli* intravenously followed by blood sample collection at different times post inoculation (PI), usually 10, 20 and 60 minutes PI. The samples are inoculated in McConkey agar plates and the amount of *E. coli* recovered measures the ability of the immune system, mainly macrophages, to clear the *E. coli* from the blood stream. This is a good method to evaluate innate cellular immune responses (Montiel et al., unpublished).

5. Comparisons of the weight of the immune organs relative to the body weight are used to evaluate immunosuppression. The bursa to body weight ratio is widely used to assess bursal atrophy [23], and other comparisons like the bursa to spleen weight ratio have been also used.
6. Response to vaccination. Stress can negatively affect the response to vaccination and vaccine protection may decrease as a consequence of stress occurring even at an early age. It has been recently demonstrated that birds subjected to various stressors at different ages had reduced protection rates after challenge. [24,47]

To evaluate immunosuppression, it is important to use a test that is appropriate for each case. If there is a disease where stress is suspected as a contributing factor, the assessment of the immune system should be directed to the type of immune response that will help in the control of that particular disease. For example, if the problem is infectious bronchitis, coccidiosis or Marek's disease, for which cell mediated immunity is essential, the test of choice must evaluate cell mediated immunity. Conversely, if there is a disease that is protected by antibodies, such as subclinical infectious bursal disease, humoral immune responses should be tested. It is important to keep in mind that the available tests might detect immunosuppression but they might not confirm that immunosuppression is due to stress. The specific mechanisms of stress-induced immunosuppression are still poorly understood. Moreover, under field conditions, it is possible to have several agents, infectious and non infectious, that can induce immunosuppression.

Stress and poultry practice

There are a variety of stressors that will be always present in the life of poultry grown for commercial purposes. Those environmental and management factors that have a negative effect on performance (e.g. nutrition) are best studied. [19] Current research focuses on the identification of deficiencies that lead to stress and the use of antioxidants, probiotics, vitamins, minerals and other compounds and chemicals to alleviate the impact of stress in commercial birds. [4,13,25,33,49,50] In addition to factors that have a direct effect on performance, it is important to evaluate neuroendocrine changes that act as immunomodulators and impair the immune status of birds and the efficacy of poultry health programs.

Further research on the mechanisms of stress-induced immunosuppression are warranted to develop better methods of diagnosis and control. In the meantime, and given the high impact of stress in immunosuppression, minimizing stress in birds will contribute to a healthier immune system and, thus, to a more efficient poultry operation.

References

1. Altan, O., Pabuccuoglu, A., Altan, A., Konyalioglu, S., and H. Bayraktar. Effects of heat stress on oxidative stress, lipid peroxidation and some stress parameters in broilers. British Poultry Science, 44: 545 – 550, 2003.
2. Blalock, J. E. A molecular basis for bidirectional communication between the immune and neuroendocrine systems. The American Physiological Society, 69: 1 – 32, 1989.
3. Campo, J. L., Gil, M. G., Davila, S. G., and I. Munoz. Influence of perches and footpad dermatitis on tonic immobility and heterophil to lymphocyte ratio of chickens. Poultry Science, 84:1004 – 1009, 2005.
4. Costantini, D. and Pape Moller, A. Does immune response cause oxidative stress in birds? A meta analysis. Comparative Biochemistry and Physiology, Part A, 153:339 – 344, 2009.
5. Davis, S. L. Environmental modulation of the immune system via the endocrine system. Domestic Animal Endocriniology, 15: 283 – 289, 1998.
6. Davison, F., Kaspers B., and K. Schat. Avian immunology. Elsevier, 2008.
7. Dennis, R. L., Fahey, A. G., and H. W. Cheng. Infrared beak treatment method compared with conventional hot-blade trimming in laying hens. Poultry Science, 88: 38 – 43, 2009.
8. Dickens, M. J., Delehanty, D. J., and M. Romero. Stress and translocation: Alterations in the stress physiology of translocated birds. Biological Sciences, 276: 2051 – 2056, 2009.
9. Dohms, J. E. and A. Metz. Stress—mechanisns of immunosuppression. Veterinary Immunology and Immunopathology, 30: 89 – 109, 1991.
10. El-Lethey, H., Aerni, V., Jungi, T. W., and B. Wechsler. Stress and feather pecking in laying hens in relation to housing conditions. British Poultry Science, 41: 22 – 28, 2000.
11. El-Lethey, H., Huber-Eicher, B., and T. W. Jungi. Exploration of stress-induced immunosuppression in chickens reveals both stress-resistant and stress-susceptible antigen response. Veterinary Immunology and Immunopathology, 95: 91 – 101, 2003.
12. Fadly A.M., Davison TF ; Payne L.N., and K Howes. Avian leukosis virus infection and shedding in brown leghorn chickens treated with corticosterone or exposed to various stressors. Avian Pathology, 18: 183-98, 1989.
13. Ghareeb K., Awad W., and J Böhm . Ameliorative effect of a microbial feed additive on infectious bronchitis virus antibody titer and stress index in broiler chicks fed deoxynivalenol. Poultry Science, 91: 800-807, 2012.
14. Gross, W. B. Effects of short-term exposures of chickens to corticosterone on restistance to challenge exposure to Escherichia coli and antibody response to sheep erythrocytes. American Journal of Veterinary Research 53:291- 293, 1992.
15. Gross, W.B., and H.S.Siegel. Evaluation of the Heterophil/Lymphocyte Ratio as a Measure of Stress in Chickens. Avian Diseases, 27(4): 972-979, 1983.
16. Hall, R. D. and W. B. Gross. Effects of social stress and inherited plasma corticosterone leveles in chickens on populations of the Northern Fowl Mite, Ornitonyssus sylviarum. The Journal of Parasitology, 61: 1096 – 1100, 1975.
17. Heckert, R. A., Estevez, I., Russek-Cohen, E., and R. Pettit-Riley. Effects of density and perch availability on the immune status of broilers. Poultry Science, 81: 451 – 457, 2002.
18. Henriksen, R., Groothuis, T. G., and S. Rettenbacher. Elevated plasma corticosterone decreases yolk testosterone and progesterone in chickens; linking maternal stress and hormone-mediated maternal effects. PLoS ONE, 6(8):e23824.
19. Hocking, P. M., Maxwell, H. M., Robertson, G. W., and M. A. Mitchell. Welfare assessment of modified rearing programmes for broiler breeders. British Poultry Science, 42: 424 – 432, 2001.
20. Knowles, T. G., Warriss, P. D., Brown, S. N., Edwards, J. E., and M. A. Mitchell. Response of broilers to deprivation of food and water for 24 hours. British Veterinary Journal, 151: 197 – 203, 1995.
21. Koivula, M. J. and T. Eeva. Metal-related oxidative stress in birds. Environmental Pollution, 158: 2359 – 2370, 2010.
22. Lin, H., Decuypere, E., and J. Buyse. Oxidative stress induced by corticosterone administration in broiler chickens (Gallus gallus domesticus) 2. Short-term effect. Comparative Biochemistyr and Physiology, Part B, 139: 145 – 751, 2004.
23. Lucio, B., and S. B. Hitchner. Infectious bursal disease emulsified vaccine: effect upon neutralizing antibody levels in the dam and subsequent protection of the progeny. Avian Diseases, 23:,466-479. 1979.
24. Lynn, S. E., Prince, L. E., and M. Phillips. A single exposure to an acute stressor has lasting consequences for the hypothatlamo-pituitary-andrenal response to stress in free-living birds. General and Comparative Endocrinology, 166: 337 – 344, 2010.
25. McKee, J., and P. Harrison. Effects of supplemental ascorbic acid on the performance of broiler chickens exposed to multiple concurrent stressors. Poultry Science, 74: 1772 – 1785, 1995.
26. Martin II, L. B., Gilliam, J., Han, P., Lee, K., and M. Wikelski. Corticosterone suppresses cutaneous immune function in temperate but not tropical House Sparrows, Passer domesticus. General and Comparative Endocrinology, 140:126-135, 2005.
27. Martinez-de la Puente, J., Merino, S., Tomas, G., Moreno, J., Morales, J., Lobato, E., and J. Martinez. Nest ectoparasites increase physiological stress in breeding birds: an experiment. Naturwissenschaften, 98: 99-106, 2011.

28. Matsumoto, M., and H.J. Huang. Induction of Short-Term, Nonspecific Immunity Against Escherichia coli Infection in Chickens Is Suppressed by cold Stress or corticosterone Treatment. Avian Pathology, 29: 227-232, 2000.
29. Mashaly, M. M., Trout, J. M., and G. L. Hendricks III. The endocrine function of the immune cells in the initiation of humoral immunity. Poultry Science, 72: 1289 – 1293, 1993.
30. Moe, R. O., Guemene, D., Bakken, M., Larsen, H. J. S., Shini, S., Lervik, S., Skjerve, E., Michel, V., and R. Tauson. Effects of housing conditions during the rearing and laying period on adrenal reactivity, immune response and heterophil to lymphocyte (H/L) ratios in laying hens. Animal, 4(10): 1709 – 1715, 2010.
31. Nathanson, R.M. Transformation of Chickens Lymphocytes Stimulated by Concanavalin A: Response Parameters. Canadian Journal of comparative Medicine, 46: 57-59. 1982
32. Pandiri, A. R., Gimeno, I. M., Mays, J. K., Reed, W. M, and A. M. Fadly. Reversion to subgroup J avian Leukosis Viremia in seroconverted adult meat-type chickens exposed to chronic stress by adrenocorticotrophin treatment. Avian Diseases, 56: 578 – 582, 2012.
33. Peng, X., Cui, H., Fang, J., Zuo, Z., Deng, J., Pan, K., Lai, W., and Y. Zhou. Low selenium diet alters cell cycle phase, apaptotic population and modifies oxidative stress markers of spleens in broilers. Biol Trace Elem Res, 148: 182 – 186, 2012.
34. Post, J., Rebel, M. J. and A. A. H. M. ter Huurne. Physiological Effects of Elevated Plasma Corticosterone Concentrations in Broiler Chickens. An Alternative Means by Which to Assess the Physiological Effects of Stress. Poultry Science, 82: 1313–1318. 2003.
35. Powell, P. C. and T. F. Davison. Induction of Marek's disease in vaccinated chickens by treatment with betamethasone or corticosterone. Israel Journal of Veterinary Medicine, 42: 73–78, 508, 1986.
36. Puvadolpirod and J.P. Thaxton. Model of Physiological Stress in Chickens Temporal Patterns of Response. Poultry Science, 79: 377–382, 2000.
37. Quinteiro-Filho, W. M., Ribeiro , A., Ferraz-de-Paula, V., Pinheiro, M. L., Sakai, M., Sa., L. R. M., J. Palermo-Neto. Heat stress impairs performance parameters, induces intestinal injury and decreases macrophage activity in broiler chickens. 2010 Poultry Science, 89: 1905–1914. 2010.
38. Quinteiro-Filho, M.V., Rodrigues, M.V., Ribeiro, A., Ferraz-De-Paula, V., Pinheiro, L.R. Sa., Ferreira, A.J.P., and J. Palermo-Neto. Acute Heat stress Impairs Performance Parameters and Induces Mild Intestinal Enteritis in Broiler chickens: Role of Acute Hypthalamic-Pituitary-Adrenal Axis Activation. J ANIM SCI, 90(6): 1986-1994. 2012.
39. Regnier J.A., and K.W. Kelley. Heat- and cold-stress suppresses in vivo and in vitro cellular immune responses of chickens. Ammerican Journal of Veterinary Research, 42: 294-9, 1981.
40. Regnier, J., Kelley, K., and C. Gaskins. Acute thermal stressors and synthesis of antibodies in chickens. Poultry Science, 59: 985-990. 1980.
41. Shini, S and P. Kaiser. Effects of stress, mimicked by administration of corticosterone in drinking water, on the expression of chicken cytokine and chemokine genes in lymphocytes. Stress, 12(5): 388-399. 2009.
42. Spencer, K. A., Evans, N. P., and P. Monaghan. Postnatal stress in birds: A novel model of glucocorticoid programming of the hypothalamic-pituitary-adrenal axis. Endocrinology, 150:1931 – 1934, 2009.
43. Thompson, D. L., Elgert, K. D., Gross, W. B., and P. B. Siegel. Cell-mediated immunity in Marek's disease.virus-infected chickens genetically selected for high and low concentrations of plasma corticosterone. American Journal of Veterinary Research, 41: 91 – 96, 1980.
44. Toivanen, P., and A Toivanen. Selective Activation of Chicken T Lymphocytes by Concanavalin A. J Immunol, 111: 1602-1603, 1973.
45. Virden, W. S., Lilburn, M. S., Thaxton, J. P., Corzo, A., Hoehler, D., and M. T. Kidd. The effect of corticosterone-induced stress on amino acid digestibility in Ross broilers. Poultry Science, 86:338 – 342, 2007.
46. Virden, W. S., Thaxton, J. P., Corzo, A., Dozier, W. A., and M. T. Kidd. Evaluation of models using corticosterone and adrenocorticotropin to induce conditions mimicking physiological stress in commercial broilers. Poultry Science, 86: 2485 – 2491, 2007.
47. Walstra, I., ten Napel, J., Kemp, B., Schipper, H., and H. van der Brand. Early life experience affects the adaptive capacity of rearing hens during infectious challenges. Animal, 4: 1688 – 1696, 2010.
48. Yoder, H.W., Drury, L.N., and S. R. Hopkins. Influence of Environment on Airsacculitis: Effects of Relative Humidity and Air Temperature on Broilers Infected with Mycoplasma synoviae and Infectious Bronchitis. Avian Diseases, 21: 195-208. 1977.
49. Zhang, W. H., Gao, F., Zhu, Q. F., Li, C., Jiang, Y., Dai, S. F., and G. H. Zhou. Dietary sodium butyrate alleviates the oxidative stress induced by corticosterone exposure and improves meat quality in broiler chickens. Poultry Science, 90: 2592 – 2599, 2011.
50. Zhang, Z, Wang, Q, Zhang, J, Li, S, Wang, X, and S. Xu. Effects of oxidative stress on immunosuppression induced by selenium deficiency in chickens. Biological Trace Element Research, 149: 352-361, 2012.

CHAPTER 3

VIRUS-INDUCED IMMUNOSUPPRESSION: INFECTIOUS BURSAL DISEASE

Roser Dolz and Natàlia Majó

Introduction

Infectious bursal disease (IBD) is an acute highly contagious viral disease in young chickens characterized by the destruction of B lymphocytes within the bursa of Fabricius, causing severe lesions in this organ. Since its first report at the early 60s in USA, IBD (also named Gumboro disease because first outbreaks occurred in this area of Delaware) has become widely distributed over the world and endemic in the major poultry producer areas.[15,160] A survey conducted in 1995 by the *Office International des Épizooties* (OIE) revealed that approximately 61 out of 65 of the countries inquired about declared cases of IBD.[150]

Despite major research efforts, IBD is still one of the major threats in the poultry industry with a significant economic impact by direct and indirect economic losses. Direct economic losses are mainly due to mortality induced by acute infection which will depend on the virus strain involved in the outbreak, as well as the age, breed and presence or absence of maternal antibodies. On the other hand, indirect economic losses are caused by secondary infections favored by the immunosuppressive status induced by the viral infection, which reduces flock performance and increases mortality, carcasses condemnation at slaughterhouses, and antibiotic usage. Economic impact estimations of IBD outbreaks in Northern Ireland showed an 11 % reduction in yield in clinical IBD affected flocks.[104] Also simulations of introducing a variant IBD within an integrated broiler operation in USA estimated that production costs would increase in 10 %.[128]

The aim of this chapter is to review the main aspects of this disease, and support poultry veterinarians and diagnosticians in understanding infectious bursal disease virus (IBDV) infection, the repercussions of the different clinical forms, and the methods of detection and control.

The etiological agent: Infectious Bursal Disease Virus

Taxonomy and genome organization

The infectious bursal disease virus, the causative agent of IBD, belongs to the *Birnaviridae* family within the genus *Avibirnavirus*, which is not assigned to any order.[56]

IBDV genome is formed by two double-stranded RNA (dsRNA) segments of 3.2 kbp (segment A) and 2.8 kbp (segment B)[55,81] and it only encodes five mature polypeptides. Segment A has two partially overlapping open-reading frames (ORFs).[137] The short ORF encodes for VP5, whereas the long ORF encodes for a polyprotein that is co- and post-translationally self-cleaved, yielding three polypeptides: pVP2, VP3 and VP4. A major proportion of pVP2 is further processed, throughout virion maturation and mediated by VP4, into the protein VP2 and several C-terminal segments.[22] Segment B contains one ORF that encodes VP1.

Viral structure and proteins

IBDV is a non-enveloped virus with, contrary to most dsRNA viruses, a single-shelled icosahedral capsid of 55 to 60 nm of diameter. VP2 (41 kDa) and VP3 (32 kDa) are the major structural proteins in the mature virion, constituting 51 % and 40 % of the protein in infectious virions, respectively.[25] The capsid has been demonstrated to be a relative complex icosahedron formed only by VP2 subunits, clustered as 260 trimers of outer protruding structures, with a triangulation number of T = 13.[13] Directly associated with the capsid are 200 Y-shaped trimeric structures of VP3 and four C-terminal peptides (pep46, pep7a, pep7b and pep11) yielded from the maturation process of pVP2, which have been demonstrated to be involved in the viral entry mechanism by promoting the disruption of host cell membranes.[19,22,42] A detailed description of the VP2 structure and functions is included further on.

- The VP3 protein (32 kDa) has been proposed to be a multitasking protein that can carry out multiple, apparently unrelated functions.[99] Some studies demonstrated a scaffolding activity of the VP3 C-terminal region mainly involved in the control of capsid assembly by interacting with the pVP2 and VP1 and stabilization of both segments of dsRNA.[20,21,101,116] In addition, it has also been shown that VP3 acts as transcriptional activator of the VP1 by promoting a conformational change on the VP1 that removes an inherent structural blockade of the RdRp active site.[44] Finally, VP3 participates in the recruitment of VP1 into the capsid through protein interaction forming ribonucleoprotein complexes.[99]

- The VP4 protein (28 kDa) is the viral protease that mediates the polypeptide precursor NH2- pVP2-VP4-VP3-COOH cleavage and the subsequent pVP2 maturation.[2,21] However, this viral protease has been poorly characterized and it has only been suggested to be a non-canonical RNA viral Lon proteinase.[7]
- The VP5 protein (17 kDa) is a highly basic, cysteine rich, non-essential, non-structural viral protein whose functional properties are not yet totally known.[110,111] VP5 has been demonstrated to be a class II membrane protein with an intracellular N-terminal tail and an extracellular C-terminal region that associates with the plasma membrane (PM). Moreover, it has been hypothesized that accumulation of VP5 in the PM leads to progressive alteration of the PM that would induce cell lysis and facilitate virus release.[97] In addition, some studies indicated the potential role of VP5 in the induction of apoptosis during IBDV infection, via interaction with voltage-dependent anion channel 2.[90,169] It has been demonstrated that an IBDV VP5 knockout mutant isolate was able to replicate but failed to induce any pathological lesions or clinical signs of disease.[168] Therefore, VP5 seems to play a key role in virulence, virus release and dissemination and virus-induced apoptosis.
- The VP1 protein (95 kDa) is the RNA-dependent RNA-polymerase (RdRp) responsible for the transcription (plus-strand or mRNA synthesis) and replication (minor-strand synthesis) of the genome and it is present in the virion as a free protein or covalently linked to the 5' ends of the two genome segments.[118,155] Three functional regions are identified in the VP1: the N-terminus (aa 1-167), the central polymerase domain (aa 168-658) and the C-terminus (aa 659-878). The central domain contains all structural motifs of RdRp, whereas, the N-terminus domain is responsible for protein priming and the C-terminus domain may prevent back-primed RNA synthesis during protein priming.[44,118]

The capsid of IBDV is formed only by VP2 subunits, which are considered the main host-protective antigens that elicit neutralizing antibodies.

Cell infection, genome replication and transcription

IBDV serotype 1 isolates have a selective tropism for surface immunoglobulin M (sIgM)-bearing B lymphocytes and the entry process is triggered by the specific binding of the VP2 with cellular receptors.[50,98,114] Nowadays, IBDV cell receptor has not been fully identified. Early studies suggested that N-glycosilated proteins within surface IgM-bearing B lymphocytes could be the attachment molecule for virulent IBDV strains.[114] More recently, chicken heat shock protein 90 (cHsp90) and $\alpha4\beta1$ integrin have been suggested to be functional components of a putative cellular receptor complex that mediates IBDV infection.[23,92,172] Available data suggest that interaction between IBDV particles and the $\alpha4\beta1$ integrin might allow virus-cell binding, and that this step could be followed by the interaction with cHsp90α protein and, probably, other cellular polypeptides.[23]

In the case of birnaviruses, the single-shell capsid is competent for both transcription and membrane translocation.[138] In the case of IBDV, a multi-step entry model based on the use of an endocytic pathway has been proposed. The virus is endocytosed in the presence of calcium.[170] Then, the low calcium concentration of the endosome allows pep46, a membrane-interacting peptide, to be released from the virus particles, which deforms the cell membrane, leading to the formation of pores and to the total destabilization of the membrane.[42] However, membrane pores are smaller than viral particles. Very recently, it has been suggested IBDV RNA transcription to occur within ribonucleoprotein complexes (RNP).[99] Therefore, a model was proposed in which IBDV RNPs would be extruded from the pierced-endosomes and associated to the limiting of this organelles, through VP3 targeting ability, where viral genome replication occurs. Afterward, the RNPs associated to the endocytic vesicles could traffic along microtubules to reach the perinuclear region. There, after physical contact with the Golgi complex occurred, viral replication would initiate and viral assembly would take place.[24]

Birnavirus VP1 RdRp initiates RNA synthesis via a template-independent protein-priming mechanism.[107] IBDV RNA synthesis has been proposed to follow a "copy-back" mechanism, in which the template's 3' end primes the synthesis of antisense strand that falls back to form an RNA hairpin.[118,155] During transcription, freshly synthesized transcripts have been suggested to be extruded across viral capsid pores into the cell cytoplasm to be translated.[16]

In the IBDV assembly model, most of the viral proteins have been suggested to be involved. The VP3 scaffold polypeptide interacts with pVP2, VP1 and the viral genome, and plays a key role on controlling morphogenesis and encapsidation.[20,21,96,140] The IBDV capsid protein is synthesized as precursor, pVP2 and its final maturation occurs through proteolytic steps controlled by viral and host proteases in addition to the participation of a scaffolding protein. [61]

As previously mentioned, it has been hypothesized that accumulation of VP5 in the host plasma membrane induces cell lysis and contribute to virus release. [97]

Virus properties

The absence of envelope and its simple structure confer IBDV stability and high resistance to the environment, favoring persistent viral survival in poultry houses even after thorough cleaning and disinfection.

IBDV is sensitive to:

- Sodium hydroxide at high pH.
- Iodinated and chlorinated derivatives.
- Aldehydes (formaldehyde).

IBDV is affected by:

- Phenolic derivatives.
- Quaternary ammonium. [105,150]

IBDV antigenicity and immunogenicity

Serotypes and antigenic subtypes

Two serotypes of IBDV, serotype 1 and 2, exist based on virus neutralization assays. [103] Serotype 1 is pathogenic in chickens, whereas serotype 2 was isolated from turkeys and despite being infectious and transmissible, it is considered to be non virulent for turkeys and chickens. [66,70,103]

> Only IBDV serotype 1
> is considered virulent in chickens,
> its natural host.

However, in the early 80s, antigenic variation within serotype 1 IBDV isolates was identified in USA, with the emergence of the so-called variant strains. These strains were able to cause disease in broiler flocks vaccinated with classical strains. Furthermore, variant viruses were capable of breaking through maternal immunity against classical IBDV strains, causing disease in infected chickens. Based on virus neutralization tests new variant viruses were demonstrated to be antigenically distinct to the classical virulent IBDV strains. [66] A panel of monoclonal antibodies, including R63, B69, 10, 57 and 67, was developed to differentiate classical and antigenic variant strains. [136,153] In the late 80s, new IBDV strains related with high mortality IBD emerged in Europe, and were named very virulent IBDV (vvIBDV) strains. [18,151] However, from an antigenic point of view, no differences exist between vvIBDV and classical IBDV strains. Antigenic variant strains have also been identified in Australia. However, Australian IBDV isolates are also distinct antigenically from the American variant strains. [127] Finally, in recent years, new strains have been isolated in Europe and demonstrated to be also antigenically different to classical strains and similar to American variant strains. [29,71,89]

Molecular basis of antigenicity

The VP2 protein, the unique capsid component, is considered the main host-protective antigen which carries major dominant neutralizing epitopes responsible for eliciting neutralizing antibodies. [3,16,40,48] Specifically, a major conformational dependent neutralizing antigenic domain was identified between amino acid positions 206 and 350. [2,4,165] Moreover, most of the amino acid changes among IBDV isolates, and those related with antigenic variation, are clustered within this domain, called a variable domain or hypervariable region (HVR). [4,55] This domain contains a central hydrophobic region flanked by two major hydrophilic peaks A (212-224) and B (314-325). Two smaller hydrophilic peaks between amino acids 248-252 and 279-290 were also identified within the hydrophobic region. [152]

More recently, the crystal structure of the VP2 shows three domains: base (B), shell (S) and projection (P), which contains 5 loops. [16] The HVR is located within the projection and loops P_{BC} and P_{HI} coincide with the two hydrophilic peaks A and B. Several studies have assessed the contribution of specific amino acid changes on the antigenicity of IBDV. [30,36,37,39,48,68,72,89,148] However, still some controversy exists regarding the effect of specific amino acid positions on the antigenicity. Whereas some studies restrict the ability to control the antigenic pattern to few amino acids located in the two major hydrophilic projections (loops P_{BC} and P_{HI}) [89], other studies have suggested that changes located outside the previously described loops also influence the antigenicity of IBDV, complicating prediction of antigenic changes based on sequence data. [30,72]

Despite being also a viral immunogen, VP3 only elicits non-protective non-neutralizing antibodies. [5] Four antigenic domains have been identified within the VP3, but all of them contain group-specific epitopes and two also contain serotype-specific epitopes. [100,165]

IBDV pathogenicity

Three field pathotypes are recognized within IBDV serotype 1 strains: classical, vvIBDV and variant strains. Each pathotype has different characteristics:

- The early classical strains cause a strong inflammation in the bursa of Fabricius, which induces clinical signs in the infected chickens. [15,129,159]
- Variant strains are characterized by inducing rapid atrophy of the bursa of Fabricius in the absence of inflammatory changes in the bursa and of clinical signs in the infected birds. [129]
- vvIBDV isolates cause a clinical form, similar to classical strains, but with higher mortality. [151]

Extensive passages of wild-type IBDV either in embryo eggs or in cell culture lead to adaptation to tissue culture and to attenuation of field isolates, reducing its ability to induce clinical disease or significant immunosuppression. [45,126,166] With the advent of new molecular systems, particularly reverse genetics, molecular basis of virulence and attenuation have been thoroughly investigated. [8-10,33,76,95,109,112,154,171] It seems clear that VP2 plays a key role in tissue culture adaptation and virus attenuation. [10,109,154] Indeed, site-directed mutagenesis studies showed that amino acid substitutions 253 Q→H, 279 D→N, 284 A→T and/or 330 R→S are responsible of the attenuated phenotype. [10,91,109,154] However, the failure of a cell-culture adapted strain expressing vvIBDV VP2 to induce a very virulent phenotype indicates that VP2 is not the sole determinant of IBDV virulence. [9] Actually, several more recent studies with constructed reassortant viruses containing segments derived from vvIBDV and attenuated strains indicate that VP1 also contributes to the virulent phenotype. [8,95,112] In this sense, distinct amino acid positions within the VP1 have been proposed to be involved on increased pathogenicity. Yu et al. have recently demonstrated that a single amino acid substitution in the N-terminal domain of VP1, 4 V→I leads to increased polymerase activity in cell culture and to attenuated in vivo behavior of vvIBDV. [171] Also, Escaffre et al. showed that amino acid substitution 276 A→T was responsible for the reduced pathogenicity of an IBDV isolate with genome sequences related with vvIBDV but exhibiting atypical antigenicity and pathogenicity features. [33]

From all data available up to now, it is likely that both genome segments, A and B, contribute to the very virulent phenotype of IBDV and that several amino acid substitutions at distinct regions of VP2 and VP1 can probably lead to variations in pathogenicity.

IBDV genetic diversity

RNA viruses are generally considered rapid evolving viruses due to fast replication, large populations and particularly high mutation rates associated to the lack of a proof reading RNA polymerase which leads to point mutations. Hence, antigenic drift in IBDV, attributed to substitution mutations in the loops of the projection domain of the VP2, is thought to be responsible for the formation of antigenic variant strains of the virus. [48,89] In the case of IBDV, some of these mutations can be unique to specific geographic regions suggesting phylogeographic distribution and spatially restricted evolution of IBDV within that region. [14,77] However, genetic variability in IBDV occurs not only associated to point mutations but also to homologous recombination and genome segment reassortment. Evidences of naturally-occurring homologous recombination within IBDV exist based on phylogenetic studies and recombination detection programs. [46,52,67] Putative recombination events have been detected in both genome segments, and in some cases vaccine strains were involved as putative parents. [46,156] Similarly, natural reassortment has been suggested based on phylogenetic analyses by several groups. [88,156,167] Indeed, natural reassortment seems to be involved in the emergence of vvIBDV. It has been proposed that reassortment of a vvIBDV genome B segment probably favored the expansion of vvIBDV, whereas the segment A had been acquired previously. [52,62] This hypothesis would be consistent with a significant role of VP1 within IBDV pathogenicity.

VIRAL PROTEINS ARE OF THE MOST IMPORTANCE

- VP1 seems to play a significant role in IBDV pathogenicity.
- Routine diagnostic for IBDV classification is based on VP2 sequencing.

Genotyping of IBDV field isolates has been mainly done through gene sequencing of the VP2 HVR, where molecular markers of virulence, attenuation and antigenicity have been identified. [149] Early comparisons of VP2 sequences among vvIBDV, classic and attenuated viruses pointed out several amino acid substitutions, including 222, 256, 294, 299, 330 that could be used as molecular markers, but they were not molecular determinants of the very virulent phenotype.[35,149,152,173] Also, by using reverse genetics, three amino acid positions have been suggested to be responsible of cell-culture adaptation and in vivo attenuation of IBDV. Nevertheless, these genetic markers should be taken with care as exceptions occur. For instance, some isolates can show these substitutions and not being very virulent, and contrarily some isolates lacking some of these substitutions can show a very virulent phenotype.[39,88]

Even though reassortments can occur and amino acid substitutions within VP2 should be considered only as molecular markers, nowadays, routine diagnostic for IBDV classification is based on VP2 sequencing, which usually correlates with main IBDV pathotypes and antigenotypes: classical, vvIBDV, variant, Australian, attenuated and poorly attenuated strains. However, the emergence of new strains points out the necessity of standardizing the establishment of new genotypes.

Epidemiology

Hosts and transmission

Natural and experimental hosts

Chickens are the only natural host for serotype 1 IBDVs, whereas turkeys are the natural host for IBDV serotype 2 strains.[64,103] Hence, only chickens develop disease after IBDV infection.

SUSCEPTIBILITY TO IBDV INFECTION

- Highest susceptibility to IBDV infection is between 3 and 6 weeks of age, when the bursa is at maximum development.
- When chickens are infected younger than 3 weeks of age, the infection is subclinical but induces severe immunosuppression in the infected chickens.

Antibodies against IBDV serotype 1 strains have been detected in several species of wild or captive birds. Recently, vvIBDV strains were isolated from distinct wild bird species, including waterfowl, in Korea. Highly virulence of the isolated strains was further confirmed in SPF chickens.[78] Therefore, these findings suggest that wild birds may play a role within IBDV epidemiology as reservoirs or vectors.[43,113,157]

Transmission

IBDV is horizontally transmitted by the oral or respiratory routes by direct contact with infected chickens or by indirect contact with contaminated vectors. As stated before, the virus is highly resistant to the external environment, what favors the indirect transmission. It has been demonstrated that the virus can survive between 54 and 122 days in contaminated houses after removing infected birds.[6]

Carriers and vectors

IBDV was demonstrated to survive in water, feed and droppings from infected pens until 52 days from exposure.[6]

Very few reports exist regarding the role of insects as reservoirs of IBDV. One IBDV isolate obtained from a mosquito was unable to reproduce a clinical form of IBD when inoculated in SPF chickens.[53] Adult forms of *Alphitobius diaperinus*, a darkling beetle, have been suggested to act as a reservoir up to 14 days after virus exposure (contaminated feed) despite virus isolation was erratic during this period.[102] The only data regarding the role of rodents as carriers of IBDV is based on positive serology against IBDV on rats from infected IBDV houses.[38]

Finally, viable vvIBDV was shed in faeces by dogs feeded with carcasses from vvIBDV infected chickens until 2 days post-infection (dpi).[117]

Geographic distribution of IBDV

vvIBDV strains were first reported in United Kingdom.[18] Since then, they have been reported in most of the countries of Europe, South America, Central America, Middle East, Asia and Africa.[12,18,28,34,49,58,63,71,86,94,123,124,133,144,147,149,173] Sporadic outbreaks have been reported in USA and Finland.[139,149] No reports of vvIBDV isolates exist in New Zealand, Australia or Canada.[17,57,115]

Antigenic variant strains are the predominant IBDV isolates in USA. Variant genotypes have also been reported in South America, Canada, South Africa, Asia and Europe.[12,58,71] However, these variant isolates have to be in most cases further characterized to determine its pathological behavior.

Pathogenesis and host immune response

After IBDV entry into the chicken by the oral cavity, there is a primary replication in macrophages and lymphocytes of the cecum at 4 hours post infection (hpi). Then, it reaches the liver by the portal circulation and an early viremia is established. By the hematogenous route, the virus arrives at 11 hpi to the bursa of Fabricius, the main target organ, where it replicates extensively. Then, following a secondary viremia, distributes to other lymphoid organs.[108]

In the bursa of Fabricius, the virus replicates in immature and mature B lymphocytes present in the lymphoid follicles, causing apoptosis and necrosis of these cell populations. [141,142,158] In experimental studies carried out with vvIBDV, it was demonstrated that the first B cells to be infected and depleted are the medullary Bu-1$^+$ B cells (B cell precursors), followed by the medullary IgM$^+$ and IgG$^+$-bearing B cells and their cortical counterparts. [158] Bursal population of IgM$^+$ and IgG$^+$-bearing B cells are completely depleted and do not start to recover after 14 days. In addition, bursal repopulation at 14 dpi is mainly achieved through Bu-1$^+$ B cells, which are likely to be non-functional, because they do not express a surface immunoglobulin that allows them to colonize bursal follicles. [158] Further studies on bursal recovery after IBDV infection in neonatal chicks described two types of follicles during the recovery process: small follicles lacking a distinct cortex and medulla and apparently unable to produce antigen-responsive B cells and larger follicles with normal structure and rapidly proliferating B cells originated from bursal stem cells. The emergence of these large follicles correlates with partial recovery of humoral immune response. [162]

T cells also play a key role in the pathogenesis and control of IBDV infection. Replication of IBDV in B cells is followed by an influx of activated T cells to the bursa of Fabricius. [130,158] CD4$^+$ T cells are increased by 7 dpi and their location is restricted to the cortico-medullary boundary of the lymphoid follicles, while CD8$^+$ T cells are detected throughout the bursal follicles. [158] These T cells do not serve as targets for infection and replication of IBDV but they are involved in viral clearance and bursal recovery following infection. [82,83,158] Increased expression of cytokine genes of both Th1 (IFN-γ, IL-2 and IL-12) and Th2 (IL-4, IL-5, IL-13 and IL-10) has been demonstrated in the bursa of Fabricius after a vvIBDV strain challenge [93,122] further demonstrating the relevance of T cell-mediated immune response in the pathogenesis of IBDV infection. In addition, studies comparing the immune response to classical and vvIBDV strains showed that both strains induced a pro-inflammatory response, evidenced by increased mRNA transcription of IL-1β , IL-6, and CXCLi2, and down-regulation of TGF-β4, of similar magnitude and timing. Interestingly, IFN-γ mRNA was induced by both strains, although to a greater degree by the vvIBDV strain, suggesting that the expression of this cytokine may be affected by the increased virulence of vvIBDV. [32]

In addition, it has been suggested that T cells may also play a central role in the stimulation of bursal macrophages through IFN-γ production. [59] Bursal macrophages support viral replication [142] and are activated during the acute phase of IBDV infection, and there is an enhanced expression of IL-6, IL-1β and IL-8 cytokines and iNOS mRNA, that can explain the important inflammatory response seen in acute IBDV infections. [80,82]

Although the involvement of lymphoid organs other than the bursa of Fabricius in the pathogenesis of IBDV infection has been suggested as an important event that correlates with IBDV pathogenicity [59,122], there are few detailed studies describing such changes. IBDV replication in lymphocytes and macrophages in the thymus, spleen, cecal tonsil and bone marrow associated to cell depletion in all these organs has been shown from 12 hpi to 7 dpi. [142] In a more recent study, Williams and Davidson described vvIBDV replication in the thymus from 4 to 7 dpi associated to thymic lymphoid depletion. [158] However, these authors suggest that thymic B cells are the ones which are supporting viral replication and that it seems unlikely that IBDV directly infects and replicates within T cells in the thymus.

The pathogenesis of the hemorrhages often observed in IBDV-infected animals was studied by several authors, but the origin of these lesions has not been fully elucidated. A hypersensitivity type III reaction with immune complexes formation and deposition was suspected but it was not entirely demonstrated. [134,135] Furthermore, increased clotting times were detected in IBDV-infected chickens and an acquired coagulopathy as result of the viral infection has been suggested as one of the factors involved in the pathogenesis of the hemorrhages. [84,135] However, the mechanism by which IBDV is causing the acquired coagulopathy still remains unknown.

Regarding comparative immunopathogenesis of classical and variant IBDV infection, it has been shown that classical and variant IBDV viruses caused extensive gross and histologic lesions in the bursa of Fabricius. [129] However, bursal necrosis induced by the classical isolate was accompanied by an inflammatory response, whereas the inflammatory component was lacking in the lesion induced by the variant isolate. Furthermore, the classical isolate induced extensive lesions in the thymus, but the variant isolate did not. In a more recent study, it has been demonstrated that there are marked differences between classical and variant IBDV not only on the bursal damage, but also in the T cell infiltration and expression of cytokines, chemokines and TLRs in the bursa of Fabricius. Classical IBDV infection induces a higher expression of innate cytokines (IFN-γ, IFN-β), proinflammatory cytokines and mediators (IL-6 and iNOS) and chemokines (IL-8 and MIP-α) than infection with the variant IBDV strain. [121]

The effect of the genetic background on the immunopathogenesis of IBDV infection has also been evaluated. Stronger stimulation of innate immune reactions especially after vvIBDV infection in the early phase may lead to faster and more severe clinical outcome, lesion and mortality rate in layer-type chickens compared to broiler-type chickens. [1]

Immunosuppression

IBDV interacts with several immune cells (B cells, T cells, macrophages) causing a complex disarrangement of the chicken immune system and an immunosuppressive effect on the chicken. Increased susceptibility of IBDV-infected chickens to other diseases, such as inclusion body hepatitis, coccidiosis, infectious bronchitis, has been extensively demonstrated (reviewed in Eterradossi et al.). [38]

IBDV replication in the mature and immature B cells of the bursa of Fabricius results in a reduction of the circulating IgM^+ B cells and an impairment of the humoral immune responses. [38,59] Early studies postulated that suppression of humoral immune response was greatest if IBDV infection occurred in young birds (until seven-day-old), but had lower effects when birds were infected at an older age. [41] Interference on the humoral responses after immunization with several viruses, such as infectious bronchitis virus, Marek's disease virus or Newcastle disease virus has been largely reported, suggesting disruption of the B-cell system (reviewed in Hoerr et al.). [51] Interestingly, even in one-day-old IBDV-infected chicks, the humoral immune response against IBDV itself is adequate. [134]

There are several studies demonstrating the effect of IBDV in cell-mediated immunity. IBDV induces bursal T lymphocytes to inhibit normal splenic T cell mitogenic response. [82,122] In addition, a downregulation of the T cell immune response in the recovery phase of the IBDV infection linked to a reduced expression of IFN-γ has been suggested. [59] Bursal macrophages support viral replication, and their phagocytic activity as well as their cytokine gene expression is modified following IBDV infection, probably influencing the normal responsiveness of the affected birds. [80] On the contrary, NK cells, another important effector cells of the innate immune system are not influenced by the IBDV infection. [131]

Comparison of the humoral and cellular immune competence in birds infected with classical or variant IBDV strains resulted in that both isolates induced similar depression of the mitogenic response to T-cell mitogens and primary and secondary antibody response to sheep erythrocytes and *Brucella abortus*. [129]

Clinical signs

The clinicopathological outcome of IBDV infection greatly differs depending on the type of strain, age, genetic background and maternal immunity of the susceptible chickens.

IBDV infection by classical and vvIBDV strains is generally observed in 3-6 week-old susceptible birds. Susceptible birds younger than 3 weeks may suffer subclinical infection and severe immunosuppression as a consequence of viral replication. [38] Incubation period is short (3-4 days) and some authors have suggested that the onset of clinical signs in vvIBDV infections can be even faster (48 hours). [158]

The most relevant clinical signs are:

- Anorexia.
- Ruffled feathers.
- Watery diarrhea.
- Prostration.
- Death.

Morbidity is usually high, achieving 100 % of the flock. Mortality is more variable. In classical IBDV infections, it can be nil but can also be 20-30 %. It usually starts at 3 dpi and lasts until 5-7 dpi. [38] In vvIBDV infections, mortality is usually higher than in classical IBDV infections. When the first outbreaks by vvIDBV took place, mortalities of 90-100 % in susceptible leghorn chickens were described. [18] The origin of the differences among classical and vvIBDV in terms of onset and severity of the clinical signs and mortality is currently unknown. Different authors have suggested that the highly virulent behavior of vvIBDV is due to the more extensive viral replication and cellular damage in the bursa of Fabricius and also in other lymphoid tissues. [142,158] On the contrary, it has been recently postulated that there is no correlation between the clinicopathological outcome and the extent of the bursal damage, since some birds that survive to the IBDV infection have extensive bursal damage while others die with mild bursal lesions. [59] Host immune response and, more specifically, the levels of some cytokines, notably IFN-γ, may have a crucial role in the enhanced virulence of vvIBDV. [32]

Regarding infections with variant IBDV strains, outbreaks are generally reported in vaccinated birds younger than three weeks without any evidence of clinical disease or mortality. [38] Experimental infection with American variant E/Del IBDV strain in one-day-old chickens did not result in any clinical sign. [31] Similarly, experimental infection of four-day-old chickens with American variant AL2 IBDV strain induced neither overt clinical signs nor mortality. [145]

Gross and microscopic lesions

The most relevant gross lesion in IBDV infected animals is observed in the bursa of Fabricius, the target organ. In the early stages of the infection by classical or vvIBDV (2-3 dpi), a marked increase in size of the bursa due to acute inflammation can be observed. Edema of the bursal serosal surface is sometimes evident (Fig. 1) and small petechia in the mucosal surface of the bursa (Fig. 2) or extensive hemorrhages throughout the entire organ may be seen at this stage. At 5 to 8 dpi, animals that survive show marked bursal atrophy. [38]

> Whereas at early stages the bursa a Fabricius increases in size due to inflammation and edema, the animals that survive after 8 days post-infection with classical and vvIBDV strains show bursal atrophy.

In addition, birds infected with classical or vvIBDV may show macroscopic lesions in other organs. Dehydration and hemorrhages in the thigh and pectoral muscles are very often observed (Fig. 3). Hemorrhages in the proventricular mucosa can also be seen, especially in vvIBDV-infected animals. Kidneys may also be secondarily affected, due to dehydration, and show paleness, a marked lobular pattern, and even urate deposition in the parenchyma and ureters (Fig. 4). [38] As regards

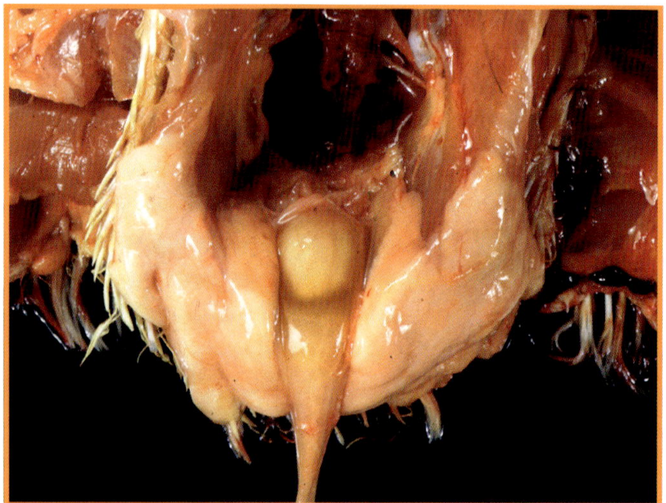

Fig. 1 | Marked peribursal edema in a broiler chicken with acute IBDV infection.

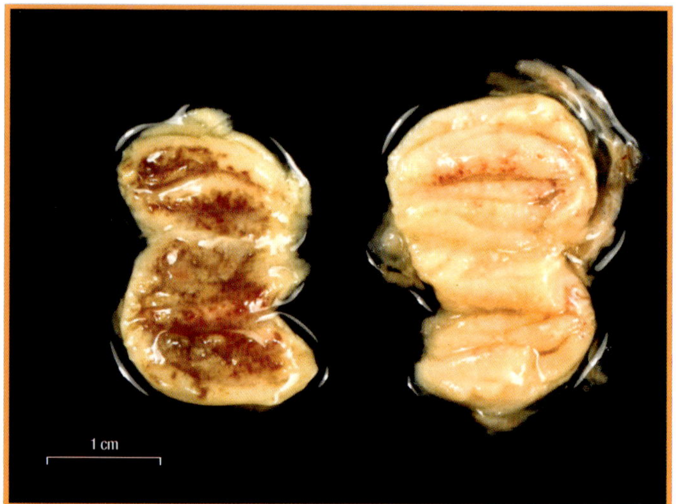

Fig. 2 | Multiple petechiae in the bursa of Fabricius in a broiler chicken with acute IBDV infection.

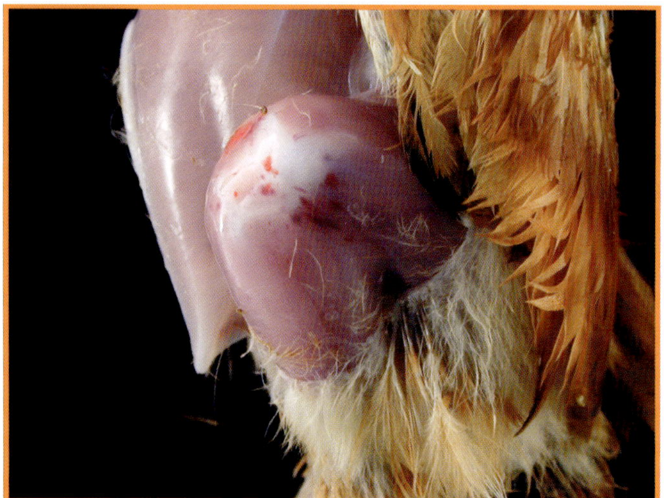

Fig. 3 | Multiple petechiae and ecchymosis in the thigh muscles of a broiler chicken infected with IBDV.

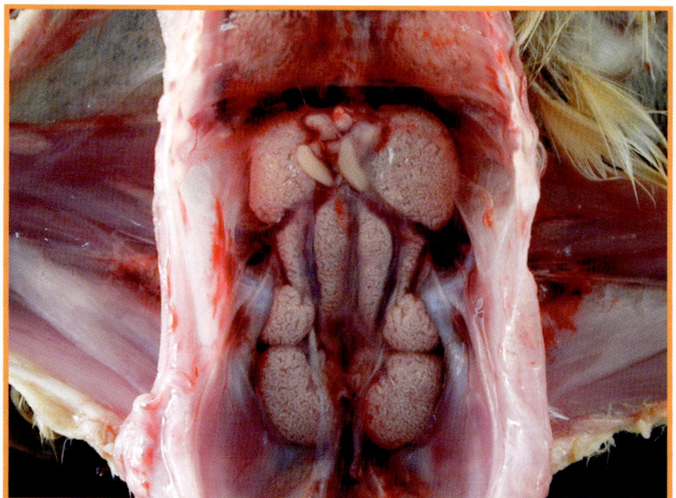

Fig. 4 | Severe nephropathy with marked intraparenchymal urate deposition, probably secondary to dehydration, in an IBDV-infected broiler chicken.

to other lymphoid organs, mild thymus atrophy [158] and mottling of the spleen [122] are the macroscopic lesions that have been more frequently described associated to classical and vvIBDV infection.

Experimental infection with variant E/Del IBDV strain resulted in bursal atrophy from 2 weeks post infection (wpi) that persisted until 6 wpi, without any evidence of acute inflammatory reaction. [31] Likewise, infection of four-day-old chickens with variant AL2 IBDV strain induced reduced bursal indices. [145]

More relevant microscopic lesions in IBDV-infected animals are observed in the bursa of Fabricius. In the acute stage, lymphocytolysis of follicular medullary lymphocytes, associated to marked interstitial edema, heterophilic and macrophage influx is the hallmark lesion of acute IBDV infection (Figs. 5a and 6a). Interstitial hemorrhages can also be frequently seen. Microscopic lesions tend to be diffuse, affecting all the follicles of the bursa and viral antigens are widely detected following immunohistochemical staining (Figs. 5b and 6b). At 4-5 dpi, a reduction in size of the lymphoid follicles with evident loss of follicular lymphocytes and replacement by macrophages containing cellular debris is observed. At more chronic stages, reduction of the size of the follicles due to lymphocyte depletion is more evident with shrinkage of the corticomedullary junction. Cystic cavities may develop in the medullary areas of the follicles, lined by a

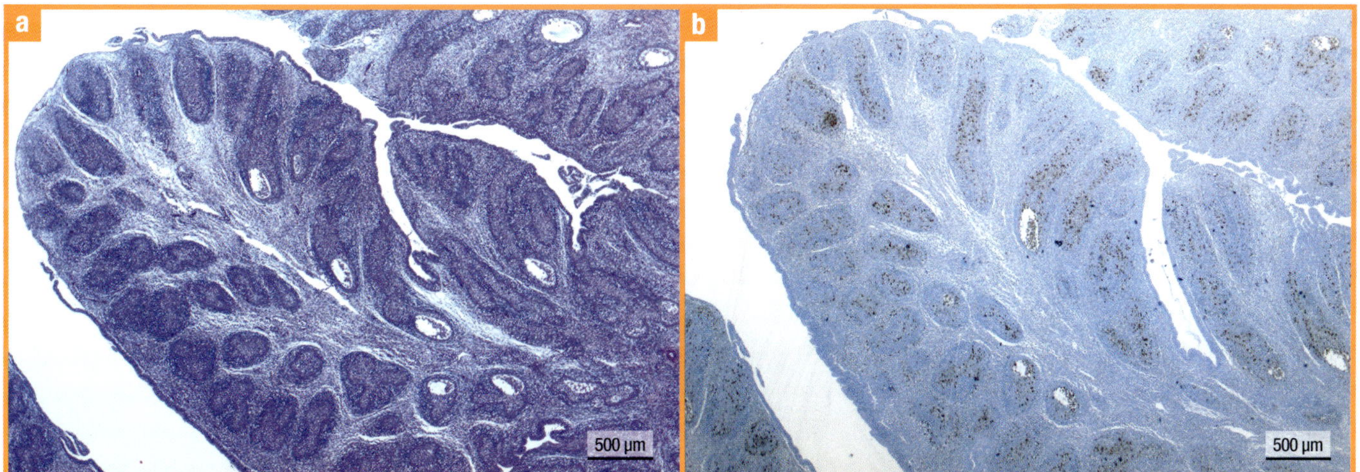

Fig. 5 | Microscopic image of a bursa of Fabricius from a broiler chicken with acute IBDV infection. (a) Diffuse lymphocytolysis associated to marked interfollicular edema and heterophilic and macrophagic influx is observed. HE staining. Bar = 500 µm. (b) Viral antigen widely distributed in follicular cells. Immunohistochemical staining with VP2 antibody. Bar = 500 µm.

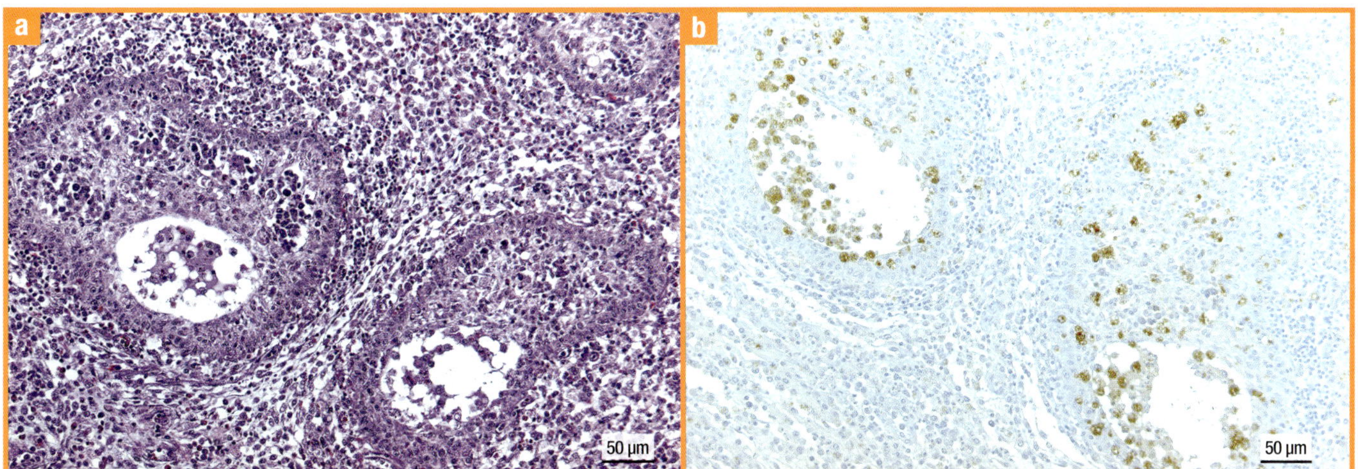

Fig. 6 | Microscopic image of a bursa of Fabricius from a broiler chicken with acute IBDV infection. (a) Marked lymphocytolysis of follicular medullary lymphocytes associated to marked interfollicular edema and heterophilic and macrophagic influx. HE staining. Bar = 50 µm. (b) Viral antigen in the cytoplasm of follicular cells. Immunohistochemical staining with VP2 antibody. Bar = 50 µm.

columnar epithelium, and often filled with granular basophilic material resembling mucus. Marked interfollicular fibrosis as well as plicae formation in the superficial bursal epithelium is also frequently observed at late stages of infection (Fig. 7).

The evolution of microscopic bursal lesions in chickens experimentally infected with American E/Del variant IBDV strain is as follows. The lesions start at 2 wpi as mild to moderate diffuse lymphoid depletion and necrosis of the bursal follicles with complete absence of inflammatory reaction. By 4 wpi, there is severe follicular lymphoid depletion with cyst formation and plical atrophy. At 6 wpi, follicular cyst formation and bursal atrophy persist, but there is a narrow zone of repopulating lymphocytes at the periphery of some follicles. [31]

Moreover, infection of four-day-old chickens with American variant AL2 IBDV strain also induces bursa lymphocyte depletion. [145]

Microscopic lesions associated to IBDV infection in other organs are mild and non-specific. Cortical lymphocyte depletion in the thymus due to lymphocyte apoptosis has been associated to classical and vvIBDV infection. [60,142,158] In addition, slight lymphocyte depletion of the peri-ellipsoid sheath of the spleen and enlargement of reticular cells around sheated arteries has been described, as well as decreased numbers of lymphoid cells in the cecal tonsil and myelocytes in the extrasinusoidal space of the bone marrow. [142] Reduction of the plasma cell population of the Harderian gland after IBDV infection has also been reported. [26] Variant strains (E/Del) do not cause any lesions in the thymus, but diffuse lymphoid depletion in the germinal centers and around the peri-ellipsoid and peri-arteriolar sheaths in the spleen are observed at 4 and 6 wpi. [31]

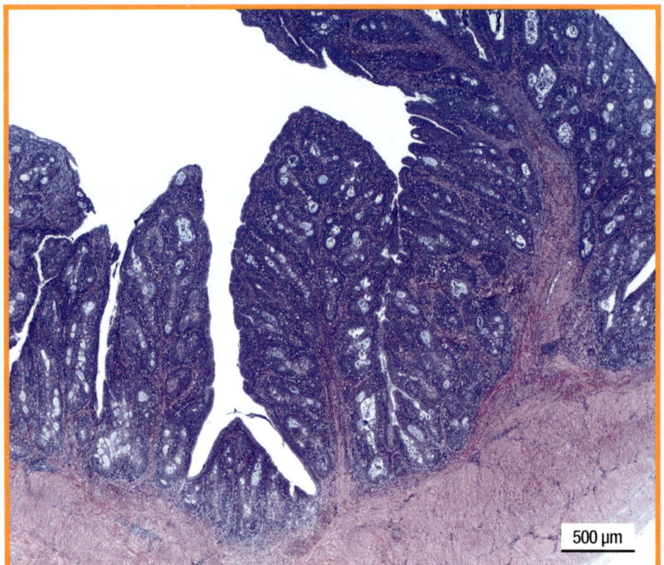

Fig. 7 | Microscopic image of a bursa of Fabricius from a broiler chicken with chronic IBDV infection. Marked follicular lymphoid depletion, with follicular cyst formation and interfollicular fibrosis are evident. HE staining. Bar = 500 µm.

HALLMARK LESIONS OF CLASSICAL AND VIRULENT IBD IN THE BURSA OF FABRICIUS

- Lymphocytolysis of follicular medullary lymphocytes.
- Marked interstitial edema.
- Heterophilic and macrophage influx.

Diagnosis

Presumptive diagnosis of IBD infection is usually made on the basis of the clinical signs, mortality and bursa of Fabricius gross lesions. However, particularly if subclinical infection is suspected, further confirmation of IBDV infection by laboratory techniques is strongly recommended. In addition, it has to be pointed out that several of the gross lesions described in IBDV can also be associated to other pathological conditions (Table 1).

Nowadays, a number of diagnostic techniques to detect and classify IBDV from clinical samples are available and will be further presented and discussed in this chapter. In addition, diagnosis of IBDV infection can also be achieved by serological techniques.

Viral detection

There are several techniques that allow detection of IBDV in the target organ, the bursa of Fabricius.

RECOMMENDATIONS FOR VIRAL DETECTION

- It is important to sample animals suffering the acute phase of the disease.
- If subclinical infection is suspected, regular sampling along the fattening or rearing period is indicated.

Viral isolation

Isolation of IBDV either in embryonated specific-pathogen-free (SPF) eggs or primary cell cultures is a highly sensitive method of viral detection. [38] However, it is time-consuming and expensive and it is not routinely used for IBDV diagnosis.

IBDV field viruses can be isolated in 9-11 day-old embryonated SPF eggs inoculated by the chorioallantoic membrane or the yolk route. Death of infected embryos usually happens at 3-5 dpi. Isolation and replication of field viruses in primary cell cultures (B cells derived from cloacal bursa, chicken embryo fibroblasts, or chicken embryo kidney cells) is not straightforward and can only be achieved after adaption by serial passages in these cell cultures that may induce changes in the genome of these viruses. [166]

Histology and viral detection by immunohistochemistry

As said, microscopic lesions associated to classical or vvIBDV infections in the bursa of Fabricius of animals suffering the acute stage of the disease are specific and distinctive of this viral process. In these cases, further confirmation of IBDV infection following immunofluorescence or immunoperoxidase staining with polyclonal or monoclonal antibodies in tissues is advisable. These detection techniques are highly specific but sensitivity is lower than the molecular techniques.

It is worth mentioning that non-specific follicular lymphoid depletion can be microscopically observed in:

- Variant IBDV infections.
- Chronic stages of classical or vvIBDV infections.
- Use of poorly attenuated vaccines.

Viral genome detection by molecular methods

In the last years, molecular diagnosis of IBDV infection has become the most widely used system to detect and classify IBDV strains circulating in a farm. Different reverse transcription-polymerase chain reaction (RT-PCR) techniques targeting the hypervariable region of the VP2 of any IBDV isolate have been developed. [27,69,163] This technique is fast and very sensitive and could be performed on fresh or frozen bursal samples (minimum 5 bursas/flock) or even from tissues collected in FTA® cards that can be stored at room temperature. Multiplex RT-PCR [85] or real-time RT-PCR [75] aimed to detect and differentiate IBDV strains and microarrays coupled with RT-PCR [143] have also been developed.

IBDV genotyping

Detection of IBDV by RT-PCR in a field sample is usually followed by some molecular techniques that allow differentiate field and vaccine strains of IBDV. There are two main techniques used for this purpose:

1. The Restriction Fragment Length Polymorphism technique (RFLP).
2. The sequencing of the RT-PCR amplified fragment.

Table 1. Differential diagnoses of IBDV infection, based on gross lesions.

DISEASE OR CONDITION	LESION			
	Enlarged, edematous and/or hemorrhagic bursa	Atrophic bursa	Muscular and proventricular hemorrhages	Nephropathy
Infectious bursal disease	✓	✓	✓	✓
Mycotoxicosis		✓	✓	✓
Marek's disease		✓		
Infectious bronchitis				✓
Avian influenza			✓	
Newcastle disease			✓	
Water deprivation				✓

In the RFLP, the amplified RT-PCR product is cut by different restriction enzymes and fragments obtained are visualized by electrophoresis. [74] The RFLP pattern (length and number of fragments) of the field strain is then compared with that of the reference strains and endorsed to one particular molecular group. The main disadvantage of this technique is that it only gives information about a very limited number of nucleotides of the VP2 gene and new patterns are often reported based on few nucleotide changes.

Nowadays, the most used system to genotype IBDV strains is the sequencing of the RT-PCR amplified fragment. [14,73] By sequencing the fragment, detailed information on the nucleotide changes in the VP2 gene region is obtained. Phylogenetic comparison of the amplified gene fragment with reference strains found in the Genbank allows clustering the field strain in a particular genotype group (Fig. 8). It is worth mentioning that nucleotide mutations do not always imply antigenic changes in the viral protein. Furthermore, sporadically, IBDV strains with VP2 gene

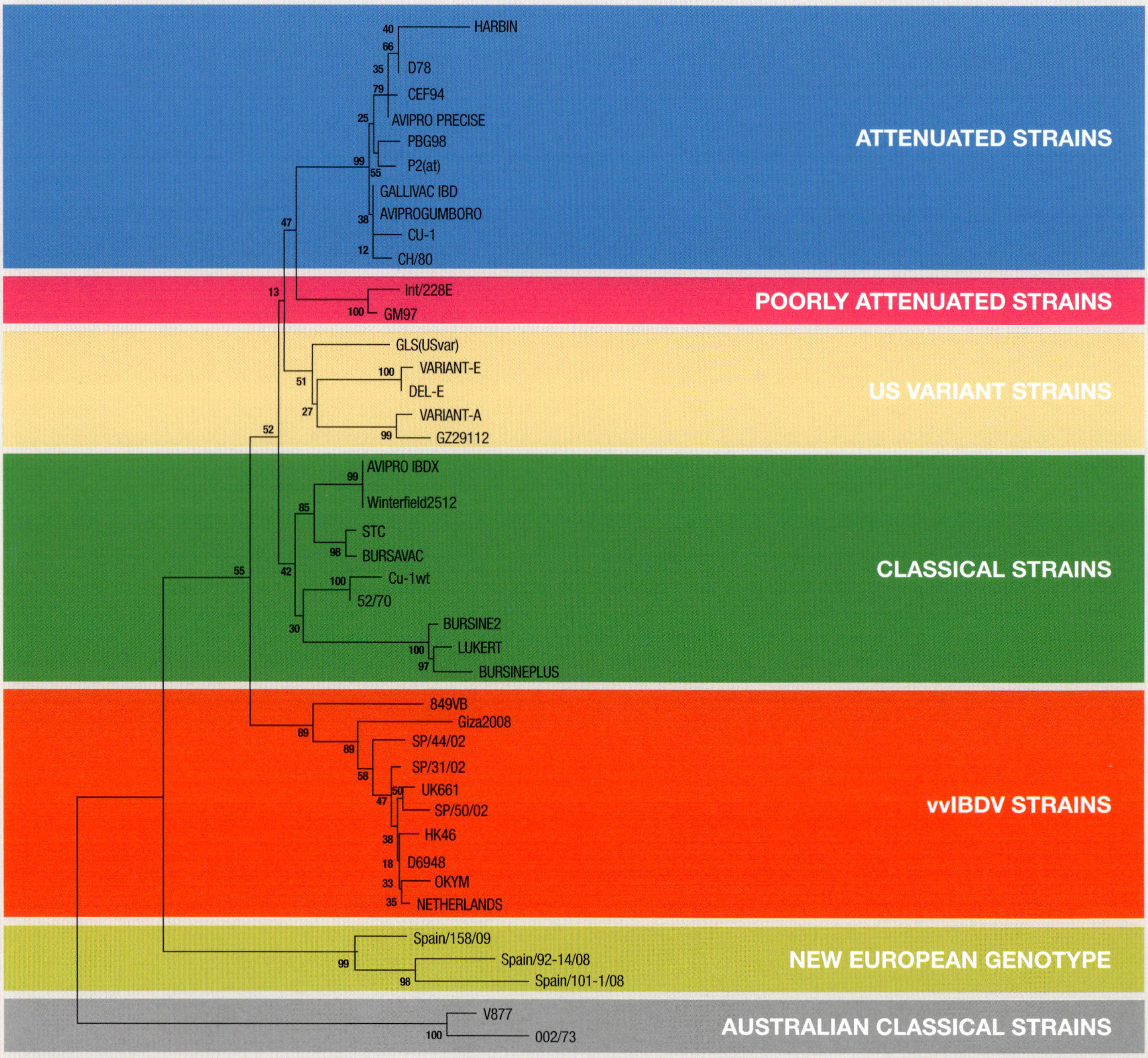

Fig. 8 | Phylogenetic analysis of the nucleotide sequences of reference and vaccine IBDV isolates based on a 480 bp region of the VP2 gene. Sequences from reference strains were obtained from Genbank. A neighbor-joining method using 1000 bootstrapping replicates was conducted.

clustering within vvIBDV isolates have been reported to have a reduced virulence. [88] Therefore, pathogenic and protection studies are advisable if the results of the molecular techniques do not match with the field observations.

Antibody detection

Detection and quantification of antibodies against IBDV is mainly useful to:

- Measure the maternal antibody levels of day-old chicks to further calculate the day of vaccination.
- Detect subclinical infections.
- Assess the immune response to IBDV vaccination at the end of the productive period.

> **A critical point when interpreting serological results is the number of samples used. A minimum of 18 serum samples are recommended to obtain reliable results.**

ELISA

Several commercial ELISA are currently available to assess the level of IBDV antibodies in field samples.

They are specific, consistent, quick and non-expensive techniques that allow detecting the humoral response against IBDV from 7 to 10 days after infection or vaccination. However, ELISA kits may present intra and inter-laboratorial variation so care should be taken when comparing results obtained by different ELISA kits. [38]

Viral neutralization assay

This is the gold standard assay to detect antibodies against IBDV. [134] This technique is serotype-specific and detects neutralizing antibodies as soon as 7 dpi or vaccination. Although it is highly sensible and specific, it is a very time-consuming technique and therefore is not routinely used for serological IBDV diagnosis. In addition, it has been proven very difficult to standardize among different laboratories.

Prevention and control

IBDV is usually endemic within areas of intensive poultry production probably due to its high resistance to physical conditions and chemical products, which confers the virus with a strong persistence in the environment. Nonetheless, high biosecurity and hygienic standards are essential in order to control the disease together with vaccination.

Vaccination success depends on distinct factors but mostly on the choice of:

- Vaccine strain.
- Age of vaccination.
- Schedule of vaccination.

The schedule of vaccination will change depending on the field strain and field pressure. It is critical to know the field strains circulating and involved in IBD outbreaks, as antigenic and pathogenic changes in the strains can affect vaccine efficacy. Several types of vaccines and vaccine strains are available. Complete revisions of this topic have been recently published, including those vaccines only reported in literature. [106] Therefore, a summary of only the main vaccines currently available will be included in this chapter.

Inactivated vaccines

IBDV commercial inactivated vaccines are mostly based on inactivated whole viruses or viral subunits, which lack replicating abilities. Although they are very secure, as no live virus is included, they are less immunogenic than live vaccines. Therefore, in order to increase the immunogenic potential, they should be mixed with adjuvants, mostly water-in-oil emulsions. [106] For this reason, these kinds of vaccines are mainly restricted to breeders, in order to induce high and homogenous levels of antibodies against IBDV that will provide passive immunity to the offspring by means of maternally derived antibodies.

> **INACTIVATED VACCINES**
>
> They are regularly used as a booster in birds previously primed with live attenuated vaccines.

Conventional live attenuated virus vaccines

After serial passage in embryonated SPF eggs, IBDV ability to cause clinical disease or significant immunosuppression is attenuated, whereas they still induce an immune response. [125,126] The main problem with live vaccines is the interference with maternal antibodies. In order to protect chickens from early infections (during the two first weeks of age), a common practice is to induce high levels of maternal immunity. However, these antibodies can also neutralize live attenuated vaccines. To avoid this effect, distinct degrees of attenuation can be produced depending on the number of serial passages carried out. IBDV live vaccine strains are classified as mild, intermediate, intermediate plus or hot vaccines depending on the attenuation degree, from more attenuated to poor attenuated. [150] The poorer the degree of vaccine attenuation, the higher its capacity to break through higher levels of maternal antibodies and to induce bursal lesions and immunosuppression.

Therefore, one of the critical decisions within the vaccination program design is the age at which birds should be vaccinated: [150]

- On one hand, the vaccine cannot be administered whereas levels of maternal antibodies able to neutralize the vaccine are present in the birds.
- On the other hand, vaccine should be administered early enough to protect against field infection.

In this sense, vvIBDV are characterized by breaking through higher levels of maternal antibodies, therefore, intermediate to hot vaccines are used. However, balance should be found to use the more attenuated virus that can prevent field virus and induce the minimum lesions in the bursa of Fabricius.

Formulas to calculate the right age of vaccination based on the levels of maternal antibodies at one day of age have been proposed. However, these formulas are often impractical when field isolates are vvIBDV because the resulting age of vaccination will be too late, leading to vaccine failure. [161] To avoid vaccination failures it is critical to keep in mind proper practical on-farm procedures for vaccination in drinking water. The critical factors affecting the vaccination success are:

- Vaccine storage conditions.
- Elution of the vaccine.
- Quality of drinking water in which vaccine is administered.
- Husbandry techniques to vaccinate a large number of birds in a short period of time.

With the advent of in ovo vaccination techniques, new IBDV vaccine technologies able to be also applied in ovo were developed and commercialized.

Vector vaccines

IBDV vector vaccines are based on inserting one gene of IBDV, mainly VP2 gene, within the genome of another organism, mainly another virus (the vector). [106] When the vector virus replicates in the chicken, it also expresses the inserted gene of IBDV, and therefore, it elicits a protection against both viruses: IBDV and the vector virus. Several viruses have been reported to be used as vector viruses for VP2 gene. [47,54,120,132,146,164] However, as far as the authors know, only IBDV-VP2 vectored vaccines based on turkey herpesvirus (HVT) as vector have been commercialized until now. [87] Several studies have been published regarding the efficacy of these vaccines against vvIBDV and variant IBD viruses. [11,87,119]

One of the main advantages of vector vaccines is that protection against IBDV is afforded without the undesired effects of IBDV replication within the bursa of Fabricius.

Immune complex vaccines

Immune complex (Icx) vaccines are based on a mixture of live attenuated IBDV vaccines and anti-IBDV antibodies produced by hyperimmunization of SPF chickens. With this technology, live attenuated IBD viruses can be used in presence of high levels of maternal antibodies, as they are coated and protected with specific antibodies. Therefore, Icx vaccines can be administered in ovo or subcutaneously at one day of age. The working mechanism of Icx was investigated in SPF chickens, and it could be shown that virus complexing with specific antibodies induced a delay in virus replication when compared with inoculation of virus alone. [79] However, Icx virus could not be detected before virus replication occurred, and therefore, the place where Icx virus allocates after injection could not be demonstrated. Studies with chickens with maternal antibodies have also been carried out, and after in ovo vaccination with Icx vaccine, IBDV can only be detected by real time PCR in the bursa of Fabricius from 21 days of age onwards. [65]

References

1. Aricibasi M, Jung A, Heller ED, and Rautenschlein S. Differences in genetic background influence the induction of innate and acquired immune responses in chickens depending on the virulence of the infecting infectious bursal disease virus (IBDV) strain. Vet Immunol Immunopathol 135: 79-92, 2010.
2. Azad AA, Fahey KJ, Barrett SA, Erny KM, and Hudson PJ. Expression in Escherichia coli of cDNA fragments encoding the gene for the host-protective antigen of infectious bursal disease virus. Virology 149: 190-198, 1986.
3. Azad AA, Jagadish MN, Brown MA, and Hudson PJ. Deletion mapping and expression in Escherichia coli of the large genomic segment of a birnavirus. Virology 161: 145-152, 1987.
4. Bayliss CD, Spies U, Shaw K, Peters RW, Papageorgiou A, Muller H, and Boursnell ME. A comparison of the sequences of segment A of four infectious bursal disease virus strains and identification of a variable region in VP2. J Gen Virol 71 (Pt 6): 1303-1312, 1990.
5. Becht H, Muller H, and Muller HK. Comparative studies on structural and antigenic properties of two serotypes of infectious bursal disease virus. J Gen Virol 69 (Pt 3): 631-640, 1988.
6. Benton WJ, Cover MS, Rosenberger JK, and Lake RS. Physicochemical properties of the infectious bursal agent (IBA). Avian Dis 11: 438-445, 1967.
7. Birghan C, Mundt E, and Gorbalenya AE. A non-canonical lon proteinase lacking the ATPase domain employs the ser-Lys catalytic dyad to exercise broad control over the life cycle of a double-stranded RNA virus. EMBO J 19: 114-123, 2000.
8. Boot HJ, and Pritz-Verschuren SB. Modifications of the 3'-UTR stem-loop of infectious bursal disease virus are allowed without influencing replication or virulence. Nucleic Acids Res 32: 211-222, 2004.
9. Boot HJ, ter Huurne AA, Hoekman AJ, Peeters BP, and Gielkens AL. Rescue of very virulent and mosaic infectious bursal disease virus from cloned cDNA: VP2 is not the sole determinant of the very virulent phenotype. J Virol 74: 6701-6711, 2000.
10. Brandt M, Yao K, Liu M, Heckert RA, and Vakharia VN. Molecular determinants of virulence, cell tropism, and pathogenic phenotype of infectious bursal disease virus. J Virol 75: 11974-11982, 2001.
11. Bublot M, Pritchard N, Le Gros FX, and Goutebroze S. Use of a vectored vaccine against infectious bursal disease of chickens in the face of high-titred maternally derived antibody. J Comp Pathol 137 Suppl 1: S81-84, 2007.
12. Cao YC, Yeung WS, Law M, Bi YZ, Leung FC, and Lim BL. Molecular characterization of seven Chinese isolates of infectious bursal disease virus: classical, very virulent, and variant strains. Avian Dis 42: 340-351, 1998.
13. Caston JR, Martinez-Torrecuadrada JL, Maraver A, Lombardo E, Rodriguez JF, Casal JI, and Carrascosa JL. C terminus of infectious bursal disease virus major capsid protein VP2 is involved in definition of the T number for capsid assembly. J Virol 75: 10815-10828, 2001.
14. Cortey M, Bertran K, Toskano J, Majo N, and Dolz R. Phylogeographic distribution of very virulent infectious bursal disease virus isolates in the Iberian Peninsula. Avian Pathol 41: 277-284, 2012.
15. Cosgrove AS. An apparently new disease of chickens-Avian nephrosis. Avian Dis 6: 385-389, 1962.
16. Coulibaly F, Chevalier C, Gutsche I, Pous J, Navaza J, Bressanelli S, Delmas B, and Rey FA. The birnavirus crystal structure reveals structural relationships among icosahedral viruses. Cell 120: 761-772, 2005.
17. Chai YF, Christensen NH, Wilks CR, and Meers J. Characterisation of New Zealand isolates of infectious bursal disease virus. Arch Virol 146: 1571-1580, 2001.
18. Chettle N, Stuart JC, and Wyeth PJ. Outbreak of virulent infectious bursal disease in East Anglia. Vet Rec 125: 271-272, 1989.
19. Chevalier C, Galloux M, Pous J, Henry C, Denis J, Da Costa B, Navaza J, Lepault J, and Delmas B. Structural peptides of a nonenveloped virus are involved in assembly and membrane translocation. J Virol 79: 12253-12263, 2005.
20. Chevalier C, Lepault J, Da Costa B, and Delmas B. The last C-terminal residue of VP3, glutamic acid 257, controls capsid assembly of infectious bursal disease virus. J Virol 78: 3296-3303, 2004.
21. Chevalier C, Lepault J, Erk I, Da Costa B, and Delmas B. The maturation process of pVP2 requires assembly of infectious bursal disease virus capsids. J Virol 76: 2384-2392, 2002.
22. Da Costa B, Chevalier C, Henry C, Huet JC, Petit S, Lepault J, Boot H, and Delmas B. The capsid of infectious bursal disease virus contains several small peptides arising from the maturation process of pVP2. J Virol 76: 2393-2402, 2002.
23. Delgui L, Ona A, Gutierrez S, Luque D, Navarro A, Caston JR, and Rodriguez JF. The capsid protein of infectious bursal disease virus contains a functional alpha 4 beta 1 integrin ligand motif. Virology 386: 360-372, 2009.
24. Delgui LR, Rodriguez JF, and Colombo MI. The endosomal pathway and the Golgi complex are involved in the Infectious Bursal Disease Virus life cycle. J Virol 2013.
25. Dobos P. Peptide map comparison of the proteins of infectious bursal disease virus. J Virol 32: 1047-1050, 1979.
26. Dohms JE, Lee KP, Rosenberger JK, and Metz AL. Plasma cell quantitation in the gland of Harder during infectious bursal disease virus infection of 3-week-old broiler chickens. Avian Dis 32: 624-631, 1988.

27. Dolz R, Majó N, Ordóñez G, and Porta R. Viral genotyping of infectious bursal disease viruses isolated from the 2002 acute outbreak in Spain and comparison with previous isolates. Avian Dis 49: 332-339, 2005.
28. Dolz R, Majó N, Ordóñez G, Ponsa F, Biarnès M, and Porta R. Molecular charatcerization of Infectious Bursal Disease Viruses isolated in Spain. In: XXII World's poultry Congress. Istanbul, Turkey: 2004, p. 707.
29. Dolz R, Strauss J, Bertran K, Bobi J, Pérez M, and Majo N. Dinámica de la infección por un nuevo genotipo de virus de Gumboro en pollos de engorde comerciales de 7 y 21 días de edad. In: XLVIII Simposio Científico de Avicultura, edited by WPSA AEdCA-SE. Santiago de Compostela, Spain: 2011, p. 201-206.
30. Durairaj V, Sellers HS, Linnemann EG, Icard AH, and Mundt E. Investigation of the antigenic evolution of field isolates using the reverse genetics system of infectious bursal disease virus (IBDV). Arch Virol 156: 1717-1728, 2011.
31. Elankumaran S, Heckert RA, and Moura L. Pathogenesis and tissue distribution of a variant strain of infectious bursal disease virus in commercial broiler chickens. Avian Dis 46: 169-176, 2002.
32. Eldaghayes I, Rothwell L, Williams A, Withers D, Balu S, Davison F, and Kaiser P. Infectious bursal disease virus: strains that differ in virulence differentially modulate the innate immune response to infection in the chicken bursa. Viral Immunol 19: 83-91, 2006.
33. Escaffre O, Le Nouen C, Amelot M, Ambroggio X, Ogden KM, Guionie O, Toquin D, Muller H, Islam MR, and Eterradossi N. Both genome segments contribute to the pathogenicity of very virulent infectious bursal disease virus. J Virol 87: 2767-2780, 2013.
34. Eterradossi N. Progress in the Diagnosis and Prophylaxis of Infectious Bursal Disease in Poultry. In: Comprehensive reports on technical items presented to the International Committee or to regional Commissions, edited by Epizooties OId. Paris: 1995, p. 75-82.
35. Eterradossi N, Arnauld C, Tekaia F, Toquin D, Coq HL, Rivallan G, Guittet M, Domenech J, Van den Berg TP, Skinner MA, and le Coq H. Antigenic and genetic relationships between European very virulent infectious bursal disease viruses and an early West African isolate. Avian Pathol 28: 36-46, 1999.
36. Eterradossi N, Arnauld C, Toquin D, and Rivallan G. Critical amino acid changes in VP2 variable domain are associated with typical and atypical antigenicity in very virulent infectious bursal disease viruses. Arch Virol 143: 1627-1636, 1998.
37. Eterradossi N, Rivallan G, Toquin D, and Guittet M. Limited antigenic variation among recent infectious bursal disease virus isolates from France. Arch Virol 142: 2079-2087, 1997.
38. Eterradossi N, and Saif YM. Infectious Bursal Disease. In: Diseases of Poultry, edited by Saif YM. Iowa: Blackwell Publishing, 2008, p. 185-208.
39. Eterradossi N, Toquin D, Rivallan G, and Guittet M. Modified activity of a VP2-located neutralizing epitope on various vaccine, pathogenic and hypervirulent strains of infectious bursal disease virus. Arch Virol 142: 255-270, 1997.
40. Fahey KJ, Erny K, and Crooks J. A conformational immunogen on VP-2 of infectious bursal disease virus that induces virus-neutralizing antibodies that passively protect chickens. J Gen Virol 70 (Pt 6): 1473-1481, 1989.
41. Faragher JT, Allan WH, and Wyeth PJ. Immunosuppressive effect of infectious bursal agent on vaccination against Newcastle disease. Vet Rec 95: 385-388, 1974.
42. Galloux M, Libersou S, Morellet N, Bouaziz S, Da Costa B, Ouldali M, Lepault J, and Delmas B. Infectious bursal disease virus, a non-enveloped virus, possesses a capsid-associated peptide that deforms and perforates biological membranes. J Biol Chem 282: 20774-20784, 2007.
43. Gardner H, Kerry K, Riddle M, Brouwer S, and Gleeson L. Poultry virus infection in Antarctic penguins. Nature 387: 245, 1997.
44. Garriga D, Navarro A, Querol-Audi J, Abaitua F, Rodriguez JF, and Verdaguer N. Activation mechanism of a noncanonical RNA-dependent RNA polymerase. Proc Natl Acad Sci U S A 104: 20540-20545, 2007.
45. Hassan MK, al-Natour MQ, Ward LA, and Saif YM. Pathogenicity, attenuation, and immunogenicity of infectious bursal disease virus. Avian Dis 40: 567-571, 1996.
46. He CQ, Ma LY, Wang D, Li GR, and Ding NZ. Homologous recombination is apparent in infectious bursal disease virus. Virology 384: 51-58, 2009.
47. Heine HG, and Boyle DB. Infectious bursal disease virus structural protein VP2 expressed by a fowlpox virus recombinant confers protection against disease in chickens. Arch Virol 131: 277-292, 1993.
48. Heine HG, Haritou M, Failla P, Fahey K, and Azad A. Sequence analysis and expression of the host-protective immunogen VP2 of a variant strain of infectious bursal disease virus which can circumvent vaccination with standard type I strains. J Gen Virol 72 (Pt 8): 1835-1843, 1991.
49. Hernandez M, Banda A, Hernandez D, Panzera F, and Perez R. Detection of very virulent strains of infectious bursal disease virus (vvIBDV) in commercial broilers from Uruguay. Avian Dis 50: 624-631, 2006.
50. Hirai K, and Calnek BW. In vitro replication of infectious bursal disease virus in established lymphoid cell lines and chicken B lymphocytes. Infect Immun 25: 964-970, 1979.
51. Hoerr FJ. Clinical aspects of immunosuppression in poultry. Avian Dis 54: 2-15, 2010.

52. Hon CC, Lam TY, Drummond A, Rambaut A, Lee YF, Yip CW, Zeng F, Lam PY, Ng PT, and Leung FC. Phylogenetic analysis reveals a correlation between the expansion of very virulent infectious bursal disease virus and reassortment of its genome segment B. J Virol 80: 8503-8509, 2006.
53. Howie RI, and Thorsen J. Identification of a strain of infectious bursal disease virus isolated from mosquitoes. Can J Comp Med 45: 315-320, 1981.
54. Huang Z, Elankumaran S, Yunus AS, and Samal SK. A recombinant Newcastle disease virus (NDV) expressing VP2 protein of infectious bursal disease virus (IBDV) protects against NDV and IBDV. J Virol 78: 10054-10063, 2004.
55. Hudson PJ, McKern NM, Power BE, and Azad AA. Genomic structure of the large RNA segment of infectious bursal disease virus. Nucleic Acids Res 14: 5001-5012, 1986.
56. ICTV. Virus taxonomy: classification and nomenclature of viruses: Ninth Report of the International Committee on Taxonomy of Viruses. San Diego: Elsevier, 2012.
57. Ignjatovic J, and Sapats S. Confirmation of the existence of two distinct genetic groups of infectious bursal disease virus in Australia. Aust Vet J 80: 689-694, 2002.
58. Ikuta N, El-Attrache J, Villegas P, Garcia EM, Lunge VR, Fonseca AS, Oliveira C, and Marques EK. Molecular characterization of Brazilian infectious bursal disease viruses. Avian Dis 45: 297-306, 2001.
59. Ingrao F, Rauw F, Lambrecht B, and van den Berg T. Infectious Bursal Disease: A complex host-pathogen interaction. Dev Comp Immunol 2013.
60. Inoue M, Fukuda M, and Miyano K. Thymic lesions in chicken infected with infectious bursal disease virus. Avian Dis 38: 839-846, 1994.
61. Irigoyen N, Caston JR, and Rodriguez JF. Host proteolytic activity is necessary for infectious bursal disease virus capsid protein assembly. J Biol Chem 287: 24473-24482, 2012.
62. Islam MR, Zierenberg K, Eterradossi N, Toquin D, Rivallan G, and Muller H. Molecular and antigenic characterization of Bangladeshi isolates of infectious bursal disease virus demonstrate their similarities with recent European, Asian and African very virulent strains. J Vet Med B Infect Dis Vet Public Health 48: 211-221, 2001.
63. Islam MT, Le TH, Rahman MM, and Islam MA. Molecular characterization of two Bangladeshi infectious bursal disease virus isolates using the hypervariable sequence of VP2 as a genetic marker. J Vet Sci 13: 405-412, 2012.
64. Ismail NM, and Saif YM. Differentiation between antibodies to serotypes 1 and 2 infectious bursal disease viruses in chicken sera. Avian Dis 34: 1002-1004, 1990.
65. Ivan J, Velhner M, Ursu K, German P, Mato T, Dren CN, and Meszaros J. Delayed vaccine virus replication in chickens vaccinated subcutaneously with an immune complex infectious bursal disease vaccine: quantification of vaccine virus by real-time polymerase chain reaction. Can J Vet Res 69: 135-142, 2005.
66. Jackwood DH, and Saif YM. Antigenic diversity of infectious bursal disease viruses. Avian Dis 31: 766-770, 1987.
67. Jackwood DJ. Molecular epidemiologic evidence of homologous recombination in infectious bursal disease viruses. Avian Dis 56: 574-577, 2012.
68. Jackwood DJ, Jackwood RJ, and Sommer SE. Identification and comparison of point mutations associated in classic and variant infectious bursal disease viruses. Virus Res 49: 131-137, 1997.
69. Jackwood DJ, and Nielsen CK. Detection of infectious bursal disease viruses in commercially reared chickens using the reverse transcriptase/polymerase chain reaction-restriction endonuclease assay. Avian Dis 41: 137-143, 1997.
70. Jackwood DJ, Saif YM, and Moorhead PD. Immunogenicity and antigenicity of infectious bursal disease virus serotypes I and II in chickens. Avian Dis 29: 1184-1194, 1985.
71. Jackwood DJ, and Sommer-Wagner S. Genetic characteristics of infectious bursal disease viruses from four continents. Virology 365: 369-375, 2007.
72. Jackwood DJ, and Sommer-Wagner SE. Amino acids contributing to antigenic drift in the infectious bursal disease Birnavirus (IBDV). Virology 409: 33-37, 2011.
73. Jackwood DJ, and Sommer-Wagner SE. Molecular epidemiology of infectious bursal disease viruses: distribution and genetic analysis of newly emerging viruses in the United States. Avian Dis 49: 220-226, 2005.
74. Jackwood DJ, and Sommer SE. Restriction fragment length polymorphisms in the VP2 gene of infectious bursal disease viruses. Avian Dis 41: 627-637, 1997.
75. Jackwood DJ, Spalding BD, and Sommer SE. Real-time reverse transcriptase-polymerase chain reaction detection and analysis of nucleotide sequences coding for a neutralizing epitope on infectious bursal disease viruses. Avian Dis 47: 738-744, 2003.
76. Jackwood DJ, Sreedevi B, LeFever LJ, and Sommer-Wagner SE. Studies on naturally occurring infectious bursal disease viruses suggest that a single amino acid substitution at position 253 in VP2 increases pathogenicity. Virology 377: 110-116, 2008.
77. Jackwood DJ, and Stoute ST. Molecular evidence for a geographically restricted population of infectious bursal disease viruses. Avian Dis 57: 57-64, 2013.
78. Jeon WJ, Lee EK, Joh SJ, Kwon JH, Yang CB, Yoon YS, and Choi KS. Very virulent infectious bursal disease virus isolated from wild birds in Korea: epidemiological implications. Virus Res 137: 153-156, 2008.

79. Jeurissen SH, Janse EM, Lehrbach PR, Haddad EE, Avakian A, and Whitfill CE. The working mechanism of an immune complex vaccine that protects chickens against infectious bursal disease. Immunology 95: 494-500, 1998.
80. Khatri M, Palmquist JM, Cha RM, and Sharma JM. Infection and activation of bursal macrophages by virulent infectious bursal disease virus. Virus Res 113: 44-50, 2005.
81. Kibenge FS, Jackwood DJ, and Mercado CC. Nucleotide sequence analysis of genome segment A of infectious bursal disease virus. J Gen Virol 71 (Pt 3): 569-577, 1990.
82. Kim IJ, and Sharma JM. IBDV-induced bursal T lymphocytes inhibit mitogenic response of normal splenocytes. Vet Immunol Immunopathol 74: 47-57, 2000.
83. Kim IJ, You SK, Kim H, Yeh HY, and Sharma JM. Characteristics of bursal T lymphocytes induced by infectious bursal disease virus. J Virol 74: 8884-8892, 2000.
84. Kosters J, Becht H, and Rudolph R. Properties of the infectious bursal agent of chicken (IBA). Med Microbiol Immunol 157: 291-298, 1972.
85. Kusk M, Kabell S, Jorgensen PH, and Handberg KJ. Differentiation of five strains of infectious bursal disease virus: development of a strain-specific multiplex PCR. Vet Microbiol 109: 159-167, 2005.
86. Kwon HM, Kim DK, Hahn TW, Han JH, and Jackwood DJ. Sequence of precursor polyprotein gene (segment A) of infectious bursal disease viruses isolated in Korea. Avian Dis 44: 691-696, 2000.
87. Le Gros FX, Dancer A, Giacomini C, Pizzoni L, Bublot M, Graziani M, and Prandini F. Field efficacy trial of a novel HVT-IBD vector vaccine for 1-day-old broilers. Vaccine 27: 592-596, 2009.
88. Le Nouen C, Rivallan G, Toquin D, Darlu P, Morin Y, Beven V, de Boisseson C, Cazaban C, Comte S, Gardin Y, and Eterradossi N. Very virulent infectious bursal disease virus: reduced pathogenicity in a rare natural segment-B-reassorted isolate. J Gen Virol 87: 209-216, 2006.
89. Letzel T, Coulibaly F, Rey FA, Delmas B, Jagt E, van Loon AA, and Mundt E. Molecular and structural bases for the antigenicity of VP2 of infectious bursal disease virus. J Virol 81: 12827-12835, 2007.
90. Li Z, Wang Y, Xue Y, Li X, Cao H, and Zheng SJ. Critical role for voltage-dependent anion channel 2 in infectious bursal disease virus-induced apoptosis in host cells via interaction with VP5. J Virol 86: 1328-1338, 2012.
91. Lim BL, Cao Y, Yu T, and Mo CW. Adaptation of very virulent infectious bursal disease virus to chicken embryonic fibroblasts by site-directed mutagenesis of residues 279 and 284 of viral coat protein VP2. J Virol 73: 2854-2862, 1999.
92. Lin TW, Lo CW, Lai SY, Fan RJ, Lo CJ, Chou YM, Thiruvengadam R, Wang AH, and Wang MY. Chicken heat shock protein 90 is a component of the putative cellular receptor complex of infectious bursal disease virus. J Virol 81: 8730-8741, 2007.
93. Liu H, Zhang M, Han H, Yuan J, and Li Z. Comparison of the expression of cytokine genes in the bursal tissues of the chickens following challenge with infectious bursal disease viruses of varying virulence. Virol J 7: 364, 2010.
94. Liu HJ, Huang PH, Wu YH, Lin MY, and Liao MH. Molecular characterisation of very virulent infectious bursal disease viruses in Taiwan. Res Vet Sci 70: 139-147, 2001.
95. Liu M, and Vakharia VN. VP1 protein of infectious bursal disease virus modulates the virulence in vivo. Virology 330: 62-73, 2004.
96. Lombardo E, Maraver A, Cast n JR, Rivera J, Fernandez-Arias A, Serrano A, Carrascosa JL, and Rodriguez JF. VP1, the putative RNA-dependent RNA polymerase of infectious bursal disease virus, forms complexes with the capsid protein VP3, leading to efficient encapsidation into virus-like particles. J Virol 73: 6973-6983, 1999.
97. Lombardo E, Maraver A, Espinosa I, Fernandez-Arias A, and Rodriguez JF. VP5, the nonstructural polypeptide of infectious bursal disease virus, accumulates within the host plasma membrane and induces cell lysis. Virology 277: 345-357, 2000.
98. Luo J, Zhang H, Teng M, Fan JM, You LM, Xiao ZJ, Yi ML, Zhi YB, Li XW, and Zhang GP. Surface IgM on DT40 cells may be a component of the putative receptor complex responsible for the binding of infectious bursal disease virus. Avian Pathol 39: 359-365, 2010.
99. Luque D, Saugar I, Rejas MT, Carrascosa JL, Rodriguez JF, and Caston JR. Infectious Bursal disease virus: ribonucleoprotein complexes of a double-stranded RNA virus. J Mol Biol 386: 891-901, 2009.
100. Mahardika GN, and Becht H. Mapping of cross-reacting and serotype-specific epitopes on the VP3 structural protein of the infectious bursal disease virus (IBDV). Arch Virol 140: 765-774, 1995.
101. Maraver A, Ona A, Abaitua F, Gonzalez D, Clemente R, Ruiz-Diaz JA, Caston JR, Pazos F, and Rodriguez JF. The oligomerization domain of VP3, the scaffolding protein of infectious bursal disease virus, plays a critical role in capsid assembly. J Virol 77: 6438-6449, 2003.
102. McAllister JC, Steelman CD, Newberry LA, and Skeeles JK. Isolation of infectious bursal disease virus from the lesser mealworm, Alphitobius diaperinus (Panzer). Poult Sci 74: 45-49, 1995.
103. McFerran JB, McNulty MS, McKillop ER, Connor TJ, McCracken RM, Collins DS, and Allan GM. Isolation and serological studies with infectious bursal disease viruses from fowl, turkeys and ducks: demonstration of a second serotype. Avian Pathol 9: 395-404, 1980.

104. McIlroy SG, Goodall EA, and McCracken RM. Economic effects of subclinical infectious bursal disease on broiler production. Avian Pathol 18: 465-480, 1989.
105. Meulemans G, and Halen P. Efficacy of some disinfectants against infectious bursal disease virus and avian reovirus. Vet Rec 111: 412-413, 1982.
106. Muller H, Mundt E, Eterradossi N, and Islam MR. Current status of vaccines against infectious bursal disease. Avian Pathol 41: 133-139, 2012.
107. Muller H, and Nitschke R. The two segments of the infectious bursal disease virus genome are circularized by a 90,000-Da protein. Virology 159: 174-177, 1987.
108. Muller R, Kaufer I, Reinacher M, and Weiss E. Immunofluorescent studies of early virus propagation after oral infection with infectious bursal disease virus (IBDV). Zentralbl Veterinarmed B 26: 345-352, 1979.
109. Mundt E. Tissue culture infectivity of different strains of infectious bursal disease virus is determined by distinct amino acids in VP2. J Gen Virol 80 (Pt 8): 2067-2076, 1999.
110. Mundt E, Beyer J, and Muller H. Identification of a novel viral protein in infectious bursal disease virus-infected cells. J Gen Virol 76 (Pt 2): 437-443, 1995.
111. Mundt E, Kollner B, and Kretzschmar D. VP5 of infectious bursal disease virus is not essential for viral replication in cell culture. J Virol 71: 5647-5651, 1997.
112. Nouen CL, Toquin D, Muller H, Raue R, Kean KM, Langlois P, Cherbonnel M, and Eterradossi N. Different domains of the RNA polymerase of infectious bursal disease virus contribute to virulence. PLoS One 7: e28064, 2012.
113. Ogawa M, Wakuda T, Yamaguchi T, Murata K, Setiyono A, Fukushi H, and Hirai K. Seroprevalence of infectious bursal disease virus in free-living wild birds in Japan. J Vet Med Sci 60: 1277-1279, 1998.
114. Ogawa M, Yamaguchi T, Setiyono A, Ho T, Matsuda H, Furusawa S, Fukushi H, and Hirai K. Some characteristics of a cellular receptor for virulent infectious bursal disease virus by using flow cytometry. Arch Virol 143: 2327-2341, 1998.
115. Ojkic D, Martin E, Swinton J, Binnington B, and Brash M. Genotyping of Canadian field strains of infectious bursal disease virus. Avian Pathol 36: 427-433, 2007.
116. Ona A, Luque D, Abaitua F, Maraver A, Caston JR, and Rodriguez JF. The C-terminal domain of the pVP2 precursor is essential for the interaction between VP2 and VP3, the capsid polypeptides of infectious bursal disease virus. Virology 322: 135-142, 2004.
117. Pages-Mante A, Torrents D, Maldonado J, and Saubi N. Dogs as potential carriers of infectious bursal disease virus. Avian Pathol 33: 205-209, 2004.
118. Pan J, Vakharia VN, and Tao YJ. The structure of a birnavirus polymerase reveals a distinct active site topology. Proc Natl Acad Sci U S A 104: 7385-7390, 2007.
119. Perozo F, Villegas AP, Fernandez R, Cruz J, and Pritchard N. Efficacy of single dose recombinant herpesvirus of turkey infectious bursal disease virus (IBDV) vaccination against a variant IBDV strain. Avian Dis 53: 624-628, 2009.
120. Perozo F, Villegas P, Estevez C, Alvarado IR, Purvis LB, and Williams S. Protection against infectious bursal disease virulent challenge conferred by a recombinant avian adeno-associated virus vaccine. Avian Dis 52: 315-319, 2008.
121. Rauf A, Khatri M, Murgia MV, Jung K, and Saif YM. Differential modulation of cytokine, chemokine and Toll like receptor expression in chickens infected with classical and variant infectious bursal disease virus. Vet Res 42: 85, 2011.
122. Rautenschlein S, Yeh HY, and Sharma JM. Comparative immunopathogenesis of mild, intermediate, and virulent strains of classic infectious bursal disease virus. Avian Dis 47: 66-78, 2003.
123. Razmyar J, and Peighambari SM. Molecular characterization of Iranian infectious bursal disease viruses. Avian Dis 52: 665-669, 2008.
124. Remorini P, Calderon MG, Aguirre S, Periolo O, La Torre J, and Mattion N. Characterization of infectious bursal disease viruses from Argentina. Avian Dis 50: 245-251, 2006.
125. Rodriguez-Chavez IR, Rosenberger JK, and Cloud SS. Characterization of the antigenic, immunogenic, and pathogenic variation of infectious bursal disease virus due to propagation in different host systems (bursa, embryo, and cell culture). I. Antigenicity and immunogenicity. Avian Pathol 31: 463-471, 2002.
126. Rodriguez-Chavez IR, Rosenberger JK, Cloud SS, and Pope CR. Characterization of the antigenic, immunogenic, and pathogenic variation of infectious bursal disease virus due to propagation in different host systems (bursa, embryo, and cell culture). III. Pathogenicity. Avian Pathol 31: 485-492, 2002.
127. Sapats SI, and Ignjatovic J. Antigenic and sequence heterogeneity of infectious bursal disease virus strains isolated in Australia. Arch Virol 145: 773-785, 2000.
128. Shane SM, Lasher HN, and Paxton KW. Economic impact of Infectious Bursal Disease. In: International Symposiumon Infectious Bursal Disease and Chicken Infectious Anemia, edited by Kaleta EF. Rauischholzhausen, Germany: Institut für Geflügelkrankheiten, Justus-Ilebig-Universität, 1994, p. 196-205.
129. Sharma JM, Dohms JE, and Metz AL. Comparative pathogenesis of serotype 1 and variant serotype 1 isolates of infectious bursal disease virus and their effect on humoral and cellular immune competence of specific-pathogen-free chickens. Avian Dis 33: 112-124, 1989.

130. Sharma JM, Kim IJ, Rautenschlein S, and Yeh HY. Infectious bursal disease virus of chickens: pathogenesis and immunosuppression. Dev Comp Immunol 24: 223-235, 2000.
131. Sharma JM, and Lee LF. Effect of infectious bursal disease on natural killer cell activity and mitogenic response of chicken lymphoid cells: role of adherent cells in cellular immune suppression. Infect Immun 42: 747-754, 1983.
132. Shaw I, and Davison TF. Protection from IBDV-induced bursal damage by a recombinant fowlpox vaccine, fpIBD1, is dependent on the titre of challenge virus and chicken genotype. Vaccine 18: 3230-3241, 2000.
133. Singh A, Bedekar MK, Sharma R, Sarkhel BC, Singh S, and Jain SK. Detection of very virulent infectious bursal disease virus from a field outbreak in Central India. Acta Vet Hung 60: 165-174, 2012.
134. Skeeles JK, Lukert PD, De Buysscher EV, Fletcher OJ, and Brown J. Infectious bursal disease viral infections. II. The relationship of age, complement levels, virus-neutralizing antibody, clotting, and lesions. Avian Dis 23: 107-117, 1979.
135. Skeeles JK, Slavik M, Beasley JN, Brown AH, Meinecke CF, Maruca S, and Welch S. An age-related coagulation disorder associated with experimental infection with infectious bursal disease virus. Am J Vet Res 41: 1458-1461, 1980.
136. Snyder DB, Lana DP, Cho BR, and Marquardt WW. Group and strain-specific neutralization sites of infectious bursal disease virus defined with monoclonal antibodies. Avian Dis 32: 527-534, 1988.
137. Spies U, Muller H, and Becht H. Nucleotide sequence of infectious bursal disease virus genome segment A delineates two major open reading frames. Nucleic Acids Res 17: 7982, 1989.
138. Spies U, Muller H, and Becht H. Properties of RNA polymerase activity associated with infectious bursal disease virus and characterization of its reaction products. Virus Res 8: 127-140, 1987.
139. Stoute ST, Jackwood DJ, Sommer-Wagner SE, Cooper GL, Anderson ML, Woolcock PR, Bickford AA, Senties-Cue CG, and Charlton BR. The diagnosis of very virulent infectious bursal disease in California pullets. Avian Dis 53: 321-326, 2009.
140. Tacken MG, Peeters BP, Thomas AA, Rottier PJ, and Boot HJ. Infectious bursal disease virus capsid protein VP3 interacts both with VP1, the RNA-dependent RNA polymerase, and with viral double-stranded RNA. J Virol 76: 11301-11311, 2002.
141. Tanimura N, and Sharma JM. In-situ apoptosis in chickens infected with infectious bursal disease virus. J Comp Pathol 118: 15-27, 1998.
142. Tanimura N, Tsukamoto K, Nakamura K, Narita M, and Maeda M. Association between pathogenicity of infectious bursal disease virus and viral antigen distribution detected by immunohistochemistry. Avian Dis 39: 9-20, 1995.
143. Tao Q, Wang X, Bao H, Wu J, Shi L, Li Y, Qiao C, Yakovlevich SA, Mikhaylovna PN, and Chen H. Detection and differentiation of four poultry diseases using asymmetric reverse transcription polymerase chain reaction in combination with oligonucleotide microarrays. J Vet Diagn Invest 21: 623-632, 2009.
144. To H, Yamaguchi T, Nguyen NT, Nguyen OT, Nguyen SV, Agus S, Kim HJ, Fukushi H, and Hirai K. Sequence comparison of the VP2 variable region of infectious bursal disease virus isolates from Vietnam. J Vet Med Sci 61: 429-432, 1999.
145. Toro H, Effler JC, Hoerr FJ, and van Ginkel FW. Pathogenicity of infectious bursal disease virus variant AL2 in young chickens. Avian Dis 53: 78-82, 2009.
146. Tsukamoto K, Saito S, Saeki S, Sato T, Tanimura N, Isobe T, Mase M, Imada T, Yuasa N, and Yamaguchi S. Complete, long-lasting protection against lethal infectious bursal disease virus challenge by a single vaccination with an avian herpesvirus vector expressing VP2 antigens. J Virol 76: 5637-5645, 2002.
147. Tsukamoto K, Tanimura N, Hihara H, Shirai J, Imai K, Nakamura K, and Maeda M. Isolation of virulent infectious bursal disease virus from field outbreaks with high mortality in Japan. J Vet Med Sci 54: 153-155, 1992.
148. Vakharia VN, He J, Ahamed B, and Snyder DB. Molecular basis of antigenic variation in infectious bursal disease virus. Virus Res 31: 265-273, 1994.
149. Van den Berg TP. Acute infectious bursal disease in poultry: a review. Avian Pathol 29: 175-194, 2000.
150. van den Berg TP, Eterradossi N, Toquin D, and Meulemans G. Infectious bursal disease (Gumboro disease). Rev Sci Tech 19: 509-543, 2000.
151. Van den Berg TP, Gonze M, and Meulemans G. Acute infectious bursal disease in poultry: isolation and characterisation of a highly virulent strain. Avian Pathol 20: 133-143, 1991.
152. Van den Berg TP, Gonze M, Morales D, and Meulemans G. Acute infectious bursal disease in poultry: immunological and molecular basis of antigenicity of a highly virulent strain. Avian Pathol 25: 751-768, 1996.
153. Van der Marel P, Snyder D, and Lutticken D. Antigenic characterization of IBDV field isolates by their reactivity with a panel of monoclonal antibodies. Dtsch Tierarztl Wochenschr 97: 81-83, 1990.
154. Van Loon AA, de Haas N, Zeyda I, and Mundt E. Alteration of amino acids in VP2 of very virulent infectious bursal disease virus results in tissue culture adaptation and attenuation in chickens. J Gen Virol 83: 121-129, 2002.
155. Von Einem UI, Gorbalenya AE, Schirrmeier H, Behrens SE, Letzel T, and Mundt E. VP1 of infectious bursal disease virus is an RNA-dependent RNA polymerase. J Gen Virol 85: 2221-2229, 2004.
156. Wei Y, Li J, Zheng J, Xu H, Li L, and Yu L. Genetic reassortment of infectious bursal disease virus in nature. Biochem Biophys Res Commun 350: 277-287, 2006.

157. Wilcox GE, Flower RL, Baxendale W, and Mackenzie JS. Serological survey of wild birds in Australia for the prevalence of antibodies to egg drop syndrome 1976 (EDS-76) and infectious bursal disease viruses. Avian Pathol 12: 135-139, 1983.
158. Williams AE, and Davison TF. Enhanced immunopathology induced by very virulent infectious bursal disease virus. Avian Pathol 34: 4-14, 2005.
159. Winterfield RW, Fadly AM, and Bickford A. Infectivity and distribution of infectious bursal disease virus in the chicken. Persistence of the virus and lesions. Avian Dis 16: 622-632, 1972.
160. Winterfield RW, and Hitchner SB. Etiology of an infectious nephritis-nephrosis syndrome of chickens. Am J Vet Res 23: 1273-1279, 1962.
161. Wit JJd, and de Wit JJ. Gumboro disease: optimising vaccination. Int Poultry Prod 7: 19, 21, 1999.
162. Withers DR, Davison TF, and Young JR. Diversified bursal medullary B cells survive and expand independently after depletion following neonatal infectious bursal disease virus infection. Immunology 117: 558-565, 2006.
163. Wu CC, Lin TL, Zhang HG, Davis VS, and Boyle JA. Molecular detection of infectious bursal disease virus by polymerase chain reaction. Avian Dis 36: 221-226, 1992.
164. Xu XG, Tong DW, Wang ZS, Zhang Q, Li ZC, Zhang K, Li W, and Liu HJ. Baculovirus virions displaying infectious bursal disease virus VP2 protein protect chickens against infectious bursal disease virus infection. Avian Dis 55: 223-229, 2011.
165. Yamaguchi T, Iwata K, Kobayashi M, Ogawa M, Fukushi H, and Hirai K. Epitope mapping of capsid proteins VP2 and VP3 of infectious bursal disease virus. Arch Virol 141: 1493-1507, 1996.
166. Yamaguchi T, Ogawa M, Inoshima Y, Miyoshi M, Fukushi H, and Hirai K. Identification of sequence changes responsible for the attenuation of highly virulent infectious bursal disease virus. Virology 223: 219-223, 1996.
167. Yamaguchi T, Ogawa M, Miyoshi M, Inoshima Y, Fukushi H, and Hirai K. Sequence and phylogenetic analyses of highly virulent infectious bursal disease virus. Arch Virol 142: 1441-1458, 1997.
168. Yao K, Goodwin MA, and Vakharia VN. Generation of a mutant infectious bursal disease virus that does not cause bursal lesions. J Virol 72: 2647-2654, 1998.
169. Yao K, and Vakharia VN. Induction of apoptosis in vitro by the 17-kDa nonstructural protein of infectious bursal disease virus: possible role in viral pathogenesis. Virology 285: 50-58, 2001.
170. Yip CW, Hon CC, Zeng F, and Leung FC. Cell culture-adapted IBDV uses endocytosis for entry in DF-1 chicken embryonic fibroblasts. Virus Res 165: 9-16, 2012.
171. Yu F, Ren X, Wang Y, Qi X, Song J, Gao Y, Qin L, Gao H, and Wang X. A single amino acid V4I substitution in VP1 attenuates virulence of very virulent infectious bursal disease virus (vvIBDV) in SPF chickens and increases replication in CEF cells. Virology 440: 204-209, 2013.
172. Yuan W, Zhang X, Xia X, and Sun H. Inhibition of infectious bursal disease virus infection by artificial microRNAs targeting chicken heat-shock protein 90. J Gen Virol 93: 876-879, 2012.
173. Zierenberg K, Nieper H, Van den Berg TP, Ezeokoli CD, Voss M, and Muller H. The VP2 variable region of African and German isolates of infectious bursal disease virus: comparison with very virulent, "classical" virulent, and attenuated tissue culture-adapted strains. Arch Virol 145: 113-125, 2000.

CHAPTER 4

VIRUS-INDUCED IMMUNOSUPPRESSION: CHICKEN INFECTIOUS ANEMIA

Joan A. Smyth and Karel A. Schat

Introduction

Chicken infectious anemia is caused by chicken anemia virus (CAV). This virus, and the fact that it caused aplastic anemia and thymic atrophy, was first discovered during investigations into problems caused by a Marek's disease (MD) vaccine contaminated with a reticuloendotheliosis virus (REV). [181] The virus is currently the sole member of the Genus *Gyrovirus* of the family *Circoviridae* (http://ictvonline.org/virusTaxonomy.asp?version=2012). Since its discovery, CAV or antibodies to it have been found in chickens in many countries throughout the world. In addition to causing anemia and mortality, CAV causes immunosuppression, enhancing the ability of other agents to cause disease as well as interfering with the immune response to vaccines. The pathogenicity of CAV is enhanced in chickens infected with other immunosuppressive agents such as infectious bursal disease virus (IBDV). Both clinical and subclinical infections are economically important. [95,104]

Etiology

Virus structure, composition and classification

CAV is a small (~ 25 nm in diameter, range 19.1-26 nm depending on the preparation method) [103], non-enveloped, icosahedral virus. It contains a single-stranded, negative-sense circular DNA [8] of approximately 2.3 kb. The DNA has three partially overlapping open reading frames (ORFs), which code for three proteins: VP1, VP2 and VP3.

VP1 (52 kDa) is a structural protein, and is the only protein found in the viral capsid. Under conditions of natural infection, virus neutralizing (VN) antibodies produced by the host only react with VP1. [36,118] VP1 is first detected in infected cell cultures at 30 hours post-infection. [36]

VP2 (28 kDa) has both serine/threonine and tyrosine phosphatase activity [127], and is important for efficient viral replication. [128] VP2 co-localizes with VP1 in infected cells and is thought to function as a scaffold protein. [82,118] This function is very important in the context of development of subunit vaccines (see Subunit and DNA vaccines). VP2 is also associated with the ability of CAV to reduce expression of major histocompatibility complex (MHC) class I molecules in vitro. [129] It is not currently known whether expression of MHC class 1 molecules is affected in vivo. VP2 can be detected in infected cell cultures by 12 hours post-infection. [36]

VP3, which is also known as 'apoptin' (13.8 kDa), can be detected in infected cell cultures by 12 post-infection. [36] Noteborn et al. suggested in 1994 [117] that VP3 is important to virus replication, and it was later confirmed that VP3 is indeed essential for virus replication (Schat, unpublished data). [133] It has been the most extensively studied CAV protein because it can induce apoptosis in neoplastically transformed but not in normal mammalian cells [29], making it of substantial interest to medical researchers as a potential anti-cancer chemotherapeutic.VP3 also has anti-neoplastic effects on Rous sarcoma virus-induced tumors in chickens. [114]

Until recently, it was thought that these three virus proteins were produced exclusively from a single 2 kB polycistronic mRNA. However, lesser quantities of spliced mRNAs have been demonstrated, one of which also codes for VP2 and VP3. [80] A further splice variant has three additional ORFs, but proteins corresponding to these ORFs have not been identified. The importance of these spliced mRNAs has not yet been established.

Classification

CAV is currently classified by the International Committee on Taxonomy of Viruses (ICTV) as the sole member of the genus *Gyrovirus* of the family *Circoviridae*. (http://ictvonline.org/virusTaxonomy.asp?version=2012). However, the ICTV is considering a proposal to include the *Gyrovirinae* with one genus (*Gyrovirus*) in the family *Anelloviridae* (Maggio, ICTV personal communication). New members of the *Gyrovirus* genus have recently been proposed but are not yet accepted by the ICTV: avian gyrovirus 2 [138] and three human gyroviruses. [9,25,131,143] It has been suggested that two of the proposed human gyroviruses may be derived from CAV. [131,193] The proposed avian gyrovirus 2, which was found to be widespread in chickens [35], has about 40 % identity with CAV. The importance of these new gyroviruses as avian and/or human pathogens is currently unknown. These new viruses will not be further discussed in this chapter.

Genotypes

CAV isolates show comparatively little genetic variability [39,168], with about 4.4 % diversity worldwide in VP1 at the nucleotide level. [39] Depending on the approaches used to DNA-based typing, CAV isolates have been classed into between 3 and 7 genetic groups. Based on the VP1 sequences of CAV isolates from different parts of the world, isolates were grouped into three major clusters: I, II and III.

Cluster III was further subdivided into two subgroups, IIIa and IIIb. [39] However, this clustering system did not hold when 74 VP1 CAV sequences from China were included. [40] Based on DNA sequence of VP1, VP2 and VP3, four genogroups [24,42], and five subgroups were reported. [42] The clinical and pathologic significance of such genetic groups is currently unknown. He et al. [61] found evidence of two mosaic CAV isolates and suggested that homologous recombination plays a role in generating genetic diversity in natural populations of CAV. Since then, additional naturally occurring recombinant strains have been reported. [41,115]

Serotypes

With the exception of one isolate (CIAV-7) [156], all isolates of CAV are closely related antigenically and are considered to belong to one serotype. CIAV-7 is antigenically quite distinct from the Del-Ros strain of CAV and antibodies to these viruses do not cross neutralize CIAV-7 and Del-Ros, respectively. Antibodies to CIAV-7 were not detected by a commercial CAV ELISA test. Furthermore, antiserum to CIAV-7 did not react with CAV in immunofluorescence assays or in Western blots. It has subsequently been suggested that CIAV-7 may be a novel virus rather than a new serotype of CAV. [144] Its relationship to avian gyrovirus 2 is currently unknown.

Stability

CAV is non-enveloped and is very resistant to chemical and physical treatments.

CAV is resistant to:

- 70 °C for 1 hour.
- 80 °C for 15 minutes.
- pH 3.0 for 3 hours.

Infectivity is destroyed or inactivated by treatment with:

- 50 % phenol for 5 minutes.
- 10 % hypochlorite solution for 2 hours at 37 °C.
- 5 % formaldehyde at room temperature for 24 hours. [181,192]

Infectivity is reduced but not destroyed by treatment with:

- Formaldehyde fumigation for 24 hours.

CAV is very resistant to treatment with acetone, and infectivity was undiminished after exposure to 90 % acetone for 24 hours. [160] This is relevant to diagnostic and research laboratories because fixation of smears or cells in acetone for 10 minutes is a common procedure. [78,105] While 100 % acetone may be used for fixation, it would be wise to assume that CAV is not inactivated by this treatment until proven otherwise.

Chicken byproducts and chickens which have died during rearing may contain CAV. CAV survives fermentation but is inactivated by heating at 95 °C (core temperature) for 30 minutes or 100 °C for 10 minutes. [166] In some regions, composting of chicken litter and fallen chickens is legal. We could not find any studies specifically examining the survivability of CAV during composting, but given the marked resistance of the virus, it may be prudent to assume that it is not inactivated. There are commercially available disinfectants with pH 2 which are effective and are frequently used by producers of specific-pathogen-free (SPF) flocks.

Epidemiology

Host range

CAV infection is widespread in chickens and there is serological evidence of CAV infecting chickens in the USA since at least 1959. [165] There is evidence of CAV-induced anemia in 1969, when a case of anemia was originally linked to MD, but CAV was later detected in frozen tumor cells. [144]

Naturally occurring infections in turkeys by CAV strains, which are of low pathogenicity for chickens, have been reported. [148] Turkeys infected with low pathogenic strains can be identified based on the presence of neutralizing antibodies. Interestingly, turkeys inoculated intramuscularly with a pathogenic strain of CAV did not develop anemia nor did they develop antibodies. [103] Neutralizing antibodies to CAV have been found in Japanese quail, but disease due to CAV infection has not been reported in this species. Current indications are that CAV produces disease only in chickens.

Geographical distribution

CAV or antibodies to CAV have been found in chickens worldwide.

Transmission

There are some very important differences in the maintenance and transmission of CAV in SPF flocks versus flocks of the food production sector, hereafter referred to as commercial production flocks. We will first discuss transmission of CAV as it pertains to development of disease in commercial production flocks, although some of our understanding is based on studies of experimentally infected SPF birds. Then, in a separate section, we describe maintenance and transmission in SPF flocks. It is important to realize that many of the events described in the section on SPF flocks probably also occur in commercial production flocks, but likely go unrecognized.

Transmission in commercial production flocks

In commercial production flocks, CAV can be transmitted both vertically and horizontally.

Outbreaks of clinical disease most commonly occur as a result of vertical transmission, when seronegative flocks become infected during lay.[23,50,104,172,188] While early studies suggested that vertical transmission occurs for a period of up to 14 days after infection[64,187], vertical transmission can occur over a much longer time period in a flock.[23,172] This is because in horizontally infected breeding flocks, the virus will take time to spread throughout the entire flock and infected eggs may be produced by the flock as a whole for as long as 9 weeks[172] after infection is introduced. In the field situation, flocks have generally been deemed to be non-transmitting after this time. However, the virus can persist in the gonads of seropositive chickens similar to the situation in SPF chickens (see Transmission in SPF flocks) and a small percentage of embryos from antibody-positive commercial production breeders contained CAV DNA.[15,57] The importance of this in large scale commercial production is unknown but it seems likely that this low level of transmission would go un-noticed, especially since maternally derived antibody seems to be protective against infection and clinical disease.[92,104,125,126,181,182]

Horizontal transmission of CAV can also occur.[101,155,157] After experimental infection of one-day-old chickens, virus was recoverable in high titer from feces up to 49 days post-infection at which time testing stopped[186], and was recoverable from feces for 5 weeks after inoculation of laying hens.[64] The presence of infectious virus has also been demonstrated in feather shafts.[31] Thus, horizontal transmission can occur through droppings, feathers and feather picking by penmates, contaminated fomites or equipment. The outcome of horizontally acquired infection depends on the age of bird at infection and its maternal antibody status (see above and Clinical Signs). Laying hens can also be infected horizontally by insemination with semen from cockerels infected with CAV. These infected laying hens can then transmit the virus vertically.[65] If parent and grandparent breeder flocks are kept under conditions of strict hygiene, CAV infection and subsequent transmission may be delayed until close to sexual maturity[46,95], which resembles the situation observed in SPF flocks. Once egg production starts, it becomes harder to maintain biosecurity if hatching eggs have to be collected from the farm for transport to hatcheries, since this necessitates movement of vehicles, equipment and personnel onto the farms.

Transmission in SPF flocks

The SPF industry has continuously experienced problems with CAV infections in spite of maintaining the flocks in filtered air, positive pressure facilities and requiring showering in. Flocks often become seropositive during the laying period.[144] Serological studies using SPF flocks at Cornell University confirmed that in SPF flocks, seroconversion often starts around sexual maturity and the number of positive birds may increase slowly during the laying period.[19,107,146] Interestingly, chicks hatched from these flocks never showed any signs of disease irrespective of the numbers of parent birds that seroconverted[146], even though it has been shown that vertical transmission can occur from seronegative and seropositive hens. The reasons why the presence of viral DNA or virus does not cause disease in SPF flocks need to be elucidated. The fact that this phenomenon can occur in chicks hatched from eggs from antibody-negative hens rules out the neutralization of CAV by maternal antibodies. Horizontal spread of CAV is very slow at best if SPF chickens are kept in adjacent individual cages.[107] The finding by Cardona et al.[20] that SPF birds can maintain viral DNA in the gonads independently of the presence of VN antibodies, suggests that CAV can remain latent in special circumstances. Interestingly, McNulty[103] had previously suggested that latency could be an important aspect of CAV infections. The apparent link between seroconversion and the start of sexual maturity suggested possible hormonal regulation of viral transcription. Examination of the promoter enhancer region of CAV indeed indicated the presence of hormonal response elements (HRE). Using the CAV promoter enhancer, it was then shown that estrogen enhanced the expression of reporter genes in LMH2A cells, which overexpress estrogen receptors.[109] Miller et al.[110] also identified two inhibitors of transcription:

- The chicken ovalbumin upstream promoter-transcription factor 1 COUP-TF1, which binds to the promoter enhancer region.
- The delta EF1, which binds to an E-box sequence located at the transcription initiation site.

These inhibitors are important for the maintenance of latency. Transcription of CAV from the latent virus will only proceed if the balance becomes altered toward the binding of estrogen to the estrogen receptor which can then bind to the HRE of CAV. The factors regulating the expression of inhibitors are poorly understood at the present time.

The presence of CAV or CAV DNA in the gonads can lead to transmission of CAV DNA to the embryos, independently of the antibody status of the hen, and it can also be detected in many organs of 18-to-20-day-old embryos. [108] Miller et al. [108] hatched chicks from seronegative hens from the infected SPF flocks, in individual baskets, then extracted DNA from egg shell membranes and screened for the presence of CAV DNA by quantitative PCR (qPCR). They found that testing the membranes identified more positive embryos than testing pooled lymphoid organs. Such methodology could be used as part of an approach to develop small flocks of CAV-free chickens.

The phenomenon of latency with subsequent seroconversion during or after sexual maturity poses a real problem for those managing SPF flocks, especially when flocks are used for generating materials for human and poultry vaccine production. Screening of vaccines produced in chicken cells or embryonated eggs for evidence of contamination by CAV is mandatory in many countries (e.g., Europe and USA).

Pathogenesis

CAV has a very small genome and lacks the necessary genes for DNA replication. Therefore CAV needs host cell enzymes for DNA replication, and these are present only in dividing cells.

Outbreaks of clinical disease are usually seen after vertical transmission of the virus or after early horizontal infection of chicks lacking maternal antibodies to CAV. [182] Hatchability is unaffected in naturally occurring infections that resulted in diseased progeny. Experimentally, some isolates produce lesions in embryo [30,86,157] (see Embryos), while other isolates do not affect embryonal development. [16,177,181,187] In embryos of SPF flocks where vertical transmission is occurring, viral DNA can be found in the blastoderm independently of the antibody status of the hen and can also be detected in many organs of 18-to-20-day-old embryos. [108] Viral transcription was detected in the blastoderm, between embryo incubation day (EID) 4 to 7 when estrogen is produced, and between EID 10 to 12 (Miller et al., unpublished data cited in Schat). [145] Using in situ PCR, Cardona et al. [20] found CAV DNA in mesenchymal cells surrounding developing cartilaginous vertebrae of 11-day-old embryos. It was suggested that these positive cells may have been pluripotent cells that are able to migrate to tissues such as gonads, bone marrow and liver.

Since vertically infected chicks appear normal at hatch and do not usually show signs of disease until about 10-14 days of age, there are no reports on pathogenesis in the early post-hatching period in naturally infected chickens. However, early experimental studies showed that inoculation of day-old chickens intramuscularly with CAV resulted in a clinical course and pathologic changes that paralleled the characteristics of naturally occurring disease. [181,186] Therefore, much of what is known about the early pathogenesis is based on this experimental infection model.

Intra- and extra- sinusoidal hemocytoblasts in the bone marrow are an early target for CAV infection in chickens experimentally infected at one day of age. CAV replication is first detectable at around 4 days post-inoculation in these cells [85,152] (Figs. 1 and 2), which are the precursors for erythroid and myeloid cells and thrombocytes. [3] Some CAV-positive cells in the bone marrow were MHC class II positive but negative for T cell markers. [2] The precursor cells are destroyed and there is depletion of developing cells of these lineages from the bone marrow. [53,54,63,152,181] The exact mechanism leading to cell death remains to be determined (see next paragraph), but loss of these precursor cells explains the reduced number of granulocytes and erythrocytes in affected CAV infected chicks. [85,158,159] Loss of thrombocytes [159] not only explains the occurrence of hemorrhages in affected chickens, but likely also contributes to diminished phagocytosis because chicken thrombocytes are highly phagocytic. [21] Regeneration of hemopoietic bone marrow is usually evident by 16-20 days post-infection [85,152,159] and is complete at around 32 days post-infection. Apart from histologic and limited ultrastructural evaluation (see Chickens), and immunohistochemical studies of antigen distribution, mechanistic events in the hemopoietic cells have received little attention. Interestingly, only rare hemocytoblasts become infected in immunocompetent chickens inoculated with CAV after two weeks of age, and anemia does not develop, unless the immune system is impaired by infection with IBDV or by embryonal bursectomy. [67,183,191] Hu et al. [67]

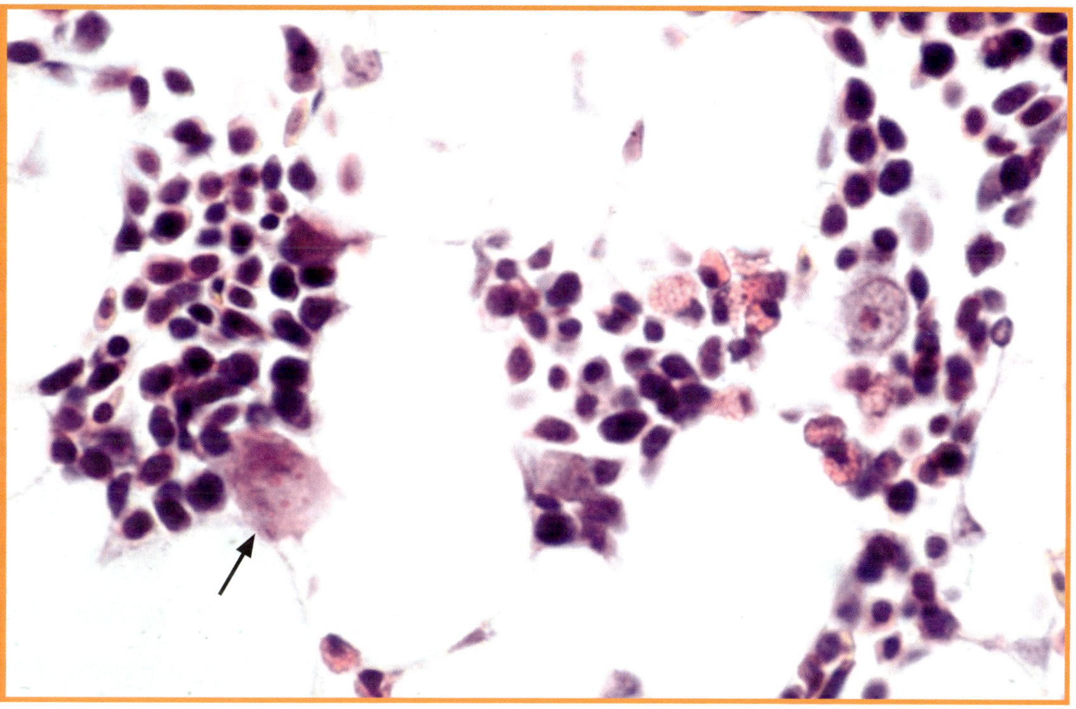

Fig. 1 | Bone marrow of a SPF chicken at day 4 post-infection after intramuscular (I/M) inoculation with the Cux-1 strain of chicken anemia virus (CAV) at one-day-old. There are two enlarged hemocytoblasts with moderate to marked karyomegaly. The nucleus of the most enlarged cell (arrow) contains multiple small eosinophilic inclusions. Hematoxylin & eosin (H&E).

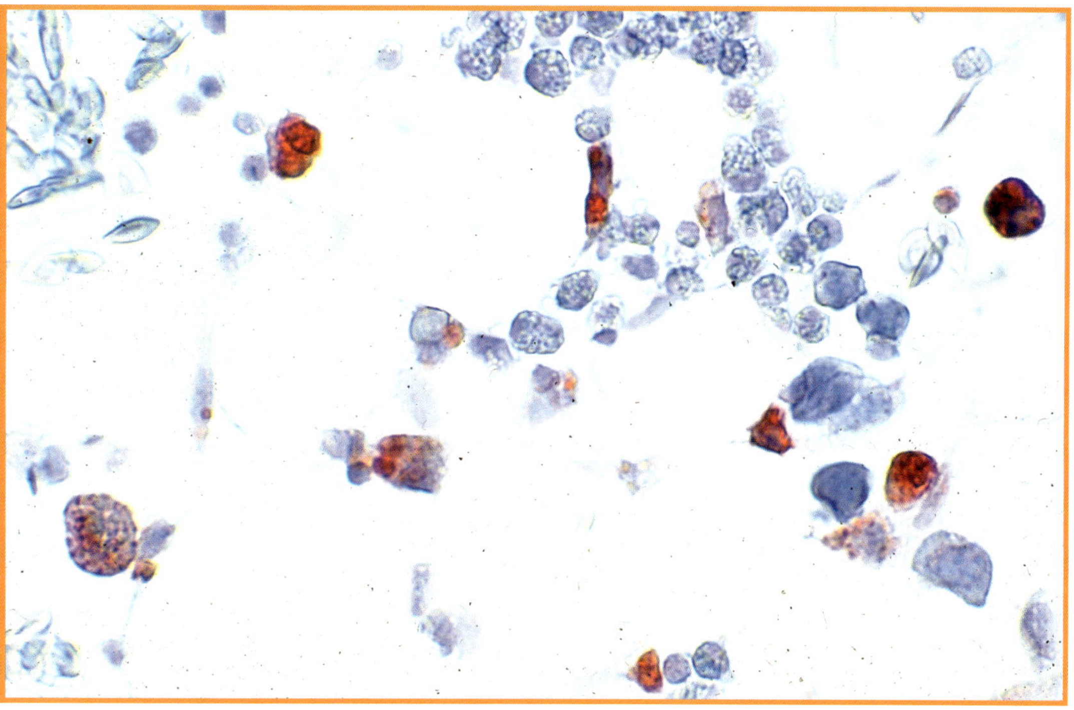

Fig. 2 | Bone marrow of an SPF chicken at day 6 post-infection after I/M inoculation with the Cux-1 strain of CAV at one-day-old. There are multiple CAV antigen positive cells (stained red). Streptavidin peroxidase (SAP) with aminoethylcarbazide (AEC) substrate and hematoxylin counterstain (for method, see Smyth et al.).[152]

infected embryonally bursectomized (EBX) chickens and intact hatchmates at 38 days of age with the CIA-1 strain of CAV. The EBX birds developed severe anemia at 14 days post-infection, while the intact hatchmates did not develop clinical evidence of infection (Fig. 3). In addition, the EBX birds showed a significant reduction in $CD4^+$ and $CD8^+$ cells and did not develop anti-CAV antibodies in contrast to the intact chickens. These experiments clearly show the importance of an intact humoral immune response for the control of CAV replication as suggested by Yuasa et al.[183,191]

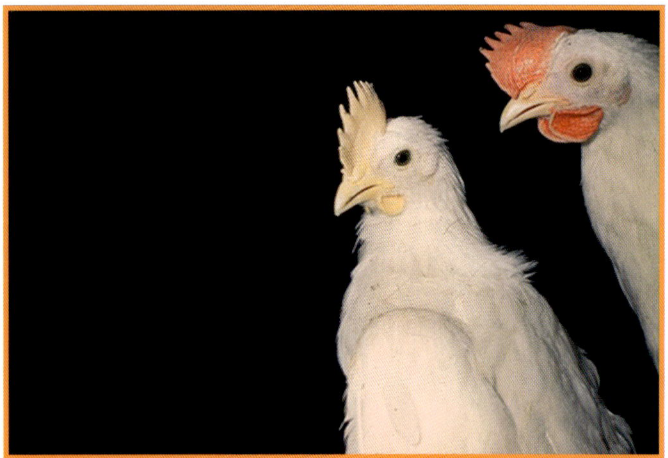

Fig. 3 | Infection of 35-day-old chickens with the CIA-1 strain of CAV. At 14 days post-infection, the embryonally bursectomized chicken developed severe anemia (left), while the intact hatchmate remained clinically normal (right).

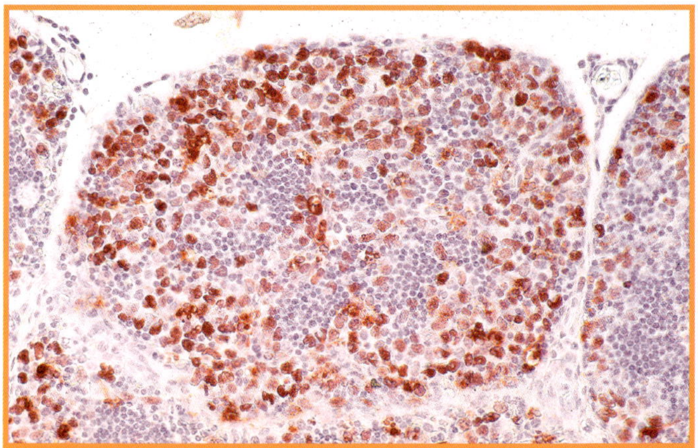

Fig. 4 | High magnification image of a thymic cortex immunostained (red) for CAV antigen. There are large numbers of infected cells in predominantly subcapsular cortex. Day 8 post-infection after I/M inoculation with the Cux-1 strain of CAV at one-day-old. SAP with AEC substrate and hematoxylin counterstain.

Fig. 5 | Spleen at day 8 post-infection after I/M inoculation with the Cux-1 strain of CAV at one-day-old. There are several very enlarged pale staining nuclei. Enlarged nucleoli are very common in such cells. In this section, two of the cells have eosinophilic nuclear inclusions of different sizes. Immunostaining of adjacent sections show that these cells [152], as well as other more normally sized cells, are positive for CAV antigen. Similar cells may be seen in lymphoid tissue throughout the body, with the possible exception of the bursa of Fabricius in which infected cells are uncommon. H&E.

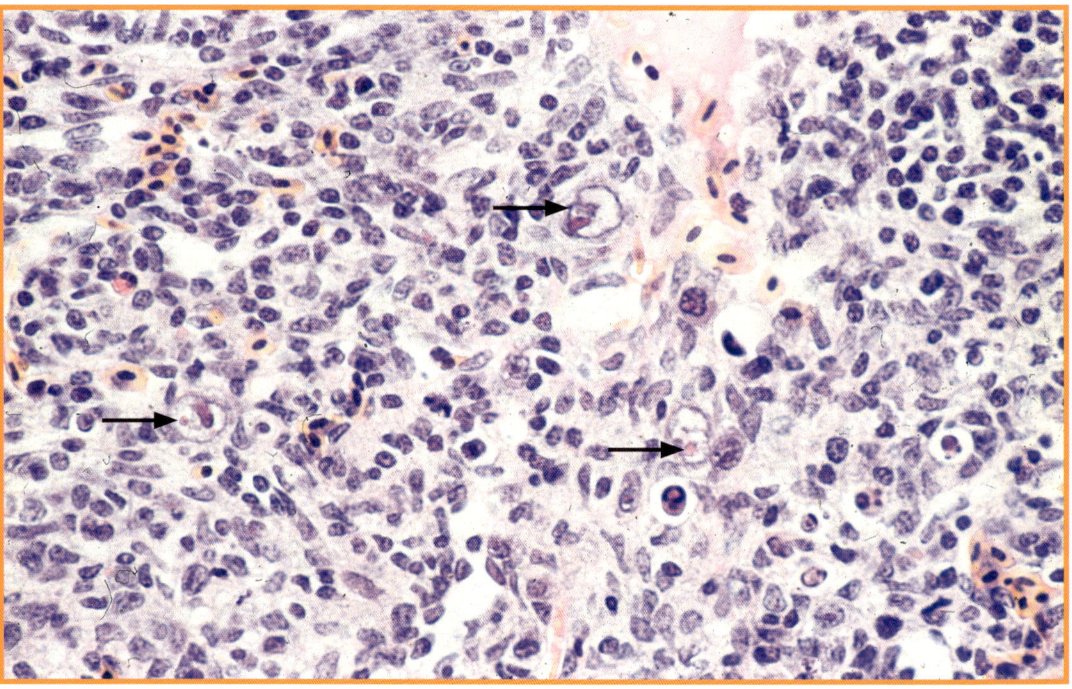

Thymocytes in the thymic cortex are an early target for CAV replication. [2,66,85,152] Viral replication, as evidenced by expression of CAV antigens, is detectable in these cells starting at around 4 days post-infection [85,152] and very large numbers of infected cells are detectable on days 5-8 post-infection (Fig. 4). The virus can also replicate in lymphoid cells in other organs albeit at a lower level (Figs. 5 and 6). Of tissues other than bone marrow and thymus that have been examined for evidence of viral antigen, spleen and lymphoid tissue in the mucosa of the proventriculus (Fig. 6) and duodenum have the most abundant viral antigen. [152] At least some of the infected spleen cells are functionally identified as antigen-committed cytotoxic T lymphocytes (CTLs) based on the decreased CTL activity against REV-transformed target cells after co-infection with CAV and REV. [92,100] CAV antigen can also be found in scattered mononuclear cells in lung, brain and heart. [152] This may represent normal cell trafficking but the exact nature of these cells has not been determined. Consequent to the viral replication, there

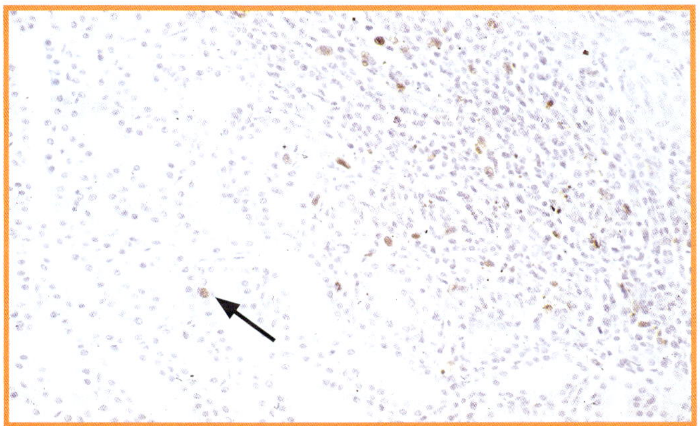

Fig. 6 | Abundant CAV antigen (brown) in proventricular mucosal lymphoid tissue (MALT) (top right quadrant). Note also a single positive cell within epithelium (arrow). Day 10 post-infection after I/M inoculation with the Cux-1 strain of CAV at one-day-old. Avidin-biotin-peroxidase-complex method with diaminobenzidine substrate and hematoxylin counterstain (ABC method) (for method, see Smyth et al.). [152]

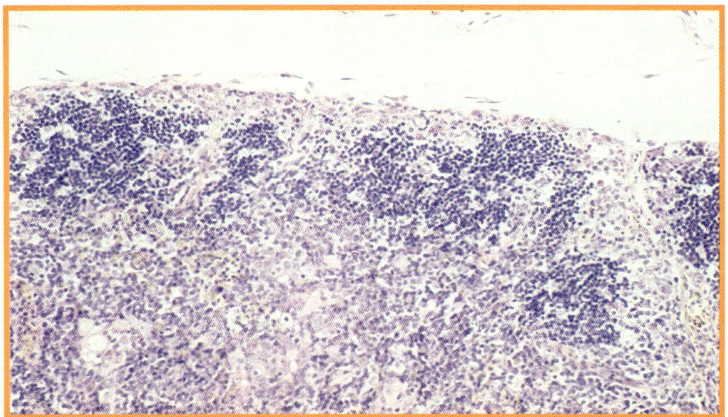

Fig. 7 | Thymus from a 36-day-old SPF chicken, which was inoculated orally with the Cux-1 strain of CAV at 21 days of age. There is marked thinning of the cortex, resulting from a marked reduction in the number of lymphocytes. Islands of lymphocytes with normal appearance remain, mainly within the deeper cortex. Such lesions can be limited in extent in older birds, making the cortical thinner and difficult to detect at the gross level. Day 15 post-infection. H&E.

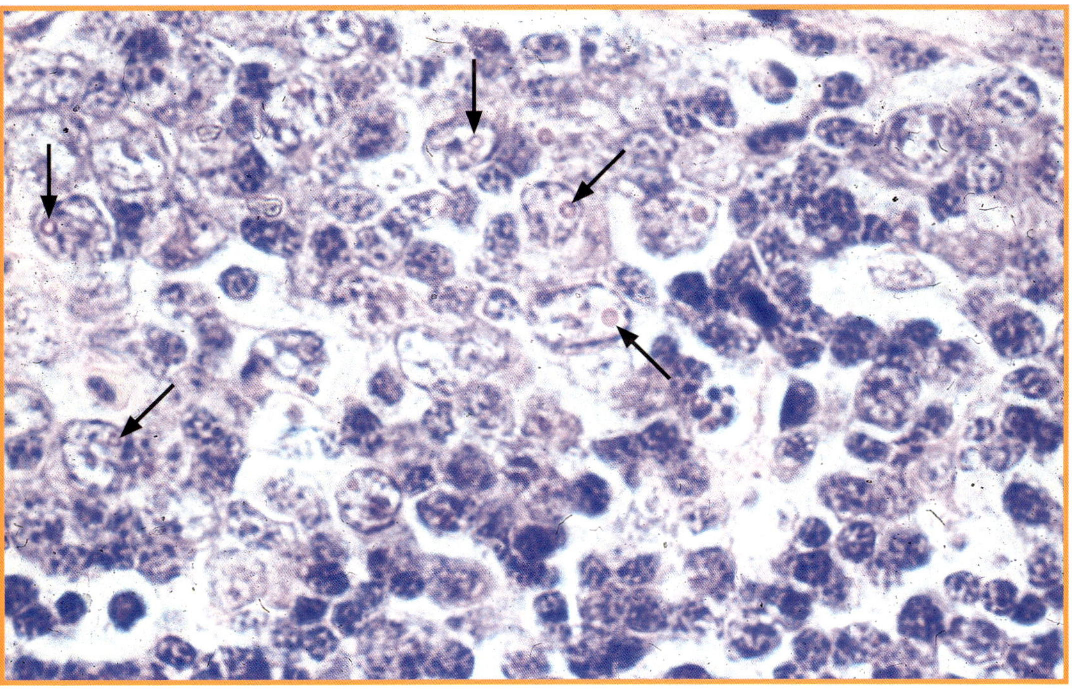

Fig. 8 | Thymic cortex. Note the numerous markedly enlarged nuclei compared to those of the normal lymphocytes. Several of these very enlarged nuclei, as well as some of the less enlarged nuclei, contain eosinophilic circular refractile inclusions (arrows) as well as some eosinophilic non-refractile inclusions. The former (circular and refractile) are characteristic of CAV infection. These cells are in the outer thymic cortex. Day 13 post-infection after oral inoculation with the Cux-1 strain of CAV at 21 days of age. H&E.

is lymphocyte depletion, which is most marked in the thymic cortex (Fig. 7), consistent with the relative abundance of viral replication at this site. It was proposed that lymphocyte depletion in the thymus is consequent to apoptosis. [73] Cells undergoing apoptosis exhibit characteristic morphologic changes including cell shrinkage, chromatin condensation into dense masses along the nuclear membrane. [83] However, CAV infected cells in chickens exhibit marked cytomegaly and karyomegaly (Figs. 1, 5, 8 and 9) and most commonly have very dispersed chromatin [152,153] (see Pathology), neither of which are features of apoptosis. While it is possible that such cells eventually undergo apoptosis, further work on the mechanism of cell death in the natural host (chickens) is indicated, especially since the studies that first led to the recognition that VP3 could induce apoptosis were all done in transformed cells. Indeed, it has been shown that VP3 could not induce apoptosis in normal mammalian cells [29] or in non-transformed avian cells (chicken embryo fibroblasts). [117]

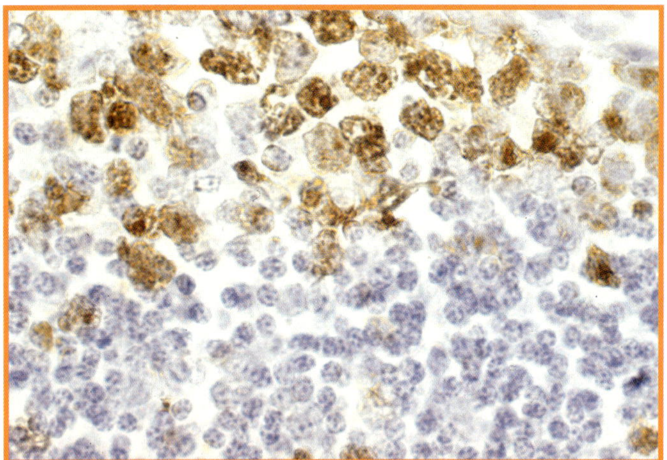

Fig. 9 | Thymus. CAV DNA labeled (brown) by in situ hybridization. Note the very large size of the nuclei of the infected cells compared to uninfected lymphocytes. Day 6 post-infection after I/M inoculation with the Cux-1 strain of CAV at one-day-old.

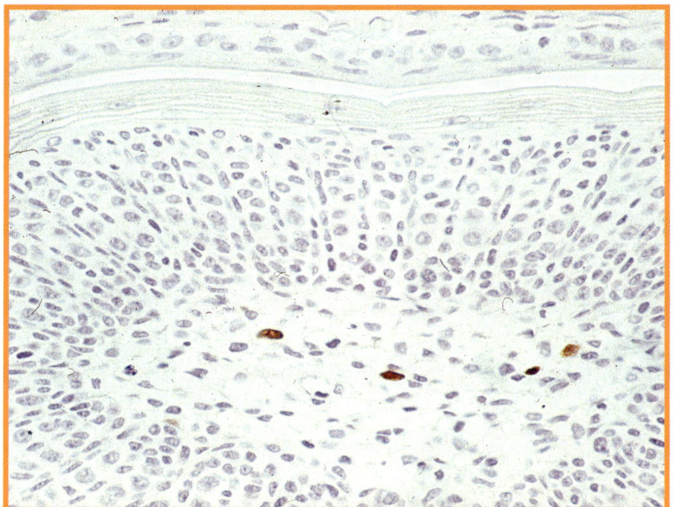

Fig. 10 | CAV antigen (brown) in feather pulp. Day 12 post-infection after I/M inoculation with the Cux-1 strain of CAV at one-day-old. ABC method.

In antigen distribution studies [55,63,66,152], infected cells were rare in the bursa of Fabricius, and these were usually in the interfollicular tissue [55,66,152] suggesting that B cells are not susceptible to CAV infection. This finding is apparently discrepant with multiple reports of notable bursal atrophy. Bursal atrophy in field cases may be the result of co-infections. However, it is more difficult to explain reports of bursal pathology in experimentally induced disease when virus inoculum has been grown in cell culture, given the facts that:

- Immunophenotyping of the target cells of CAV have suggested that the infected lymphoid cells are of T cell lineage. [3,26,66,67]
- B cell populations in bursa of Fabricius and spleen were unaffected. [26]
- B cells are considered not susceptible to infection with CAV. [3]

It has been suggested that effects on the bursa of Fabricius are the result of indirect effects of CAV mediated by destruction of other effector populations and/or disruption of cytokine networks, or enhanced pathogenicity of other agents which directly affect the bursa. [3] The former theory related to indirect effects of CAV does not explain the discrepancies fully since the listed indirect effects of CAV also occur in experimentally infected birds. In addition to the possibility of co-infecting agents targeting the bursa of Fabricius, the discrepancy could reflect differences either in the strain and/or dose of CAV. Strain and virus dose have been reported to influence other aspects of the outcome of CAV infection; e.g., severity of anemia is affected by virus dose. [66,101,140,189]

Based on studies by Joiner et al. [75], there is no evidence for genetic differences between chickens in susceptibility to CAV infection. They infected 4-week-old broilers representing 8 different MHC lines and found no significant differences in the outcome of infection.

CAV is uncommonly detected in epithelial cells [55,63,152,153], which suggests that either the virus does not replicate well in epithelia or that the relevant epithelial surface has not yet been examined. Since virus is present in large amounts in feces, it is possible that CAV excretion into feces may be the result of the passage of infected lymphoid cells or free virus particles into the lumen of the digestive tract. CAV antigen is also found in the pulp of some feathers [152] (Fig. 10) and it has now been shown that feathers contained infectious CAV particles. [31]

Clinical signs

Clinical disease is consequent to virus induced destruction of hemopoietic precursor cells and thymocytes leading to anemia (Fig. 3) and immunosuppression, respectively. Vertically infected chicks or maternal antibody-negative chicks infected horizontally during the first few days post hatching are usually asymptomatic for the first 7 to 10 days of life. Clinical signs often occur suddenly and include depression, reluctance to move, ruffled feathers, drooping wings and pallor of skin of the head, especially the comb, the beak, and mucous membranes (due to anemia), with mortality rate increases around 2-3 weeks of age. [11,23,51] Sometimes serosanguineous exudate on the wings occurs, reflecting the development of gangrenous dermatitis [11,43,45,172] (Fig. 11). Morbidity rates up to 60 % have been reported. [179] Mortality rates

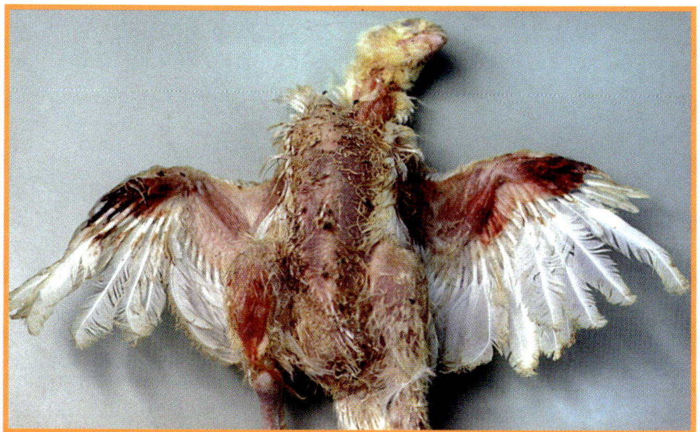

Fig. 11 | Broiler chicken naturally infected with chicken anemia virus and dying at approximately 16 days of age. Note the sanguineous exudate extending from both carpal regions to the shafts of the primary feathers, and on the cranial and medial aspect of the right tibiotarsal region. The skin overlying the breast and abdomen is markedly congested.

of 10-15 % are common [11,44,172,179], but can reach up to 60 %. [43] To understand why there can be such a wide range of morbidity and mortality, it is important to realize that an individual broiler flock may be composed of the progeny of more than one breeder flock. The larger the broiler flock, the more likely that the broilers were derived from multiple parent flocks. If one breeder flock is transmitting CAV vertically, then its progeny will form the vast majority of the clinically affected chickens. These clinically affected chicks will excrete virus which can then infect their flockmates. The outcome of this horizontally acquired infection depends on whether or not these exposed chicks are maternal antibody positive, since antibody will protect against viral replication, and also, whether there are other immunosuppressive viruses or other pathogens simultaneously infecting the flock (see Interactions with other Infectious Agents).

Clinical signs are not evident in broilers horizontally infected after about a week of age [104] or SPF chickens experimentally infected after one week of age [14,30,157], unless there are co-infecting pathogens. Clinical signs or effects on egg production, fertility or hatchability are not reported in breeding flocks which become infected during lay. [10,43,64,95,172]

Pathology

There have been no systematic sequential histologic studies of naturally or experimentally infected embryos, or of chicks hatched from naturally infected eggs. However, it was shown in early studies [181,186] that intramuscular inoculation of newly hatched chicks produced clinical signs and pathology that closely matched the naturally occurring clinical disease, with a similar time of clinical onset. Most information about the pathology produced by CAV in vertically infected chicks has been gleaned from studies of experimentally infected chickens.

Embryos

In naturally infected embryos, there is no apparent effect on hatchability [95,172] which suggests that pathology, if any, in the embryos is insignificant. Experimental infection by the yolk sac route at embryonic incubation day (EID) 5-7 may cause lesions depending on the strain and virus dose. For example, Cux-1, CAU269/7, and Gifu-1 strains did not cause lesions in chicken embryos [16,177,181,187] whereas other strains caused death of 50 % of embryos. [86,157] Lesions consisted of decreased body weight, paleness and edema of the embryos and hemorrhages often in the breast muscle. [30,86,130] Unilateral eye abnormalities were described by two groups [30,157], although the nature of these eye lesions was not reported. Davidson et al.[30] also reported the presence of urates on the chorioallantoic membrane. Lesions could be detected as early as EID 15 after yolk sac inoculation at EID 7. [30] Peters et al. [130] inoculated the yolk sac at EID 7 day with 10^4 $TCID_{50}$ of virus (with $TCID_{50}$ standing for tissue culture infectious doses 50). They reported severe CAV-specific pathology in five different experimental trials. There was mild to moderate petechiation in deep fascia and subcutaneous tissues, markedly reduced spleen size with parenchymal pallor and subcapsular hemorrhages. Thymic lobes were markedly reduced in size, and sometimes lobes had a hemorrhagic or gelatinous consistency. Bone marrow was pale and fatty or red and liquefied. In a minority of birds, the bursa of Fabricius was markedly reduced in size. Histopathological examination of tissues was not reported. The embryos were killed at the end of incubation so it is not known if they would have become sick or died within a few days of hatch, or succumbed to disease in the same manner as naturally vertically infected chicks.

Chickens

Gross pathology

Vertically infected chicks appear normal at hatch, but start to develop clinically evident anemia and increased mortality rate by 10-14 days of age. They may be smaller than normal. At necropsy, anemia may be manifest as pallor of the comb and of the organs and musculature (Fig. 12) and watery blood. Naturally

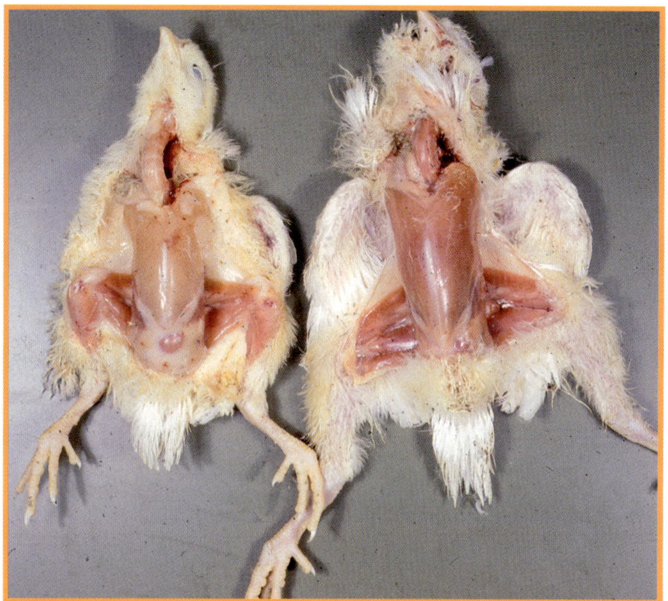

Fig. 12 Fifteen-day-old specific pathogen free (SPF) white Leghorn chickens. The bird on the left was inoculated I/M with Cux-1 strain of CAV at day-old. Note its smaller body size and the pallor of the breast muscle and lower beak (reflecting anemia) when compared to the uninfected hatchmate (right). The dark discolored focus on its left wing is a subcutaneous hemorrhage.

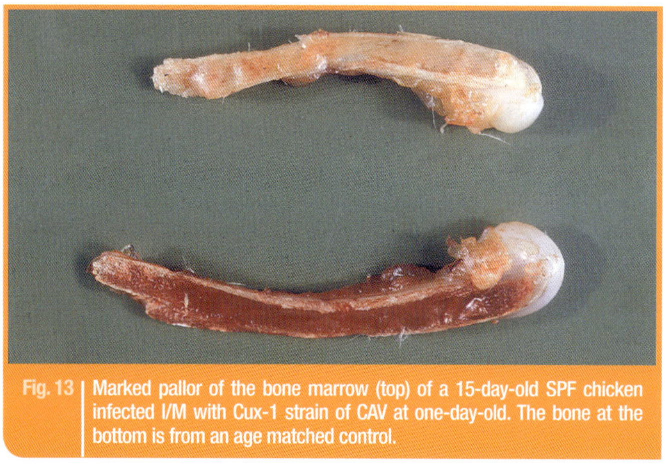

Fig. 13 Marked pallor of the bone marrow (top) of a 15-day-old SPF chicken infected I/M with Cux-1 strain of CAV at one-day-old. The bone at the bottom is from an age matched control.

infected chickens frequently have hemorrhages in the muscles, aplastic bone marrow in which hemopoietic tissue is replaced by adipocytes (Fig. 13) and there is atrophy of the thymus (Fig. 14) due to lymphocyte depletion.[190] Gangrenous dermatitis affecting the wings is commonly seen in field outbreaks[11,43,172,179] (Fig. 11) and this has resulted in names such as 'blue wing disease'[43] and 'anemia-dermatitis'[172] to describe the syndrome. Gangrenous dermatitis affecting the skin of the ventral abdomen, lateral aspects of the thorax and abdomen and of the feathered skin on the legs (Fig. 11), or severe multifocal to diffuse fungal pneumonia (Fig. 15) were common pathologic findings in sick or dead chickens during outbreaks of CAV infection in Northern Ireland (Smyth, unpublished observations), which is similar to findings in Japan[51], but often not in the same flock. When gangrenous dermatitis or other secondary infections develop, mortality rates tend to be higher.[172,179]

At necropsy examination of field material, it is important to bear in mind that lesions of CAV may easily be overlooked in the face of more fulminant lesions caused by secondary infections. Certainly where gangrenous dermatitis affects the wings, breast skins or legs, or there is extensive fungal pneumonia in birds over one week of age, the possibility of an underlying CAV infection must be considered. Gross evidence of anemia and/or moderate to severe thymic atrophy and pallor of the bone marrow were invariably present in birds dying at around two weeks of age (Smyth, unpublished observations), and such findings should increase suspicion of possible underlying CAV infection. Hoerr[62] similarly cautioned for infectious bronchitis (IB) cases with CAV infection as the underlying cause. In immunocompetent birds, which become infected after two weeks of age, the degree of thymic lymphocyte depletion is much less than that in birds inoculated at one day old, and may be hard to recognize at necropsy without the benefit of age matched control birds for direct comparison. The only noticeable gross change may

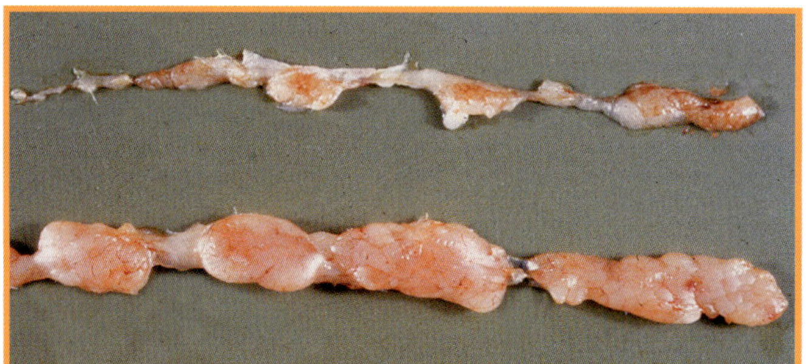

Fig. 14 Bottom: thymus from a normal 15-day-old SPF white Leghorn. Top: thymus from a hatchmate which was infected with the Cux-1 strain of CAV one-day-old. The lobes of this thymus are markedly reduced in size.

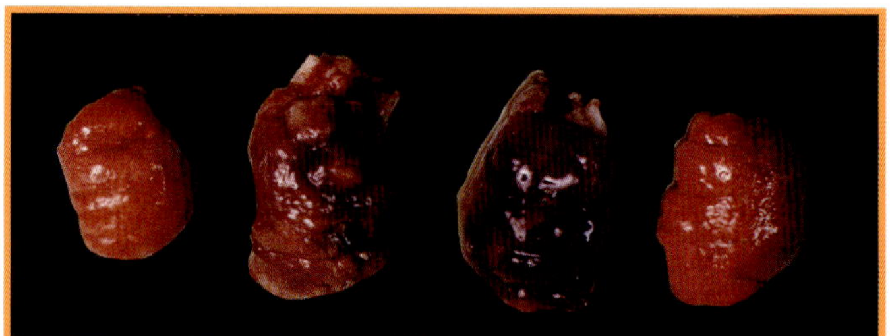

Fig. 15 Lungs from broiler chickens dying after naturally occurring vertically transmitted CAV infection. The outermost lungs are normal. The center two lungs have severe granulomatous pneumonia due to fungal infection. Fungal pneumonia is a common secondary lesion in broilers with CAV induced disease.

be less rounded thymic lobes that may be mildly to moderately reddened.[153]

Histologic findings

Since mixed infections are so common in commercial flocks, the best information on histopathologic changes caused by CAV again comes from experimentally infected chicks. The description below is based on experimental infections of SPF chicks unless otherwise specified.

Intra- and extra-sinusoidal hemocytoblasts in bone marrow, and cortical lymphoblasts in the thymus become infected as early as 3-4 days post-infection (see Pathogenesis). Characteristically, the nucleus of the infected cells become much enlarged, have dispersed or very finely stippled chromatin, or rarely margination of chromatin. In the thymus, this enlargement and dispersal of chromatin leads to reduced basophilia of the affected nuclei, which are most commonly found in the outer cortex, leading to diffuse or multifocal reduced staining of the outer cortex with hematoxylin in H&E stained sections (Fig. 16). If the nuclei in these paler staining areas are examined, then small eosinophilic, sometimes refractile circular, inclusions may be observed, particularly in the enlarged cells (Fig. 8). Sometimes nuclei can have multiple small inclusions of the non-refractile type (Figs. 1, 5 and 8). The circular refractile inclusions are very characteristic, they are CAV antigen positive[152,153], and are currently considered pathognomonic for CAV infection. The active phase of viral replication, which takes place mainly in the cortex, especially in subcapsular areas (Fig. 17) leads to marked loss of lymphoblasts and lymphocytes from the thymic cortex such that a distinct cortex may no longer be recognizable. There is also marked loss of hemopoietic cells from the bone marrow with replacement by adipocytes. If birds survive this phase of the disease, there will be partial to complete repopulation of the thymus and bone marrow (see also Pathogenesis). Nuclear changes similar to those described in the thymus can be seen in lymphoblasts in lymphoid tissue throughout the body, but they are rarely if ever reported, in the bursa of Fabricius. Next to thymus and bone marrow, spleen and lymphoid tissue in the mucosa (MALT) of the proventriculus and duodenum are the best sites for detection of viral antigen, and therefore the best sites for detection of cells with karyomegaly and nuclear inclusions should thymus and bone marrow be unavailable. However, such affected cells are infrequent.

The eosinophilic nuclear inclusions described above are very rarely seen in field material unless a concerted effort is made to acquire younger chicks hatched from transmitting flocks (Smyth, unpublished data). This is because the inclusions, which occur during the time of active viral replication in thymus, bone marrow, spleen and MALT, are transient and maximum numbers precede the onset of clinical disease, which is consequent to virus induced destruction of hemopoietic precursor cells and thymic lymphoblasts. Furthermore, the inclusions are

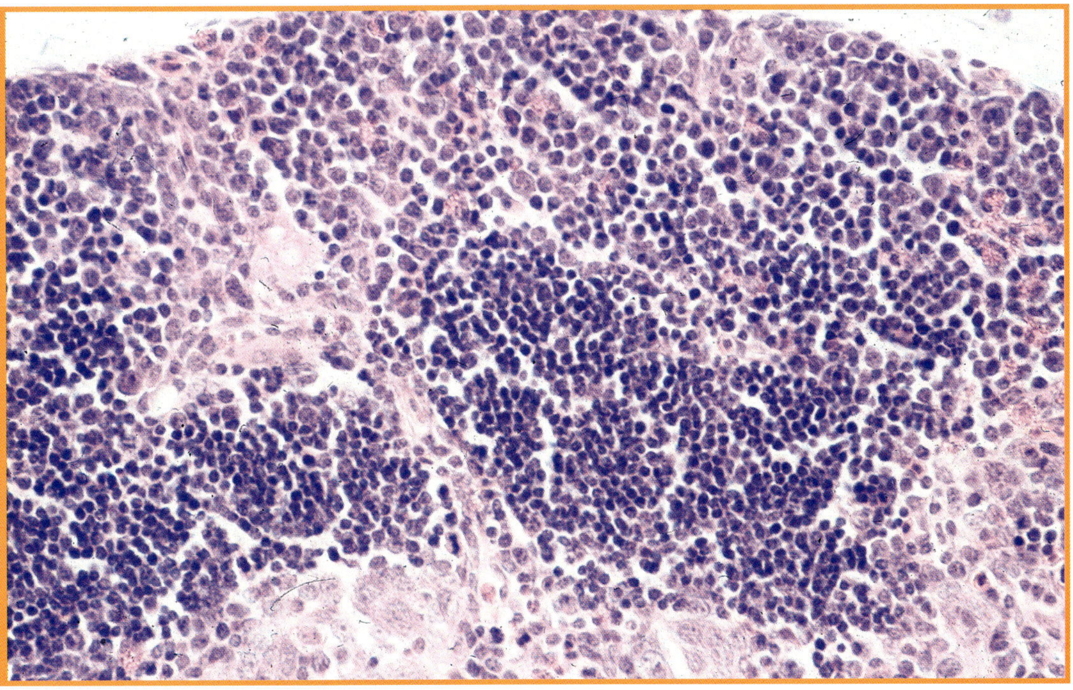

Fig. 16 Thymus of an SPF chicken at day 5 post-infection with Cux-1 strain of CAV given I/M at day-old. The outer cortex stains less intensely with hematoxylin than normal, exaggerating the difference between the inner and outer cortex. Immunoperoxidase staining of adjacent sections reveals that CAV antigen is located in the same region. (H&E).

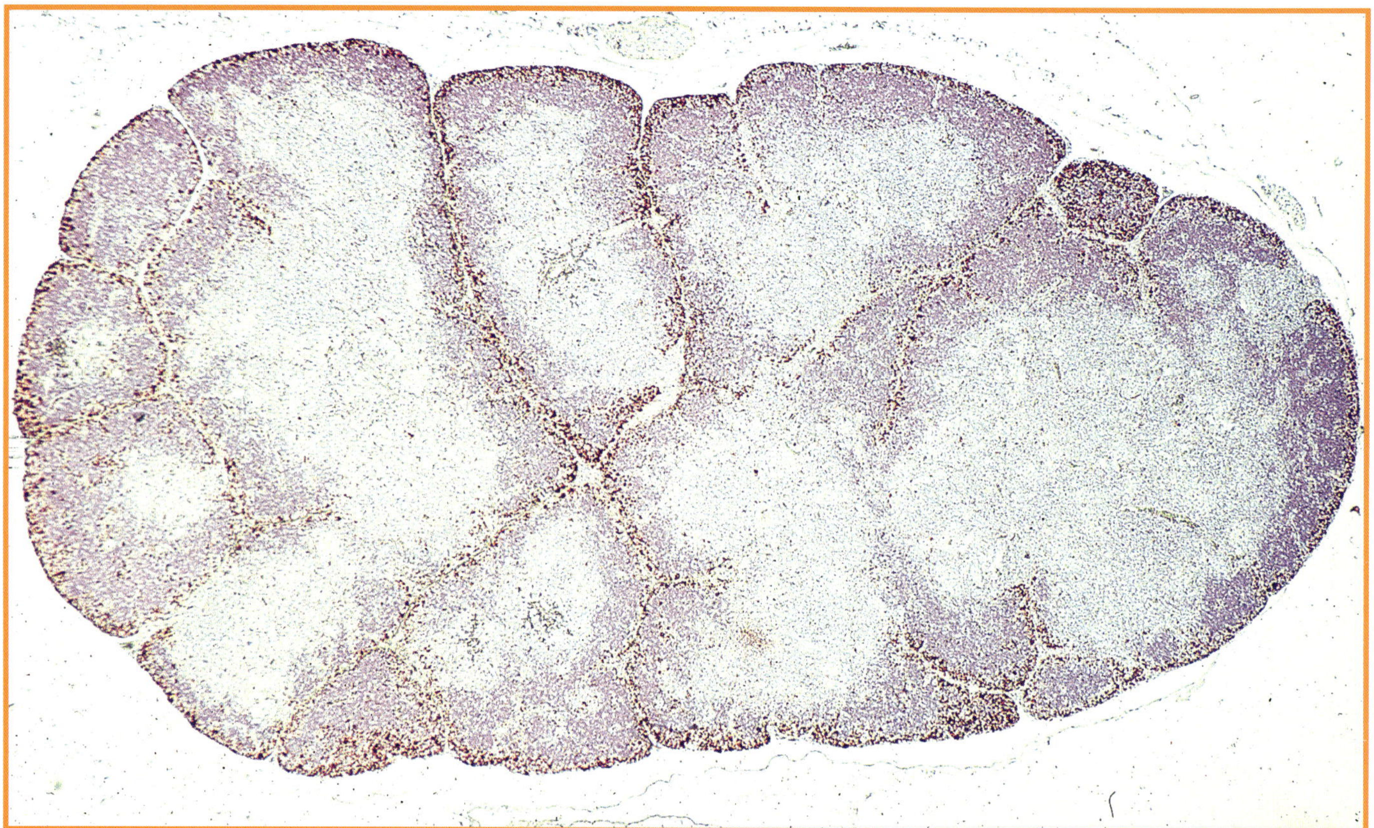

Fig. 17 | Low magnification image of a thymic lobe of eight-day-old SPF chicken, which was inoculated with the Cux-1 strain of CAV at one-day-old. CAV antigen is stained red-brown. Note antigen distribution is mainly in the subcapsular cortex. This is the region populated by immature T cells. SAP with AEC substrate.

only present in relatively large numbers in the thymus, and since they are small and may only be present in small pockets of cells, they may easily be overlooked. Collectively, these factors explain the very rare reports of finding inclusions in field cases.[11,132]

In immunocompetent chickens of three weeks and older inoculated with CAV by the oral route, which best mimics the likely route of horizontally acquired infection, viral replication and associated lesions as described above occur in thymus and, to a lesser extent, in lymphoid aggregates throughout the body.[55,152] However, the lesions are more limited in extent than those found in younger birds and accordingly may be overlooked or dismissed as insignificant. CAV antigen is rarely detected in the bone marrow, and anemia is not a feature in immunocompetent birds (see Pathogenesis). Again, the bursa of Fabricius is inconsistently affected. Mild depletion of thymic lymphocytes and absence of anemia has also been reported in older birds inoculated by intramuscular routes.[38,60,163,186]

Where there are dual infections of CAV with other agents, the time course and extent of virus replication, and therefore of histologic lesions, may be altered. For example, in birds infected with virulent Marek's disease virus (vMDV) or very virulent Marek's disease virus (vvMDV) at one day of age, and infected with CAV at four weeks of age, CAV antigens and the eosinophilic nuclear inclusions were detected in MD lymphoma cells or in lymphoproliferative lesions of some birds up to four weeks post-infection, at which point the experiments were terminated.[60] In that study, the distribution of cells with nuclear inclusions and/or antigen was very similar to that described in day-old chickens inoculated with CAV[152] except for rare inclusions that were also found in hepatocytes and CAV antigen in neural lymphomatous infiltrates, findings which have not previously been reported. This is not surprising because the MD A-type neural lesions consist mostly of transformed $CD4^+$ T cell lymphoblasts (see Chapter 5) thus providing the requirement for CAV replication: dividing T cells.

The presence of other co-infecting agents may enhance the severity of CAV induced pathology. This is particularly true in older birds, where it has been shown for example that infection of 2-week-old birds with CAV and IBDV enhances the pathogenicity of CAV, and severe thymic atrophy and bone marrow aplasia develop (see Pathogenesis and Interactions with other Infectious Agents).

> Although rarely seen in field samples, eosinophilic circular refractile inclusions in the nuclei of cells of the thymic cortex are currently considered pathognomonic for CAV infection.

Ultrastructural changes

Goryo et al. examined ultrastructural changes in thymic lymphoblasts [52] and in bone marrow. [53] They reported formation of pseudopodia and electron opaque regions in the cytoplasm and intranuclear fine granular or homogeneous inclusions in hemopoietic cells. Similar nuclear inclusions were seen, but more commonly, in thymic lymphoblasts. In addition to electron opaque regions, aggregates of microtubules and autophagosomes were present in the cytoplasm. Virus-like particles were rarely seen in either thymus or bone marrow. In immunolabeled infected MSB-1 cells and in thymic lymphocytes from experimentally infected chicks, McNulty et al. [102] found immune labeling associated with electron-dense, finely granular, non-membrane-bound nuclear inclusions, and cytoplasmic accumulations of microtubules. Aggregates of virus-like particles were sometimes observed in the nuclei of infected MSB1 cells. These authors also reported seeing many ring or doughnut like profiles of the electron-dense, finely granular, non-membrane-bound intranuclear material. It would be interesting to know if these correspond to the circular refractile inclusions seen with the light microscope. In another study, VP2 and VP3 were localized either singly or together with the nuclear inclusions, but the distribution of these proteins was not correlated with either inclusion size or electron density. [36]

CAV-induced immunosuppression

Based on the effects of CAV infection on other pathogens (for details see Interactions with other Infectious Agents), it has generally been accepted that CAV infection can cause subclinical immunosuppression. However, there are relatively few studies addressing the fundamental mechanisms causing the immunosuppression. Moreover, several of the earlier studies used methodologies that do not provide specific and detailed information based on our current knowledge of avian immunology.

Effect of infection on cell populations

There is no doubt that CAV infection impacts the thymus resulting in a severe loss of thymocytes between 7 and 28 days post-infection, especially when chicks are infected at one day of age. For example, Cloud et al. [26] and Hu et al. [66] reported a loss of $CD4^+$ and $CD8^+$ thymocytes. Because dual staining techniques for both CD markers were not possible at that time, it is not clear if the reduction in thymocyte numbers represented $CD4^+$ $CD8^+$ precursor cells, $CD4^+$ $CD8^-$ T helper (Th) cells or $CD4^-$ $CD8^+$ cytotoxic T cells (CTL) or any combination thereof. Cloud et al. [26] and Bounous et al. [12] reported lymphocytopenia in the spleen representing loss of Th and CTL subpopulations. In contrast, Hu et al. reported only a minor reduction in $CD4^+$ and $CD8^+$ cells in the spleen. In addition, Cloud et al. used an antibody against MHC class II (often called Ia antigen in 1992), which is expressed on B cells, activated T cells and subpopulations of dendritic cells and cells of the macrophage/monocyte lineage. An increase in $CD4^+$ and $CD8^+$ cells and MHC class II^+ cells was found in the bone marrow between 7 and 28 days post-infection, perhaps representing an immune response against CAV replicating in the hemocytoblasts. The importance in the reduction of CTL in the spleen was functionally examined by Markowski-Grimsrud and Schat. [92] Co-infection of 15-, 30-, and 45-day-old, CAV antibody-free chickens with CAV (CIA-1 strain) and REV resulted in high copy numbers of CAV transcripts at 7 days post-infection. A significant reduction in CTL activity against REV-transformed lymphoblastoid cells was found at the same time. In contrast, co-infection of 15- and 30-day-old chicks positive for maternal CAV antibodies at 14 days of age had no effect on the CTL activity; CAV did not replicate based on the absence of CAV transcripts. More recently, van Ginkel et al. [167] showed an effect of CAV on the Th cell population in the Harderian gland. CAV caused a reduction in the $CD4^+/CD8^+$ ratio and a reduction in IgA responses to IB virus (IBV), as measured by a reduction in IBV-specific IgA-producing B cells. The reduction is most likely the consequence of a reduction in Th cells needed to generate the switch from IgM to IgA positive cells.

Effect of infection on macrophage activity and cytokine production

McConnell et al. [93,94] examined the effects of CAV infection at 1 and 21 days of age on macrophages. Independently of the age at exposure, phagocytosis and bactericidal activity was reduced up to 43 days post exposure. Fc receptor expression was also reduced during this period.

Several groups examined the impact of CAV infection on T cell stimulation using different mitogens such as phytohemagglutin (PHA), concanavalin-A (Con-A) or pokeweed (PW). Adair et al.[1] and McConnell et al.[94] found a reduced response to stimulation of splenic lymphocytes typically between 9 and 17 days post-infection independently of infection at 1 or 21 days of age. Minor differences were reported between these studies for the duration of the reduced response to Con-A. Bounous et al.[12] also reported a reduced response to Con-A at 11 days post-infection. All three groups reported an increased response after recovery from infection although there was no agreement at which time post-infection the recovery occurred. In contrast, Cloud et al.[26] did not see an effect of CAV infection on PHA or Con-A stimulation of spleen cells, but noted an increased response to PW at 14 days post-infection and a decreased response of peripheral blood lymphocytes to PW at 17 days post-infection.

There are only a few studies addressing the impact of CAV-infection on cytokines. Bioassays for the so-called T cell growth factor, IL-1β and interferons (IFN) were used by Adair et al.[1] and McConnell et al.[93,94] In general, the bioassays showed a reduction for all three markers especially around 9 to 17 days post-infection. T cell growth factor may contain several unidentified cytokines; therefore, interpretation of these data is difficult based on our current state of knowledge about avian cytokines.[79]

Using competitive nucleic acid hybridization it was found that CAV infection at four weeks of age significantly reduced IFN-α and IFN-γ mRNA transcription in response to challenge with inactivated IBDV-IBV-NDV (potent interferon inducers) at one, two or three weeks post-infection with CAV. These data suggest that CAV causes immunosuppression, which is subclinical because birds of this age do not develop clinical disease (see Clinical signs). Markowski-Grimsrud and Schat used qRT-PCR to examine the impact of CAV infection between 15 and 45 days of age, on IL-1β, IL-2 and IFN-γ mRNA.[92] There were no significant effects on IL-1β and IL-2 at 7 and 14 days post-infection. There was a significant increase in IFN-γ mRNA transcription at 7 days post-infection when chickens were infected at 30 days of age.

Collectively, CAV infection impairs both innate immunity due to lack of granulocytes and thrombocytes caused by damage to the bone marrow and depressed macrophage functions, and adaptive immune responses due to lack of Th cells and CTLs. This immunosuppression explains the high incidence of secondary bacterial and fungal infections seen during naturally occurring outbreaks of CAV associated disease. It also explains the enhancing effect that CAV has on other viral pathogens, and its reported interference with antibody responses to vaccines (see Interactions with other Infectious Agents).

Economic effects

Economic effects of clinical CAV induced disease

In a large scale study comparing unaffected flocks with flocks exhibiting clinical disease due to CAV and elevated mortality rates of 2 %, net income was 17.3-19.6 % lower for the affected flocks. This figure included medication costs since it was deemed likely that mortality rate would have been much higher in the absence of strategic medication.[95] Depression in weight gain was of the order of 3.5 %. Higher mortality rates and greater depressions of average weight at slaughter of between 7 % and 13 % have been observed in most other outbreaks[23,43,172], so net income would likely be further reduced in such circumstances.

Economic effects of subclinical disease

Broiler flocks frequently have antibody to CAV at the time of slaughter.[34,37,77,104,155,162] This is most likely the result of infection acquired horizontally, after maternal antibodies have waned. These infections are usually subclinical[104] (see also Clinical Signs). Field-based studies investigating the effects of such infections in broilers have produced conflicting results. In one study, broiler flocks which remained seronegative achieved 13 % greater net income and a 2 % better feed conversion ratio, and were 2.5 % heavier than equivalent broiler flocks which had antibodies to CAV at the time of processing.[104] In another study, CAV infections in broilers were associated with increased condemnation rates in the slaughterhouse, although daily weight gain, feed conversion and production score were not significantly affected.[34] However, adverse effects attributable to CAV infection of broiler flocks were not found in other studies.[49,56,77] The apparently conflicting findings may reflect the presence of other factors or conditions in the examined flocks[34], especially since it has been shown experimentally that infection of immunocompetent chickens of three weeks and older causes lymphoid depletion and immunosuppression.[92,94,152]

Infection of laying flocks has not been associated with adverse effects, but there has been no comprehensive economic analysis of effects on laying flocks apart from one study which included examination of egg production, fertility and hatchability.[95] That study found no significant difference in the measured parameters.

Interactions with other Infectious Agents

CAV and infectious bursal disease virus

Concomitant infections of CAV and IBDV (infectious bursal disease virus) enhance the severity of CAV induced pathology and depression of immune effector cells.[27,141,176,183] Co-infection with IBDV abrogates the age related resistance to development of anemia in birds infected at two weeks of age and older[141,176,181] (see also Pathogenesis and Pathology). Furthermore, infection of 35-day-old chickens with very virulent IBDV followed by CAV at 40 days inhibited production of VN antibodies to CAV.[72]

In the reverse manner, development of an immune response to IBDV may be adversely affected in birds infected with CAV, since T cells (which are a target of CAV in birds of all ages) are essential for the development of IgY antibodies against IBDV. In addition, T cells are also involved in viral clearance in the bursa of Fabricius.[81,134,135]

Interactions between CAV and IBDV are particularly problematic to the poultry industry since control of IBDV infections and associated pathology remains one of the major challenges of broiler production. The major problem is achieving successful vaccination against IBDV in the face of maternal antibodies to IBDV. More virulent (hotter) strains of IBDV can break through these antibodies to create infection and disease before vaccine strains can induce immunity. In some areas and in some countries, increasingly hot vaccinal strains of IBDV are needed to control IBD caused by increasingly more virulent field strains of IBDV. These hot vaccines are capable of damaging the bursa of Fabricius and are therefore likely to enhance CAV replication leading to CAV-associated disease or immunosuppression. This, as well as poorly controlled wild type IBDV strains, will enhance the pathology and immunosuppressive effects of CAV[72,183], as well as leading to poor response to CAV vaccines. These interactions will also occur in egg laying and breeding flocks, where consequent poor response to vaccines would be problematic.

CAV and tumor viruses

There has been an abundance of published studies investigating the interactions of MDV and CAV[106,173], sometimes with apparently contradictory results. For example, one study reported significant enhancement of the lymphoproliferative lesions of MD with low doses of MDV, while co-infection of CAV with higher doses of MDV resulted in decreased lymphoproliferative lesions.[74] Depending on the virulence of the MDV strain, CAV infection can aggravate MD. Co-infection of CAV with vMDV or vvMDV strains increased MD incidence[58,106], while co-infection with the vv+MDV strain 584A did not increase MD, probably because this MDV strain already causes severe thymic atrophy.[106] Infection with the virulent JM strain of MDV or vaccination with turkey herpesvirus at one day of age followed by infection with CAV at 7 days of age aggravated the degree of thymic atrophy to that typically seen when CAV is given alone at one day-of age.[123] CAV infection can also cause MD vaccine failures.[121,122] An important consequence of CAV replication in older birds is a suboptimal vaccine protection against MD, probably by preventing a strong CTL response to MDV reactivation from latency. As a consequence, many MD vaccine breaks may not be caused by MDV strains with increased pathogenicity but by CAV-induced immunosuppression.[48]

REV-induced tumors can easily be misdiagnosed as MD.[180] Thus far, there are only a few publications on the interactions between CAV and REV. Originally, Yuasa et al.[181] isolated CAV from a disease outbreak linked to a REV-contaminated MD vaccine, but it is not clear if there was a connection between the two pathogens. Since then, synergism between CAV and REV in causing immunosuppression has been reported by two groups.[87,176]

CAV, reovirus and adenovirus

Reoviruses very commonly infect poultry flocks. Dual intra-abdominal or intramuscular inoculations of chickens with CAV and a Swedish reovirus isolated from a case of blue wing disease, resulted in more severe disease than was produced by either virus alone.[45] Furthermore, administration of some strains of reovirus, together with CAV by oral challenge, also resulted in more severe disease than in chickens inoculated with reovirus or CAV alone.[100] The severity of the effect was dependent on the strain of reovirus.

It has been shown that CAV infection in combination with fowl adenoviruses (FAVs) resulted in enhanced pathogenicity of adenovirus[175] and a much higher incidence of inclusion body hepatitis/hydropericardium syndrome.[164] These authors also showed that the degree to which CAV enhanced pathogenicity of FAVs varied during the course of the CAV infection. This is likely to be true in all dual infections.

CAV and respiratory infections

Chicks spray-vaccinated with Newcastle disease virus vaccine at either one or 10 days of age developed more severe post-vaccinal respiratory signs, conjunctivitis and growth retardation when given CAV at one day of age compared to similarly NDV vaccinated chicks that were not infected with CAV.[33] Humoral immune responses to NDV were not affected, but a breeder flock that became seropositive to CAV during rearing had lower antibody response to a killed NDV vaccine than their hatchmates which remained seronegative to CAV.[13]

Cytotoxic T cell responses are important in the clearance of IBV.[28,149] CAV reduces CTL responses to IBV and reduces the mucosal immune responses and IBV vaccine-induced B cell responses.[167] CAV administered at one day of age depressed antibody response to avian influenza virus vaccine[87], and also to Newcastle disease vaccine and infectious laryngotracheitis vaccine.[27]

CAV and bacteria or fungi

There have been many reports of secondary bacterial and fungal infections occurring with increased frequency and severity in naturally CAV infected flocks. Gangrenous dermatitis is the most commonly reported secondary bacterial infection. *Escherichia coli*, *Staphylococcus* spp. and rarely *Clostridium septicum* have been recovered from affected skin.[11,172] We are only aware of experimental studies demonstrating an enhancing effect of CAV on the development of a few bacterial diseases. During development of an experimental model of bacterial chondronecrosis (or femoral head necrosis), McNamee et al.[97] found that exposure of broilers to CAV enhanced the ability of *Staphylococcus aureus* to colonize and induce lesions in growth plates. Co-infection of CAV with *Salmonella enterica* serovar Enteritidis resulted in a decreased IgA response to *S. enterica* in the intestinal tract compared to infection with only *S. enterica*, and lesions were more severe in the combined infection than in infection with the bacteria alone.[150]

Diagnosis

General

Detection of infection by CAV is relatively straightforward. However, definitive diagnosis of disease due to CAV is more problematic since apart from the eosinophilic refractile type of inclusions (see Pathology), all other pathologic changes and clinical signs, are not specific to CAV infection. In the absence of the specific inclusions (in at least small to moderate numbers of cells) together with associated pathology, a combination of ancillary testing and examination of flock history together with pathologic findings will be needed to make a diagnosis of CAV induced disease. The degree of confidence in the diagnosis depends on the cumulative amount of supporting evidence. Co-infections of CAV with other pathogens can complicate the diagnosis. On the one hand co-infections, especially with IBDV, but also with MDV and reoviruses can exacerbate the effects of CAV (see Interactions with other Infectious Agents). On the other hand, disease caused by other pathogens may divert attention away from potential underlying CAV induced pathology; e.g., IBV, MDV and bacterial infections causing septicemia or gangrenous dermatitis.

In considering differential diagnoses, it is important to remember that infection by some of the other viruses can produce lesions that can resemble those caused by CAV. For example, IBDV strains can produce subcutaneous and/or intramuscular hemorrhages[47]; IBDV and adenovirus caused hemorrhagic-aplastic anemia[139]; vv+ MD strains can cause severe thymic atrophy long before tumors develop.[17]

Blood testing

Detection of exposure of a flock to CAV is best done by serological examination for antibodies to CAV. However, the presence or absence of antibodies at one time point does not provide sufficient information when trying to reach a diagnosis of CAV-induced disease. During any infection process, if the sample is taken too soon, antibodies will not have had time to develop. If an animal is already seropositive, then the time at which infection occurred is unknown. At minimum, two samples collected at least two weeks apart need to be tested, to look for evidence of either seroconversion or rising antibody titer (i.e., at least a four-fold increase), both of which would indicate recent infection and be supportive evidence of a CAV-associated problem. Alternatively, there may be no evidence of seroconversion or there may be declining antibody titers, which would not support a diagnosis of a CAV-associated problem.

Where vertically transmitted disease is suspected, serological examination of the parent flock(s) from which the broilers were derived, should be carried out. Thirty blood samples per parent flock have usually been found to be representative in our experience. If CAV is involved in the disease problem under investigation, then one or more of the contributing parent flocks should be seropositive at the time of testing, since at least 4-5 weeks will have passed since they produced the eggs that gave rise to the affected chickens (3 week egg incubation plus a further 1-2 weeks for clinical signs to develop in the chicks). If the parents are antibody positive, then it is important to test previously collected blood samples from the seropositive flock(s). Many large poultry producers routinely collect serum samples from chickens at around 18 weeks of age (pre- or point-of-lay samples). Such samples may be tested at the time of collection to check for example for presence of vaccinal antibodies, but importantly, aliquots are usually kept in storage. These can be very valuable samples to test when investigating disease problems that occur during the laying period since they serve as pre-disease samples which provide a baseline from which to identify seroconversion or rising titers. However, if a problem develops late in lay, and seroconversion to an agent is found, then it is important to bear in mind the possibility that seroconversion could have occurred prior to the problem under investigation.

There are many types of antibody detection systems. Originally, antibodies to CAV were detected by the classical virus neutralization test (VN) using virus growing in cell culture. [186] Neutralizing antibodies can persist for a long time in naturally infected chickens. [64,70] A few years later, indirect immunofluorescence (IFA) tests were developed and used. [174,188] There have been some reported specificity problems with the IFA test [178], although this could be reduced by screening sera at a 1:50 dilution rather than 1:10 [124] and careful titration of the secondary antibody to determine the optimal concentration. [89] These tests, especially the VN tests, are very labor intensive and therefore costly and not practical for routine use in the diagnostic laboratory. A micro-neutralization test was developed by Imai and Yuasa. [69] While less cumbersome and less costly than the conventional neutralization test, it is not suitable for routine use. The problem with these classical VN tests is that they require a large number of culture passages before definitive results are obtained. Two micro-neutralization tests that do not require the serial passage of cell cultures have been developed. One of these observes for cytopathic effects (cpe) after 3-4 days of culture [76], while the other uses qPCR analysis to determine if the virus was neutralized. [169] However, the latter test remains expensive and quite time consuming because of the need to extract DNA from all of the wells.

Enzyme linked immunoassays (ELISA) have become very popular for antibody detection in many species, including chickens, because of the comparative ease of testing many samples and the capability for high throughput laboratories to automate steps such as addition of reagents, plate washes and calculation of results. There are several commercially available CAV antibody detecting ELISA kits, which are either indirect or competitive (blocking) detection systems. In some of these tests, the corrected absorbance reading can give an indication of antibody titer. In others, the result is determined as positive/negative, but this may be the only information that is required in many cases. Using the positive/negative assays, titration of serum would be needed to get an indication of titer. Specificity, which can be a problem with some ELISA tests, is very important when testing the status of SPF birds. One approach to solve this problem could be to use ELISA for screening purposes and then to test all positive sera by another test for confirmation. As with any serological test, it is very important that serum samples are handled appropriately. For example moderate to marked hemolysis of serum samples reduced the degree of positivity as determined by ELISA. [84]

Other tests can be performed on blood such as in situ hybridization [142] and virus isolation [86], and these methodologies are discussed in the respective sections below. However, such testing is better performed on tissue samples such as thymus and spleen.

Examination of diseased chickens

To detect infection within a diseased chicken, several approaches can be used. Testing of blood samples for detection of antibody can be performed, and subject to the same qualifications as given above, this can provide potentially useful information.

Antigen detection

In our experience, one of the best confirmatory tests to employ has been immunochemical tests on tissue smears or tissue sections from diseased chickens. Such tests are designed to detect viral antigens. A major advantage of antigen detection over DNA detection is that the presence of detectable viral antigens is an indication that the virus is, or has recently been, replicating, and furthermore, the amount of antigen can be visually assessed. However, another approach which allows quantification of CAV transcription (and therefore replication) and has given excellent results, is the use of qRT-PCR to detect mRNA, which will be described in next section (CAV DNA or mRNA detection). It is likely that more modern approaches such as this, which do not require use of animals to generate reagents, will become common.

Direct or indirect immunofluorescent examination of impression smears of thymus, and bone marrow in young birds is a quick and relatively inexpensive method of demonstrating CAV antigens in tissues. [98] A same day result is very feasible. Either polyclonal or monoclonal antibodies can be used. Direct immunofluorescent examination using CAV antibody directly conjugated to a fluorochrome such as fluorescein isothiocyanate, will allow the fastest result. Cryostat sections of quench-frozen tissues can also be used very effectively, but production of cryostat sections requires more and skilled labor, and access to more expensive and specialized equipment. Freezing tissues by placing them in a freezer results in very poor quality sections and is not recommended. If a laboratory does not have a fluorescent microscope, it would also be possible to do immunohistochemical staining on tissue smears, but the authors are not aware of this approach being used for diagnosis, so such an assay would have to be developed and validated.

Immunohistochemical staining of formalin-fixed paraffin-embedded tissue sections for evidence of the antigens of pathogens has become a widely used diagnostic test for many diseases because preparation of such samples is standard in the non-clinical practice diagnostic laboratories. However, it is important to realize that the ability to detect CAV antigens in tissue sections is markedly adversely affected by prolonged fixation in 10 % neutral buffered formalin (NBF). [152] NBF is the most widely used fixative in diagnostic laboratories. Ability to detect antigen was also markedly adversely affected by the use of a standard bone decalcifying solution. [152] This is relevant if the marrow has been processed while still within the bone, which is a common practice for young poultry with small bones. For CAV antigen detection, optimum tissue fixation time in NBF was six hours. Such a short fixation time would be unusual in diagnostic laboratories. Furthermore, while short fixation allows excellent visualization of CAV antigens in tissue sections, the use of such short fixation times creates other problems, most notably non-specific binding of detection system reagents to endogenous substances in the tissues [152], a problem which is not encountered to significant degree in material fixed for longer periods of time. Therefore, it would be very important to have good controls against which the test sections can be compared. There was markedly less immunolabeling of CAV antigen after fixation in NBF for three days, and very pronounced reduction after seven days fixation. Where fixation has been prolonged, in situ hybridization can be used successfully (see below) to detect viral DNA in tissue sections (Fig. 9). As with other test methods, the results of these tests must be considered in conjunction with other information in reaching a diagnosis. For example, negative results could be due to performing the test on inappropriate sample, such as thymus that has been fixed too long in 10 % NBF.

Unfortunately, neither fluorescent antibody tests nor immunohistochemical testing for CAV are offered by many diagnostic laboratories, perhaps since to date, ready to use antibodies to CAV are not readily available. We could only find two commercial providers of CAV antibody; one antibody was developed for use in ELISA tests and has not been validated for use in immunohistochemical methods, and the other is raised in chickens and would need to be conjugated and used in a direct immunofluorescence assay.

Antigen capture ELISAs are available commercially for several viral pathogens. Such tests provide several advantages, e.g., ability to test large number of samples efficiently, and since they detect antigen, the degree of positivity of the result would give an indication as to the amount of virus present. However, we could find no published information on antigen capture ELISA detection of CAV.

CAV DNA or mRNA detection

Conventional PCR based detection of CAV DNA is probably the most widely applied test today. While PCR is very sensitive for detection of CAV DNA, there are limitations to the use of PCR as a disease diagnostic.

While the sensitivity of PCR is great for detecting evidence of exposure to CAV and indeed for detecting evidence of CAV contaminating vaccines, this same sensitivity makes interpretation as to the significance of positive results in tissues from sick or dead birds difficult for the following reasons:

- Where there has been a low level of challenge that is not causing a problem to the bird, the low levels of CAV DNA may be detectable by PCR.
- PCR may detect inactivated or incomplete, and therefore non-viable, virus material. Indeed this phenomenon was offered as an explanation for the detection of CAV DNA in the feces of dogs and cats. [131]
- Presence of CAV viral DNA does not necessarily mean that the virus is actively, or has been, replicating. [20]
- CAV DNA can persist for months after infection, and its presence may have no relevance to the current disease problem being experienced (see Transmission in SPF flocks).

Thus, while conventional PCR assays can be performed by most diagnostic laboratories, positive and negative results have to be interpreted in the context of other findings in the flock and/or within the bird. For example, finding CAV DNA in the thymus or bone marrow of a chicken with anemia or lymphocyte depletion in the thymic cortex would lend support to a diagnosis of CAV induced disease, but does not confirm it. Likewise, a negative result must also consider the possibility of sampling error, possible degradation of DNA in the tissue due for example to autolysis, a variant strain whose DNA did not anneal with the primer set employed in the PCR assay. For screening purposes, it is important to select primers that bind to highly conserved regions of the genome. The sensitivity of conventional PCR, and nested PCR which has even greater sensitivity [105,154], is of great value for the testing of vaccines for contamination by CAV (e.g., Amer et al.) [5], and for research studies such as those which were able to demonstrate CAV DNA in the Cornell SPF flocks. [20,108] Many PCR methodologies and primer sets have been published in the literature including methods for application to formalin-fixed paraffin-embedded tissue sections [71] which are likely to be available (see above) when unfixed tissues may not.

A duplex PCR for adenovirus and CAV [136] and a multiplex PCR test for simultaneous detection of avian reovirus, IBDV and group 1 avian adenoviruses [22] have been reported. The latter test needs a reverse transcription step because two of the viruses are RNA viruses. The multiplex test could be used on feces and was both sensitive and specific.There are several reasons why the ability to test for multiple pathogens in the same test reaction offers advantage:

- Several chicken pathogens can present with similar signs and overlapping pathologic features.
- The presence of other chicken pathogens may have enhanced the pathogenicity of CAV and vice versa.

Real time, quantitative PCR (qPCR) has the advantage that it gives an indication of the relative amount of DNA present, and the finding of large quantities of CAV DNA, in conjunction with lesions, provides stronger support for a diagnosis of CAV induced disease than a positive result by conventional PCR. However, qPCR is more costly to perform than conventional PCR. It is more likely to be used as a routine diagnostic test when large numbers of samples are to be analyzed. Recently, a multiplex qPCR assay for the detection of CAV and MDV has been published. [32] To identify or confirm actual virus replication, qRT-PCR to detect CAV mRNA has been developed. [91,92] The use of differential primers can distinguish between two different strains of CAV. [91] This qRT-PCR assay has been used by Schat et al. [147] to measure protection by an experimental immune complex vaccine (see Experimental vaccines, and novel approaches to CAV vaccination).

Dot blot hybridization may offer a compromise between the 'over sensitivity' of conventional PCR, and the quantitative ability of qPCR, as it is less sensitive than PCR (no PCR amplification is involved) and it is easier to perform than qPCR. Dot blot hybridization has been used on tissue extracts [161] and could detect DNA (limit of sensitivity between 1 to 10 pg) in tissue extracts of experimentally infected chickens between 5 and 42 days post-infection. It could also detect DNA in chickens with signs of anemia-dermatitis syndrome but did not detect CAV DNA in chickens from normal flocks indicating that it might be helpful as a diagnostic tool.

A new technology, loop-mediated isothermal amplification (LAMP) has been developed in the last 10 years, and a LAMP assay for rapid detection of CAV has been developed. [68] This technique does not require the use of thermal cycling, and is reported to be more sensitive than conventional PCR. There is currently much investment in development of this technology, for example with a view to make the test available in micro-chip format or applying it to RNA amplification. [6]

In situ hybridization (ISH) can be used successfully to detect CAV DNA in tissue sections (Fig. 9) and in blood smears. [142] As a diagnostic tool, ISH has two major advantages over immunohistochemistry on formalin-fixed paraffin embedded tissues:

- Length of formalin fixation does not adversely affect ability to detect CAV DNA by ISH.
- With current technology, it is easier to generate DNA hybridization probes than to generate either polyclonal or monoclonal antibodies.

It also has the advantages over the PCR based methods that:

- DNA distribution can be accurately localized
- The amount of DNA present can be assessed.
- Formalin-fixed paraffin embedded tissues are often routinely prepared by diagnostic laboratories and thus available.

There have been several published methods for performing in situ hybridization for CAV in tissues [4,96,116] and one group used ISH on blood smears to aid in reaching a diagnosis. [120,142] These papers include description of how to generate CAV specific probes. Most probes have been labeled with digoxigenin or biotin to facilitate their detection. In our experience, digoxigenin is a better label for use with avian tissues than biotin, because there can be a lot of endogenous avidin and biotin in avian tissues, especially in liver and kidney, which can bind non-specifically to reagents used to detect biotin labeled probes.

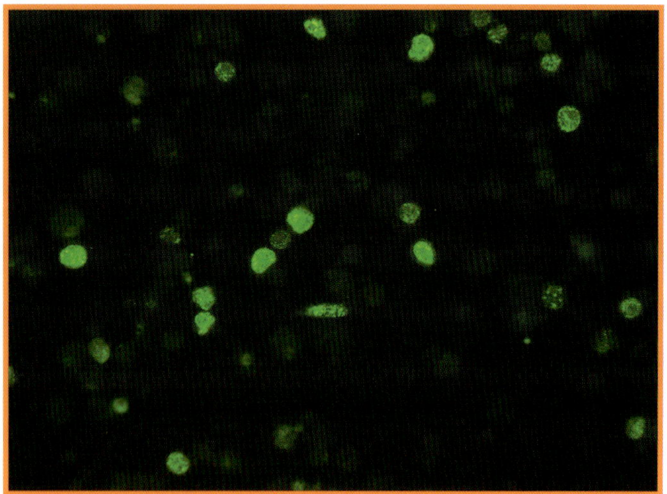

Fig. 18 | Immunofluorescently labeled CAV antigen in MDCC-MSB1 cells. Image courtesy of Virology Department, Agri-Food and Biosciences Institute, Belfast, Northern Ireland.

PCR and nested PCR have also been used successfully on extracts made from formalin fixed tissues and formalin fixed paraffin embedded tissues to detect CAV.[71]

Virus isolation

CAV is usually only propagated for reagent production (e.g., antigens for diagnostic tests), for research purposes or for vaccine production. Virus isolation is much less commonly used for diagnostic purposes given the variety of other diagnostic methodologies that can be applied.

CAV was first grown in vitro by Yuasa[185] who tested a variety of cell lines. Based on his work, MDCC-MSB-1 cells, a Marek's disease virus transformed T cell line, in which CAV produces cytopathic effects (cpe), have become the most widely used cell line for CAV isolation. Some workers have suggested that this cell line does not support the growth of some strains of CAV.[18,137] MDCC-CU147 cells are susceptible to a wider range of CAV strains and produce higher virus yields.[18] Furthermore, variability in susceptibility between sub-lines of MSB1 cells has also been reported[137] as well as loss of susceptibility after long term passage of the cells.[18,170] Inoculated cell culture material is commonly sub-cultured up to 10 times to look for cpe[105] but van Santen et al.[170] in one study passed cultures up to 30 times and found that some isolates did not produce cpe or fail until somewhere between 11 and 30 passes. Presence of CAV in the culture needs to be confirmed by immunofluorescent staining (Fig. 18) or PCR-based tests. In fact, these tests can reveal the presence of CAV growth before cpe can be recognized. It was shown that qPCR performed at 2 weeks indicated accurately with only one exception, which cultures would eventually become positive for cpe or fail due to CAV growth.[170] Thus, these authors suggested that qPCR on cultures at two weeks could replace the need for repeated culture passages. Details of the growth method for CAV in cell culture can be found in the original report by Yuasa[184] but more detailed information is provided by McNulty and Todd.[105]

Recently, it has been shown that LSCC-BK3 (BK3) cells were as sensitive as MSB-1 cells for the 2 virus strains tested.[59] It has been suggested by these authors that use of BK3 might be advantageous in some circumstances as it supports the growth of some other avian viral pathogens, e.g. REV and IBDV. However, in other circumstances such as diagnostic reagent production or use in experimental infections, the possibility of isolating or propagating CAV, IBDV and/or REV together would cause complications.

CAV can grow in mononuclear cells isolated from spleen and bone marrow, with a 10-fold increase in titer at 48 hours. However, a 100-fold increase in titer was achieved in MSB-1 cells in 72 hours.[99] It has recently been reported that CAV can be grown in peripheral blood mononuclear cells.[90] However, since virus titers did not increase on passage, these are unlikely to be used unless appropriate cell lines are unavailable. These authors speculated that stimulation of the cells with Con-A may have improved the propagation of CAV.

Virus isolation can also be achieved by yolk sac inoculation of embryonated SPF chicken eggs and this test is offered by one company as a commercial service. Inoculation of day-old SPF chicks which lack maternally derived antibody to CAV may also be used to detect the presence of the agent.[105] The use of EBX chicks can further increase the sensitivity of virus isolation.[88] Inoculated chicks can be sacrificed and examined for the presence of antigen, and the presence of typical lesions. The presence of both confirms a pathogenic strain of CAV.

Control and prevention of CAV infection and disease

General

Commercial flocks

In commercial flocks, the most effective and safest method of control is to vaccinate breeding stock during the rearing period, to ensure that they have seroconverted before the onset of lay. However, many producers rely on natural exposure of flocks to induce immunity. Barbour et al.[7] compared the effect of natural exposure of a breeder flock to CAV to that of a similar flock vaccinated with a live vaccine in the drinking water. The progeny derived from eggs collected at 35, 40 and 45 weeks of age were also examined. No significant differences were found. In at least one large UK operation and many but not all breeder farms in the USA[151], a representative sample of birds would be bled during the rearing period to check for antibodies to CAV. If antibodies were not present, or were inconsistently present, or were at low levels, then those flocks could be vaccinated well before the onset of lay. The decision to vaccinate is often based on a cost-benefit analysis especially because the current CAV vaccines are relatively expensive.

SPF flocks

For control of CAV infection in SPF flocks, a different approach is needed, especially if the flocks or their eggs are being used to produce vaccines. For SPF flocks, it is best to try to remain CAV free. If an SPF flock becomes infected, it can be very difficult to eradicate CAV given the challenges posed for example by hens remaining seronegative through rearing and seroconverting as they come into production in the absence of apparent exposure (see Transmission in SPF Flocks). A key question is how many serum samples need to be tested to be sure that the flock is seronegative. Schat and Schukken[146] found that most if not all hens could be seronegative at 18 weeks with slowly increasing numbers of seropositive hens until 60 to 65 weeks of age. Their flock sizes were approximately 100 to 135 hens and with very low seroconversion rates, detection would not be possible with sampling only 10 to 20 percent of the hens. Thus, the SPF industry needs to carefully evaluate their sampling strategy to be confident that the flocks are seronegative. Should an SPF flock become infected, it may be possible to generate a new CAV free flock by the method described (see Transmission in SPF flocks).

Vaccination using currently available vaccines

Currently, all commercially available vaccines consist of live CAV viruses. Most of these vaccines are based on attenuated strains of CAV and are intended for use in breeding flocks during the rearing period. The vaccines are administrated using a variety of methods ranging from inclusion in drinking water to injection either by wing web, subcutaneous or intramuscular routes. There have been some concerns that the live vaccines have residual pathogenicity that might adversely affect performance, especially if administered to young birds. It has recently been confirmed that one of the live attenuated vaccines has pathogenic effects (see below) but the risks posed by this are likely less when used in pullets, than the risks posed by challenge with a wild type strain.[171] While a small percentage of vaccinated birds could potentially still transmit the virus (or DNA) vertically, the percentage is so low as to be of no apparent major consequence to commercial chicken production (see Transmission).

Successful vaccination of broilers has several challenges:

- Ease of vaccine administration to large numbers.
- Vaccinating in the presence of maternal antibodies.
- Having vaccines that are not immunosuppressive.

For use in newly hatched chicks, the United States Department of Agriculture (USDA) regulations require absence of pathology after administration to one-day-old SPF chickens. Recently, Vaziry et al.[171] reported that one of the live attenuated vaccines, while not causing anemia or thymic atrophy, has residual pathogenic effects. However, the severity of the effect was not compared to that caused by wild type CAV. Ultimately, studies of the economic benefit of vaccination of broilers with the live attenuated vaccine compared to the economic performance of naturally exposed flocks would be beneficial. At least one vaccine is currently available for vaccination of broilers, but it is not clear how commonly this vaccine is used in broilers.

Experimental vaccines, and novel approaches to CAV vaccination

A variety of candidate live and inactivated vaccines, DNA vaccines and vector vaccines (*Lactobacillus*, *Baculovirus*, plant-based and herpesvirus of turkey- or MDV-based) have been developed and tested experimentally to different degrees. However, these have not been used commercially. Testing the efficacy of experimental CAV vaccines for use in young birds poses significant problems. Typically an experimental vaccine is tested first in antibody-negative, one-day-old SPF chicks followed by challenge after 7 to 14 days. However, challenge at that time produces milder lesions in non-vaccinated controls and demonstration of efficacy is much more difficult. Schat et al.[147] therefore used differential qRT-PCR analysis to demonstrate that their experimental vaccine protected against challenge with a virus which differed in sequence from the vaccine virus. It is not clear, however, that licensing authorities would accept this approach. For testing vaccines intended for use in breeding birds, the breeding birds need to be vaccinated and then progeny derived at time points representative of the entire laying period need to be challenged and examined for protection.

Inactivated vaccines

Pages-Mante et al.[126] found good protection in progeny of breeders vaccinated subcutaneously with a single dose of a water/oil adjuvant vaccine containing inactivated virus. Protection of the progeny produced by flocks up to 40 weeks of age was complete. At 50 and 60 weeks, a small proportion of progeny was not fully protected although the authors speculated that in the field situation, naturally occurring exposure to CAV would serve to boost immunity in the breeders and thus extend the period of complete protection of progeny. While this vaccine looked encouraging, inactivated vaccines are not available commercially to our knowledge, most likely because production costs are very high.

Subunit and DNA vaccines

Both VP1 and VP2 need to be expressed in the same cell for the production of VN antibodies[82], as VP2 is needed to ensure correct conformational assembly of the neutralizing epitopes on VP1.[118] Due to the partially overlapping ORFs and the need to eliminate the apoptotic activity of VP3, it will be essential to mutate the start codon of VP3. Plasmids containing the CAV genome with the mutated VP3 start codon are unable to replicate in lymphoblastoid cells or in chickens (Jia and Schat, unpublished data). A crude lysate of cells infected with baculoviruses simultaneously expressing VP1 and VP2 and adjuvanted with Freund's complete adjuvant was administered once by intramuscular injection, and was found to produce VN antibodies. It was further shown that the progeny of breeding hens vaccinated with this vaccine at 32 weeks, were protected against CAV challenge.[82] Many of the newer vaccine prototypes described below have not been tested to date by such vaccination and challenge studies.

Other genetically engineered candidates have been produced, tested for induction of immune responses and proposed as vaccine candidates. For example, a DNA vaccine generated VN antibody responses with titers between 1:256 and 1:512 as well as antigen-specific responses of splenocytes and increased serum levels of IL-2, and IFN-γ.[112] The responses were enhanced by the addition of VP22 of MDV serotype 1.[111] However, these vaccines have not been tested for longevity of the response which would be very important if for example if the vaccine is used in breeder chickens. Neither have these candidate vaccines been tested by challenge of vaccinates or their progeny. Furthermore, induction of this response required three intramuscular injections. Such requirement for multiple immunizations is a major drawback of current DNA vaccine technology as it will not be practical or cost effective for use in large scale poultry operations.

The same group have also cloned VP1 and VP2 into *Escherichia coli,* purified the expressed proteins and adsorbed them onto the surface of *Lactobacillus acidophilus.* They administered the

L. acidophilus to chickens in feed for two five-day periods starting at 21 and 35 days of age, respectively. VN antibody titers of 1:128 to 1:252 as well as VP1-specific proliferative response of splenocytes and increased serum levels of IL-2, IL-12 and IFN-γ were reported. [113] This approach is interesting because it would be a more practical administration route for poultry. However, this prototype vaccine has not been tested for duration of response, nor by challenge of vaccinated chickens or their progeny.

Jia and Schat have tried unsuccessfully to vaccinate against CAV by using a serotype 1 MDV vaccine engineered to encode for CAV VP1 and VP2 (unpublished data quoted in Schat et al.).[147]

Engineered CAV strains

A CAV strain with a mutation in the enhancer/promoter region had reduced in vitro cytopathogenicity and was able to produce a neutralizing epitope in vitro. [119] The authors suggested that this could be a candidate attenuated vaccine. However, these strains were not tested in birds. VP2 mutants [129] were tested as potential vaccines in day-old chicks. [78] Some of the strains administered subcutaneously as vaccines at day-old were able to prevent loss of thymic cortex in birds challenged with a wild type strain at day 21. However, more work is required to test the VP2 mutants for reversion to virulence [78], and to test efficacy and duration of immunity in breeder birds. Also, if mutant strains do not grow as well in vitro or in vivo, the challenge of producing adequate quantities for commercial vaccine production becomes greater.

In ovo vaccination/immune complex

The possibility of an immune complex (IC) vaccine which might ultimately be administered in ovo was investigated by Schat et al. [147] In a feasibility study, they vaccinated chicks that had no maternally derived antibody at three days of age and challenged them with wild type virus. The vaccine was able to prevent replication of the challenge virus as determined by qRT-PCR. However, as recognized by the authors, the study needs to be extended to include vaccination of chicks which have maternally derived antibody. In this study, potential adverse effects of the wild type virus contained in the IC was assessed by examination of packed cell volumes and thymus weight:body weight ratio. Since the latter were affected, future studies could usefully include evaluation of thymus and immune functions in the vaccinated chickens in order to ascertain the net effect of the immune complex.

Treatment

There is no treatment for the virus infection itself. In theory, administration of nutritional supplements may help recovery from anemia. Antibiotics have been used strategically in the face of some clinical disease outbreaks to control secondary bacterial infections, and this was offered as the reason for the low average mortality (2 %) attributed to CAV during outbreaks in Northern Ireland. [95]

References

1. Adair, B. M., F. McNeilly, C. D. McConnell, D. Todd, R. T. Nelson, and M. S. McNulty. Effects of chicken anemia agent on lymphokine production and lymphocyte transformation in experimentally infected chickens. Avian Dis. 35:783-792. 1991.
2. Adair, B. M., F. McNeilly, C. D. McConnell, and M. S. McNulty. Characterization of surface markers present on cells infected by chicken anemia virus in experimentally infected chickens. Avian Dis. 37:943-950. 1993.
3. Adair, B. M. Immunopathogenesis of chicken anemia virus infection. Dev. Comp. Immunol. 24:247-255. 2000.
4. Allan, G. M., J. A. Smyth, D. Todd, and M. S. McNulty. In situ hybridization for the detection of chicken anemia virus in formalin-fixed, paraffin-embedded sections. Avian Dis. 37:177-182. 1993.
5. Amer, H. M., H. M. Elzahed, E. A. Elabiare, A. A. Badawy, and A. A. Yousef. An optimized polymerase chain reaction assay to identify avian virus vaccine contamination with chicken anemia virus. J. Vet. Diagn.Invest. 23:34-40. 2011.
6. Asiello, P. J., and A. J. Baeumner. Miniaturized isothermal nucleic acid amplification, a review. Lab. Chip 11:1420-1430. 2011.
7. Barbour, E. K., M. T. Farran, S. K. Hamadeh, M. Bouljihad, O. Faroon, and S. Kreydiyyeh. Comparative impact of live chicken infectious anaemia virus vaccine versus natural exposure in meat chicken breeders on immunity to infectivity by CIA and inclusion body hepatitis viruses in their offspring. Vet. Res. Commun. 26:397-405. 2002.
8. Biagini, P., M. Bendinelli, S. Hino, L. Kakkola, A. Mankertz, C. Niel, H. Okamoto, S. Raidal, C. C. Teo, and D. Todd. Family Circoviridae. In: Virus Taxonomy: Ninth Report of the International Committee on Taxonomy of Viruses. A. M. Q. King, E. Lefkowitz, M. J. Adams and E. B. Carstens, eds. Elsevier Science, Burlington. pp 343-349. 2011.
9. Biagini, P., S. Bédarida, M. Touinssi, V. Galicher, and P. de Micco. Human gyrovirus in healthy blood donors, France [letter]. Emerg Infect Dis [Internet]. 2013.
10. Bisgaard, M. An age related and breeder flock associated hemorrhagic disorder in Danish broilers. Nord. Vet. Med. 35:397-407. 1983.
11. Bougiouklis, P. A., M. Sofia, G. Brellou, I. Georgopoulou, C. Billinis, and I. Vlemmas. A clinical case of chicken infectious anemia disease and virus DNA detection in naturally infected broilers in Greece. Avian Dis. 51:639-642. 2007.
12. Bounous, D. I., M. A. Goodwin, R. L. Brooks, Jr., C. M. Lamichlane, R. P. Campagnoli, J. Brown, and D. B. Snyder. Immunosuppression and intracellular calcium signaling in splenocytes from chicks infected with chicken anemia virus, CL-1 isolate. Avian Dis. 39:135-140. 1995.
13. Box, P. G., H. C. Holmes, A. C. Bushell, and P. M. Finney. Impaired response to killed Newcastle disease vaccine in chicken possessing circulating antibody to chicken anaemia agent. Avian Pathol. 17:713-723. 1988.
14. Brentano, L., N. Mores, I. Wentz, D. Chandratilleke, and K. A. Schat. Isolation and identification of chicken infectious anemia virus in Brazil. Avian Dis. 35:793-800. 1991.
15. Brentano, L., S. Lazzarin, S. S. Bassi, T. A. Klein, and K. A. Schat, Detection of chicken anemia virus in the gonads and in the progeny of broiler breeder hens with high neutralizing antibody titers. Vet. Microbiol. 105:65-72. 2005.
16. Brown, H. K., G. F. Browning, P. C. Scott, and B. S. Crabb. Full-length infectious clone of a pathogenic Australian isolate of chicken anaemia virus. Aust. Vet. J. 78:637-640. 2000.
17. Calnek, B. W., R. W. Harris, C. Buscaglia, K. A. Schat, and B. Lucio. Relationship between the immunosuppressive potential and the pathotype of Marek's disease virus isolates. Avian Dis. 42:124-132. 1998.
18. Calnek, B. W., B. Lucio-Martinez, C. Cardona, R. W. Harris, K. A. Schat, and C. Buscaglia. Comparative susceptibility of Marek's disease cell lines to chicken infectious anemia virus. Avian Dis. 44:114-124. 2000.
19. Cardona, C., B. Lucio, P. O'Connell, J. Jagne, and K. A. Schat. Humoral immune responses to chicken infectious anemia virus in three strains of chickens in a closed flock. Avian Dis. 44:661-667. 2000.
20. Cardona, C. J., W. B. Oswald, and K. A. Schat. Distribution of chicken anaemia virus in the reproductive tissues of specific-pathogen-free chickens. J. Gen. Virol. 81:2067-2075. 2000.
21. Carlson, H. C., P. R. Sweeny, and J. M. Tokaryk. Demonstration of phagocytic and trephocytic activities of chicken thrombocytes by microscopy and vital staining techniques. Avian Dis. 12:700-715. 1968.
22. Caterina, K. M., S. Frasca, Jr., T. Girshick, and M. I. Khan. Development of a multiplex PCR for detection of avian adenovirus, avian reovirus, infectious bursal disease virus, and chicken anemia virus. Mol. Cell Probes 18:293-298. 2004.
23. Chettle, N. J., R. K. Eddy, P. J. Wyeth, and S. A. Lister. An outbreak of disease due to chicken anaemia agent in broiler chickens in England. Vet. Rec. 124:211-215. 1989.
24. Chowdhury, S. M. Z. H., A. R. Omar, I. Aini, M. Hair-Bejo, A. A. Jamaluddin, B. M. Md-Zain, and Y. Kono. Pathogenicity, sequence and phylogenetic analysis of Malaysian chicken anaemia virus obtained after low and high passages in MSB-1 cells. Arch. Virol. 148:2437 - 2448. 2003.
25. Chu, D. K. W., L. L. M. Poon, S. S. S. Chiu, K. H. Chan, E. M. Ng, I. Bauer, T. K. Cheung, I. H. Y. Ng, Y. Guan, D. Wang, and

J. S. M. Peiris. Characterization of a novel gyrovirus in human stool and chicken meat. J. Clin. Virol. 55:209-213. 2012.
26. Cloud, S. S., H. S. Lillehoj, and J. K. Rosenberger. Immune dysfunction following infection with chicken anemia agent and infectious bursal disease virus. I. Kinetic alterations of avian lymphocyte subpopulations. Vet. Immunol. Immunopathol. 34:337-352. 1992.
27. Cloud, S. S., J. K. Rosenberger, and H. S. Lillehoj. Immune dysfunction following infection with chicken anemia agent and infectious bursal disease virus. II. Alterations of in vitro lymphoproliferation and in vivo immune responses. Vet. Immunol. Immunopathol. 34:353-366. 1992.
28. Collisson, E. W., Jianwu, P., Dzielawa, J., Seo, S.H. Cytotoxic T lymphocytes are critical in the control of infectious bronchitis virus in poultry. Dev. Comp. Immunol. 24:187-200. 2000.
29. Danen-Van Oorschot, A. A., D. F. Fischer, J. M. Grimbergen, B. Klein, S. Zhuang, J. H. Falkenburg, C. Backendorf, P. H. Quax, A. J. Van der Eb, and M. H. Noteborn. Apoptin induces apoptosis in human transformed and malignant cells but not in normal cells. Proc. Natl. Acad. Sci. 94:5843-5847. 1997.
30. Davidson, I., E. Loeb, A. Lublin, I. Shkoda, and K. A. Schat. Assessment of various criteria to determine the chicken anemia virus pathogenicity in embryonated eggs and in day-old chicks. Curr. Top. Virol. 6:95-111. 2007.
31. Davidson, I., N. Artzi, I. Shkoda, A. Lublin, E. Loeb, and K. A. Schat. The contribution of feathers in the spread of chicken anemia virus. Virus Res. 132:152-159. 2008.
32. Davidson, I., I. Raibshtein, and A. Al-Touri. Quantitation of Marek's disease and chicken anemia viruses in organs of experimentally infected chickens and commercial chickens by multiplex real-time PCR. Avian Dis. 57:532-538. 2013.
33. De Boer, G. F., D. J. Van Roozelaar, R. J. Moormann, S. H. M. Jeurissen, J. C. van den Wijngaard, F. Hilbink, and G. Koch. Interaction between chicken anaemia virus and live Newcastle disease vaccine. Avian Pathol. 23:263-275. 1994.
34. De Herdt, P., G. Van den Bosch, R. Ducatelle, E. Uyttebroek, and C. Schrier Epidemiology and significance of chicken infectious anemia virus infections in broilers and broiler parents under nonvaccinated European circumstances. Avian Dis. 45:706-708. 2001.
35. Dos Santos, H. F., M. B. Knak, F. L. de Castro, J. Slongo, G. A. Ritterbusch, T. A. P. Klein, P. A. Esteves, A. D. Silva, I. M. Trevisol, E. A. W. Claassen, L. A. H. M. Cornelissen, M. Lovato, A. C. Franco, P. M. Roehe, and F. A. M. Rijsewijk. Variants of the recently discovered avian gyrovirus 2 are detected in Southern Brazil and The Netherlands. Vet. Microbiol. 155:230-236. 2012.
36. Douglas, A. J., K. Phenix, K. A. Mawhinney, D. Todd, D. P. Mackie, and W. L. Curran. Identification of a 24 kDa protein expressed by chicken anaemia virus. J. Gen. Virol. 76:1557-1562. 1995.
37. Dren, C., T. Farkas, and I. Nemeth. Serological survey on the prevalence of chicken anaemia virus infection in Hungarian chicken flocks. Vet. Microbiol. 50:7-16. 1996.
38. Drén, C. N., A. Kant, D. J. Van Roozelaar, L. Hartog, M. H. Noteborn, and G. Koch. Studies on the pathogenesis of chicken infectious anaemia virus infection in six-week-old SPF chickens. Acta Vet. Hung. 48:455-467. 2000.
39. Ducatez, M. F., A. A. Owoade, J. O. Abiola, and C. P. Muller. Molecular epidemiology of chicken anemia virus in Nigeria. Arch. Virol. 151:97-111. 2006.
40. Ducatez, M. F., H. Chen, Y. Guan, and C. P. Muller. Molecular epidemiology of chicken anemia virus (CAV) in South Eastern Chinese live birds markets. Avian Dis. 52:68-73. 2008.
41. Eltahir, Y., K. Qian, W. Jin, and A. Qin. Analysis of chicken anemia virus genome: evidence of intersubtype recombination. Virol. J. 8:512. 2011.
42. Eltahir, Y., K. Qian, W. Jin, P. Wang, and A. Qin. Molecular epidemiology of chicken anemia virus in commercial farms in China. Virol. J. 8:146. 2011.
43. Engström, B. E., and M. Luthman. Blue wing disease of chickens: signs, pathology and natural transmission. Avian Pathol. 13:1-12. 1984.
44. Engström, B. E. Blue wing disease of chickens. Isolation of avian reovirus and chicken anaemia agent. Avian Pathol. 17:23-32. 1988.
45. Engström, B. E., O. Fossum, and M. Luthman. Blue wing disease of chickens: Experimental infection with a Swedish isolate of chicken anaemia agent and an avian reovirus. Avian Pathol. 17:33-50. 1988.
46. Engström, B. E. Prevalence of antibody to chicken anaemia virus (CAV) in Swedish chicken breeding flocks correlated to outbreaks of blue wing disease (BWD) in their progeny. Acta Vet. Scand. 40:97-107. 1999.
47. Eterradossi, N., and Y. M. Saif. Infectious bursal disease. In: Diseases of Poultry, 12 ed. Y. M. Saif, A. M. Fadly, J. R. Glisson, L. R. McDougald, L. K. Nolan and D. E. Swayne, eds. Wiley-Blackwell, Ames. pp 187-210. 2008.
48. Fehler, F., and C. Winter. CAV infection in older chickens: an apathogenic infection? In: Proceedings of the Second International Symposium on Infectious Bursal Disease and Chicken Infectious Anaemia. Rauischholzhausen, Germany. pp 391-394. 2001.
49. Goodwin, M. A., M. A. Smeltzer, J. Brown, T. Girshick, B. L. McMurray, and S. McCarter. Effect of so-called chicken anemia agent maternal antibody on chick serologic conversion to viruses in the field. Avian Dis. 37:542-545. 1993.

50. Goryo, M., H. Sugimura, S. Matsumoto, T. Umemura, and C. Itakura. Isolation of an agent inducing chicken anaemia. Avian Pathol. 14:483-496. 1985.
51. Goryo, M., Y. Shibata, T. Suwa, T. Umemura, and C. Itakura. Outbreak of anemia associated with chicken anemia agent in young chicks. Jpn. J. Vet. Sci. 49:867-873. 1987.
52. Goryo, M., S. Hayashi, K. Yoshizawa, T. Umemura, C. Itakura, and S. Yamashiro. Ultrastructure of the thymus in chicks inoculated with chicken anaemia agent (MSB1-TK5803 strain). Avian Pathol. 18:605-617. 1989.
53. Goryo, M., T. Suwa, T. Umemura, C. Itakura, and S. Yamashiro. Ultrastructure of bone marrow in chicks inoculated with chicken anaemia agent (MSB1-TK5803 strain). Avian Pathol. 18:329-343. 1989.
54. Goryo, M., T. Suwa, T. Umemura, C. Itakura, and S. Yamashiro. Histopathology of chicks inoculated with chicken anaemia agent (MSB1-TK5803 strain). Avian Pathol. 18:73-89. 1989.
55. Gürel, A., and B. Kusçu. Immuno-histopathologic lesions in organs other than the thymus and bone marrow during the course of experimentally-induced chicken infectious anaemia (CIA) disease. Turkish J. Vet. Animal Sci. 32:369-377. 2008.
56. Hagood, L. T., T. F. Kelly, J. C. Wright, and F. J. Hoerr. Evaluation of chicken infectious anemia virus and associated risk factors with disease and production losses in broilers. Avian Dis. 44:803-808. 2000.
57. Hailemariam, Z., A. R. Omar, M. Hair-Bejo, and T. C. Giap. Detection and characterization of chicken anemia virus from commercial broiler breeder chickens. Virol. J. 5:128-138. 2008.
58. Haridy, M., M. Goryo, J. Sasaki, and K. Okada. Pathological and immunohistochemical study of chickens with co-infection of Marek's disease virus and chicken anemia virus. Avian Pathol. 38:469-483. 2009.
59. Haridy, M., M. Goryo, J. Sasaki, and K. Okada. Comparative susceptibility of some avian and mammalian lymphoblastoid cell lines to chicken anemia virus. J. Vet. Med. Sci. 72:1637-1641. 2010.
60. Haridy, M., J. Sasaki, M. Ikezawa, K. Okada, and M. Goryo. Pathological and immunohistochemical studies of subclinical infection of chicken anemia virus in 4-week-old chickens. J. Vet. Med. Sci. 74:757-764. 2012.
61. He, C.-Q., N.-Z. Ding, W. Fan, Y.-H. Wu, J.-P. Li, and Y.-I. Li. Identification of chicken anemia virus putative intergenotype recombinants. Virology 366:1-7. 2007.
62. Hoerr, F. J. Clinical aspects of immunosuppression in poultry. Avian Dis. 54:2-15. 2010.
63. Hoop, R. K., and R. L. Reece. The use of immunofluorescence and immunoperoxidase staining in studying the pathogenesis of chicken anaemia agent in experimentally infected chickens. Avian Pathol. 20:349-355. 1991.
64. Hoop, R. K. Persistence and vertical transmission of chicken anaemia agent in experimentally infected laying hens. Avian Pathol. 21:493-501. 1992.
65. Hoop, R. K. Transmission of chicken anaemia virus with semen. Vet. Rec. 133:551-552. 1993.
66. Hu, L.-b., B. Lucio, and K. A. Schat. Abrogation of age-related resistance to chicken infectious anemia by embryonal bursectomy. Avian Dis. 37:157-169. 1993.
67. Hu, L.-b., B. Lucio, and K. A. Schat. Depletion of CD4+ and CD8+ T lymphocyte subpopulations by CIA-1, a chicken infectious anemia virus. Avian Dis. 37:492-500. 1993.
68. Huang, C. H., G. H. Lai, M. S. Lee, W. H. Lin, Y. Y. Lien, S. C. Hsueh, J. Y. Kao, W. T. Chang, T. C. Lu, W. N. Lin, and H. J. Chen. Development and evaluation of a loop-mediated isothermal amplification assay for rapid detection of chicken anaemia virus. J. Appl. Microbiol. 108:917-924. 2010.
69. Imai, K., and N. Yuasa. Development of a microtest method for serological and virological examinations of chicken anemia agent. Nippon Juigaku Zasshi 52:873-875. 1990.
70. Imai, K., S. Mase, K. Tsukamoto, H. Hihara, T. Matsumura, and N. Yuasa. A long term observation of antibody status to chicken anaemia virus in individual chickens of breeder flocks. Res. Vet. Sci. 54:392-396. 1993.
71. Imai, K., M. Mase, S. Yamaguchi, N. Yuasa, and K. Nakamura. Detection of chicken anaemia virus DNA from formalin-fixed tissues by polymerase chain reaction. Res. Vet. Sci. 64:205-208. 1998.
72. Imai, K., M. Mase, K. Tsukamoto, H. Hihara, and N. Yuasa. Persistent infection with chicken anaemia virus and some effects of highly virulent infectious bursal disease virus infection on its persistency. Res. Vet. Sci. 67:233-238. 1999.
73. Jeurissen, S. H., M. E. Janse, D. J. Van Roozelaar, G. Koch, and G. F. De Boer. Susceptibility of thymocytes for infection by chicken anemia virus is related to pre- and posthatching development. Dev. Immunol. 2:123-129. 1992.
74. Jeurissen, S. H., and G. F. de Boer. Chicken anaemia virus influences the pathogenesis of Marek's disease in experimental infections, depending on the dose of Marek's disease virus. Vet. Q. 15:81-84. 1993.
75. Joiner, K. S., S. J. Ewald, F. J. Hoerr, V. L. van Santen, and H. Toro. Oral infection with chicken anemia virus in 4-wk broiler breeders: lack of effect of major histocompatibility B complex genotype. Avian Dis. 49:482-487. 2005.
76. Jorgensen, P. H. A. micro-scale serum neutralisation test for the detection and titration of antibodies to chicken anaemia agent - prevalence of antibodies in Danish chickens. Avian Pathol. 19:583-593. 1990.
77. Jorgensen, P. H., L. Otte, O. L. Nielsen, and M. Bisgaard. Influence of subclinical infections and other factors on broiler performance. Br. Poult. Sci. 36:455-463. 1995.

78. Kaffashi, A., S. Shrestha, and G. F. Browning. Evaluation of chicken anaemia virus mutants as potential vaccine strains in 1-day-old chickens Avian Pathol. 37:109-114. 2008.
79. Kaiser, P., and P. Stäheli Avian cytokines and chemokines. In: Avian Immunology, 2 ed. K. A. Schat, B. Kaspers and P. Kaiser, eds. Academic Press/Elsevier, London. pp 189-204. 2013.
80. Kamada, K., A. Kuroishi, T. Kamahora, P. Kabat, S. Yamaguchi, and S. Hino. Spliced mRNAs detected during the life cycle of chicken anemia virus. J. Gen. Virol. 87:2227-2233. 2006.
81. Kim, I. J., S. K. You, H. Kim, H. Y. Yeh, and J. M. Sharma. Characteristics of bursal T lymphocytes induced by infectious bursal disease virus. J. Virol. 74:8884-8892. 2000.
82. Koch, G., D. J. van Roozelaar, C. A. Verschueren, A. J. van der Eb, and M. H. Noteborn. Immunogenic and protective properties of chicken anaemia virus proteins expressed by baculovirus. Vaccine 13:763-770. 1995.
83. Kumar, V., A. K. Abbas, J. C. Aster, and N. Fausto Robbins and Cotran Pathologic Basis of Disease, 8 ed. Saunders/Elsevier, Phialdelphia, PA. 2010.
84. Kurian, A., E. J. Neumann, W. F. Hall, and D. Marks. Effects of blood sample mishandling on ELISA results for infectious bronchitis virus, avian encephalomyelitis virus and chicken anaemia virus. Vet. J. 192:378-381. 2012.
85. Kuscu, B., and A. Gürel. Lesions in the thymus and bone marrow in chicks experimentally induced chciken infectious anemia disease. J. Vet. Sci. 9:15-23. 2008.
86. Lamichhane, C. M., D. B. Snyder, M. A. Goodwin, S. A. Mengel, J. Brown, and T. G. Dickson. Pathogenicity of CL-1 chicken anemia agent. Avian Dis. 35:515-522. 1991.
87. Li, Y. P. and Z. Z. Cui. Pathogenicity and genomic sequence comparison of a chicken infectious anemia virus field isolate. Wei Sheng Wu Hsueh Pao 47:894-898. 2007.
88. Lucio, B., K. A. Schat, and H. L. Shivaprasad. Identification of the chicken anemia agent, reproduction of the disease, and serological survey in the United States. Avian Dis. 34:146-153. 1990.
89. Lucio, B., K. A. Schat, and S. Taylor. Direct binding of protein A, protein G, and anti-IgG conjugates to chicken infectious anemia virus. Avian Dis. 35:180-185. 1991.
90. Manoharan, S., E. T. Jayalakshmi, and K. Kumanan. In vitro propagation of chicken anemia virus in chicken peripheral blood mononuclear cells. Acta Virol. 56:155-157. 2012.
91. Markowski-Grimsrud, C. J., M. M. Miller, and K. A. Schat. Development of strain-specific real-time PCR and RT-PCR assays for quantitation of chicken anemia virus. J. Virol. Meth. 101:135-147. 2002.
92. Markowski-Grimsrud, C. J., and K. A. Schat. Infection with chicken anemia virus impairs the generation of antigen-specific cytotoxic T lymphocytes. Immunology 109:283-294. 2003.
93. McConnell, C. D., B. M. Adair, and M. S. McNulty. Effects of chicken anemia virus on cell-mediated immune function in chickens exposed to the virus by a natural route. Avian Dis. 37:366-374. 1993.
94. McConnell, C. D., B. M. Adair, and M. S. McNulty. Effects of chicken anemia virus on macrophage function in chickens. Avian Dis. 37:358-365. 1993.
95. McIlroy, S. G., M. S. McNulty, D. W. Bruce, J. A. Smyth, E. A. Goodall, and M. J. Alcorn. Economic effects of clinical chicken anemia agent infection on profitable broiler production. Avian Dis. 36:566-574. 1992.
96. McMahon, J., and S. McQuaid. The use of microwave irradiation as a pretreatment to in situ hybridization for the detection of measles virus and chicken anaemia virus in formalin-fixed paraffin-embedded tissue. Histochem. J. 28:157-164. 1996.
97. McNamee, P. T., J. J. McCullagh, J. D. Rodgers, B. H. Thorp, H. J. Ball, T. J. Connor, D. McConaghy, and J. A. Smyth. Development of an experimental model of bacterial chondronecrosis with osteomyelitis in broilers following exposure to Staphylococcus aureus by aerosol, and inoculation with chicken anaemia and infectious bursal disease viruses. Avian Pathol. 28:26-35. 1999.
98. McNeilly, F., G. M. Allan, D. Moffett, and M. S. McNulty. Detection of chicken anaemia agent in chickens by immunofluorescence and immunoperoxidase staining. Avian Pathol. 20:125-132. 1991.
99. McNeilly, F., B. M. Adair, and M. S. McNulty. In vitro infection of mononuclear cells derived from various chicken lymphoid tissues by chicken anaemia virus. Avian Pathol. 23:547-556. 1994.
100. McNeilly, F., J. A. Smyth, B. M. Adair, and M. S. McNulty. Synergism between chicken anemia virus (CAV) and avian reovirus following dual infection of 1-day-old chicks by a natural route. Avian Dis. 39:532-537. 1995.
101. McNulty, M. S., T. J. Connor, and F. McNeilly. Influence of virus dose on experimental anaemia due to chicken anaemia agent. Avian Pathol. 19:161-171. 1990.
102. McNulty, M. S., W. L. Curran, D. Todd, and D. P. Mackie. Chicken anemia agent: an electron microscopic study. Avian Dis. 34:736-743. 1990.
103. McNulty, M. S. Chicken anemia agent: a review. Avian Pathol. 20:187-203. 1991.
104. McNulty, M. S., S. G. McIlroy, D. W. Bruce, and D. Todd. Economic effects of subclinical chicken anemia agent infection in broiler chickens. Avian Dis. 35:263-268. 1991.
105. McNulty, M. S., and D. Todd. Chicken anemia virus. In: A laboratory manual for the isolation and identification of avian pathogens 5th ed. L. Dufour-Zavala, D. E. Swayne, J. R. Glisson, J. E. Pearson, W. M. Reed, M. W. Jackwood and P. R. Woolcock,

eds. American Association of Avian Pathologists, Jacksonville, FL. pp 124-127. 2008.

106. Miles, A. M., S. M. Reddy, and R. W. Morgan. Coinfection of specific-pathogen-free chickens with Marek's disease virus (MDV) and chicken infectious anemia virus: effect of MDV pathotype. Avian Dis. 45:9-18. 2001.
107. Miller, M. M., W. B. Oswald, J. Scarlet, and K. A. Schat. Patterns of chicken infectious anemia virus (CIAV) seroconversion in three Cornell SPF flocks. In: Proceedings of the Second International Symposium on infectious bursal disease and chicken infectious anaemia. Institut fur Geflugelkrankheiten, Justus Liebig University, Giessen, Germany, Rauischholzhausen, Germany. pp 410-417. 2001.
108. Miller, M. M., K. A. Ealey, W. B. Oswald, and K. A. Schat. Detection of chicken anemia virus DNA in embryonal tissues and eggshell membranes. Avian Dis 47:662-671. 2003.
109. Miller, M. M., K. J. Jarosinski, and K. A. Schat. Positive and negative regulation of chicken anemia virus transcription. J. Virol. 79:2859-2868. 2005.
110. Miller, M. M., K. W. Jarosinski, and K. A. Schat. Negative modulation of the chicken infectious anemia virus promoter by COUP-TF1 and an E box-like element at the transcription start site binding δEF1. J. Gen. Virol. 89:2998-3003. 2008.
111. Moeini, H., A. Omar, R. Rahim, and K. Yusoff. Improving the potency of DNA vaccine against chicken anemia virus (CAV) by fusing VP1 protein of CAV to Marek's disease virus (MDV) type-1 VP22 protein. Virol. J. 8:119. 2011.
112. Moeini, H., A. R. Omar, R. A. Rahim, and K. Yusoff. Development of a DNA vaccine against chicken anemia virus by using a bicistronic vector expressing VP1 and VP2 proteins of CAV. Comp. Immunol. Microbiol. Infect. Dis. 34:227-236. 2011.
113. Moeini, H., R. Rahim, A. Omar, N. Shafee, and K. Yusoff. *Lactobacillus acidophilus* as a live vehicle for oral immunization against chicken anemia virus. Appl. Microbiol. Biotechnol. 90:77-88. 2011.
114. Natesan, S., J. M. Kataria, K. Dhama, N. Bhardwaj, and A. Sylvester. Anti-neoplastic effect of chicken anemia virus VP3 protein (apoptin) in Rous sarcoma virus-induced tumours in chicken. J. Gen. Virol. 87:2933-2940. 2006.
115. Nayabian, H., and K. Mardani. Molecular characterization of the chicken anaemia viruses isolated from broiler farms of west Azerbaijan, Iran. Avian Pathol. 42:108-113. 2013.
116. Nielsen, O. L., P. H. Jørgensen, M. Bisgaard, and S. Alexandersen. In situ hybridization for the detection of chicken anaemia virus in experimentally-induced infection and field outbreaks. Avian Pathol. 24:149-155. 1995.
117. Noteborn, M. H., D. Todd, C. A. Verschueren, H. W. de Gauw, W. L. Curran, S. Veldkamp, A. J. Douglas, M. S. McNulty, A. J. van der Eb, and G. Koch. A single chicken anemia virus protein induces apoptosis. J. Virol. 68:346-351. 1994.
118. Noteborn, M. H., C. A. Verschueren, G. Koch, and A. J. Van der Eb. Simultaneous expression of recombinant baculovirus-encoded chicken anaemia virus (CAV) proteins VP1 and VP2 is required for formation of the CAV-specific neutralizing epitope. J. Gen. Virol. 79:3073-3077. 1998.
119. Noteborn, M. H., C. A. Verschueren, H. van Ormondt, and A. J. van der Eb. Chicken anemia virus strains with a mutated enhancer/promoter region share reduced virus spread and cytopathogenicity. Gene 223:165-172. 1998.
120. Novak, R., and W. L. Ragland. In situ hybridization for detection of chicken anaemia virus in peripheral blood smears. Mol. Cell Probes 11:135-141. 1997.
121. Otaki, Y., T. Nunoya, A. Tajima, A. Kato, and Y. Nomura. Depression of vaccinal immunity to Marek's disease by infection with chicken anaemia agent. Avian Pathol. 17:333-347. 1988.
122. Otaki, Y., T. Nunoya, A. Tajima, A. Kato, K. Saito, and O. Nomura. Chicken anemia virus as a possible cause of Marek's disease vaccination failures. In: Advances in Marek's disease research. S. Kato, T. Horiuchi, T. Mikami and K. Hirai, eds. Japanese Association on Marek's Disease, Osaka. pp 364-366. 1988.
123. Otaki, Y., M. Tajima, K. Saito, and Y. Nomura. Immune response of chicks inoculated with chicken anemia agent alone or in combination with Marek's disease virus or turkey herpesvirus. Jpn. J. Vet. Sci. 50:1040-1047. 1988.
124. Otaki, Y., K. Saito, A. Tajima, and Y. Nomura. Detection of antibody to chicken anaemia agent: a comparison of three serological tests. Avian Patho.l 20:315-324. 1991.
125. Otaki, Y., K. Saito, M. Tajima, and Y. Nomura Persistence of maternal antibody to chicken anaemia agent and its effect on the susceptibility of young chickens. Avian Pathol. 21:147-151. 1992.
126. Pagès-Manté, A., N. Saubi, C. Artigas, and E. Espuña. Experimental evaluation of an inactivated vaccine against chicken anaemia virus. Avian Pathol. 26:721-729. 1997.
127. Peters, M. A., D. C. Jackson, B. S. Crabb, and G. F. Browning. Chicken anemia virus VP2 is a novel dual specificity protein phosphatase. J. Biol. Chem. 42:39566-39573. 2002.
128. Peters, M. A., B. S. Jackson, B. S. Crabb, and G. F. Browning Mutation of chicken anemia virus VP2 differentially affects serine/threonine and tyrosine protein phosphatase activities. J Gen Virol 86:623-630. 2005.
129. Peters, M. A., B. S. Crabb, E. A. Washington, and G. F. Browning. Site-directed mutagenesis of the VP2 gene of chicken anemia virus affects virus replication, cytopathology and host-cell MHC class I expression. J. Gen. Virol 87:823-831. 2006.
130. Peters, M. A., B. S. Crabb, K. A. Tivendale, and G. F. Browning. Attenuation of chicken anemia virus by site-directed mutagenesis of VP2. J. Gen. Virol. 88:2168-2175. 2007.
131. Phan, T. G., L. Li, M. G. O'Ryan, H. Cortes, N. Mamani, I. J. O. Bonkoungou, C. Wang, C. M. Leutenegger, and E. Delwart. A

third gyrovirus species in human faeces. J. Gen. Virol. 93:1356-1361. 2012.

132. Pope, C. R. Chicken anemia agent. Vet. Immunol. Immunopathol 30:51-65. 1991.

133. Prasetyo, A. A., T. Kamahora, A. Kuroishi, K. Murakami, and S. Hino. Replication of chicken anemia virus (CAV) requires apoptin and is complemented by VP3 of human torque teno virus (TTV). Virology 385:85-92. 2009.

134. Rautenschlein, S., H. Y. Yeh, M. K. Njenga, and J. M. Sharma. Role of intrabursal T cells in infectious bursal disease virus (IBDV) infection: T cells promote viral clearance but delay follicular recovery. Arch. Virol. 147:285-304. 2002.

135. Rautenschlein, S., H. Y. Yeh, and J. M. Sharma The role of T cells in protection by an inactivated infectious bursal disease virus vaccine. Vet. Immunol. Immunopathol. 89:159-167. 2002.

136. Rehman, L., B. Sultan, I. Ali, M. Bhatti, S. Khan, K. Zaman, A. Jahangiri, N. Khan, A. Iqbal, J. Bakht, Z. Swati, and M. Rehman. Duplex PCR assay for the detection of avian adeno virus and chicken anemia virus prevalent in Pakistan. Virol. J. 8:440. 2011.

137. Renshaw, R. W., C. Soine, T. Weinkle, P. H. O'Connell, K. Ohashi, S. Watson, B. Lucio, S. Harrington, and K. A. Schat. A hypervariable region in VP1 of chicken infectious anemia virus mediates rate of spread and cell tropism in tissue culture. J. Virol. 70:8872-8878. 1996.

138. Rijsewijk, F., H. dos Santos, T. Teixeira, S. Cibulski, A. Varela, D. Dezen, A. Franco, and P. Roehe. Discovery of a genome of a distant relative of chicken anemia virus reveals a new member of the genus Gyrovirus. Arch. Virol. 156:1097-1100. 2011.

139. Rosenberger, J. K., S. Klopp, R. J. Eckroade, and W. C. Krauss. The roles of the infectious bursal agent and several avian adenoviruses in the hemorrhagic-aplastic-anemia syndrome and gangrenous dermatitis. Avian Dis. 19:717-729. 1975.

140. Rosenberger, J. K., and S. S. Cloud.The effects of age, route of exposure, and coinfection with infectious bursal disease virus on the pathogenicity and transmissibility of chicken anemia agent (CAA). Avian Dis. 33:753-759. 1989.

141. Rosenberger, J. K., and S. S. Cloud. The isolation and characterization of chicken anemia agent (CAA) from broilers in the United States. Avian Dis. 33:707-713. 1989.

142. Sander, J., R. Williams, R. Novak, and W. Ragland. In situ hybridization on blood smears for diagnosis of chicken anemia virus in broiler breeder flocks. Avian Dis. 41:988-992. 1997.

143. Sauvage, V., J. Cheval, V. Foulongne, M. A. Gouilh, K. Pariente, J. C. Manuguerra, J. Richardson, O. Dereure, M. Lecuit, A. Burguiere, V. Caro, and M. Eloit. Identification of the first human gyrovirus, a virus related to chicken anemia virus. J. Virol. 85:7948-7950. 2011.

144. Schat, K. A., and V. Van Santen. Chicken infectious anemia. In: Diseases of Poultry, 12 ed. Y. M. Saif, A. M. Fadly, J. R. Glisson, L. R. McDougald, L. K. Nolan and D. E. Swayne, eds. Wiley-Blackwell. pp 211-235. 2008.

145. Schat, K. A. Chicken anemia virus. Curr.Top. Microbiol. Immunol. 331:151-184. 2009.

146. Schat, K. A., and Y. H. Schukken. An 8-year longitudinal survey for the presence of antibodies to chicken infectious anemia virus in two specific-pathogen-free strains of chickens. Avian Dis. 54:46-52. 2010.

147. Schat, K. A., N. Rodrigo da Silva Martins, P. H. O'Connell, and M. S. Piepenbrink. Immune complex vaccines for chicken infectious anemia virus Avian Dis. 55:90-96. 2011.

148. Schrier, C. C., and H. J. M. Jagt. Chicken anemia viruses of low pathogenicity. In: US patent 6,723,324. Akzo Nobel NV, USA. 2004.

149. Seo, S. H., and E. W. Collisson. Specific cytotoxic T lymphocytes are involved in in vivo clearance of infectious bronchitis virus. J. Virol. 71:5173-5177. 1997.

150. Sheela, R. R., U. Babu, J. Mu, S. Elankumaran, D. A. Bautista, R. B. Raybourne, R. A. Heckert, and W. Song. Immune responses against Salmonella enterica serovar enteritidis infection in virally immunosuppressed chickens. Clin. Diagn. Lab. Immunol. 10:670-679. 2003.

151. Smith, J. A. Impact of subclinical immunosuppression on poultry production. In: Impact of subclinical immunosuppression on poultry production. R. F.Silva, A. M. Fadly, D. J. Jackwood and K. A. Schat, eds. American Association of Avian Pathologists, Jacksonville, FL. pp 42-48. 2006.

152. Smyth, J. A., D. A. Moffett, M. S. McNulty, D. Todd, and D. P. Mackie. A sequential histopathologic and immunocytochemical study of chicken anemia virus infection at one day of age. Avian Dis. 37:324-338. 1993.

153. Smyth, J. A., D. A. Moffett, T. J. Connor, and M. S. McNulty. Chicken anaemia virus inoculated by the oral route causes lymphocyte depletion in the thymus in 3-week-old and 6-week-old chickens. Avian Pathol. 35:254-259. 2006.

154. Soiné , C., S. K. Watson, E. Rybicki, B. Lucio, R. M. Nordgren, C. R. Parrish, and K. A. Schat. Determination of the detection limit of the polymerase chain reaction for chicken infectious anemia virus. Avian Dis. 37:467-476. 1993.

155. Sommer, F., and C. Cardona. Chicken anemia virus in broilers: Dynamics of the infection in two commercial broiler flocks. Avian Dis. 47:1466-1473. 2003.

156. Spackman, E., S. S. Cloud, and J. K. Rosenberger. Comparison of a putative second serotype of chicken infectious anemia virus with a prototypical isolate. II. Antigenic and physicochemical characteristics. Avian Dis. 46:956–963. 2002.

157. Tan, J., and G. A. Tannock. Role of viral load in the pathogenesis of chicken anemia virus. J. Gen. Virol. 86:1327-1333. 2005.

158. Taniguchi, T., N. Yuasa, M. Maeda, and T. Horiuchi. Hematopathological changes in dead and moribund chicks induced by

chicken anemia agent. Natl. Inst. Anim. Health Q. (Jpn.) 22:61-69. 1982.

159. Taniguchi, T., N. Yuasa, M. Maeda, and T. Horiuchi. Chronological observations on hemato-pathological changes in chicks inoculated with chicken anemia agent. Natl. Inst. Anim. Health. Q. (Jpn.) 23:1-12. 1983.
160. Taylor, S. P. The effect of acetone on the viability of chicken anemia agent. Avian Dis. 36:753-754. 1992.
161. Todd, D., J. L. Creelan, and M. S. McNulty. Dot blot hybridization assay for chicken anemia agent using a cloned DNA probe. J. Clin. Microbiol .29:933-939. 1991.
162. Todd, D. Circoviruses: immunosuppressive threats to avian species: a review. Avian Pathol. 29:373-394. 2000.
163. Toro, H., A. M. Ramirez, and J. Larenas..Pathogenicity of chicken anaemia virus (isolate 10343) for young and older chickens. Avian Pathol. 26:485-499. 1997.
164. Toro, H., C. Gonzalez, L. Cerda, M. Hess, E. Reyes, and C. Geissea. Chicken anemia virus and fowl adenoviruses: association to induce the inclusion body hepatitis/ hydropericardium syndrome. Avian Dis. 44:51-58. 2000.
165. Toro, H., S. Ewald, and F. J. Hoerr Serological evidence of chicken infectious anemia virus in the United States at least since 1959. Avian Dis. 50:124-126. 2006.
166. Urlings, H. A., G. F. de Boer, D. J. van Roozelaar, and G. Koch. Inactivation of chicken anaemia virus in chickens by heating and fermentation. Vet. Q. 15:85-88. 1993.
167. Van Ginkel, F. W., V. L. van Santen, S. L. Gulley, and H. Toro. Infectious bronchitis virus in the chicken Harderian gland and lachrymal fluid: viral load, infectivity, immune cell responses, and effects of viral immunodeficiency. Avian Dis. 52:608-617. 2008.
168. van Santen, V. L., L. Li, F. J. Hoerr, and L. H. Lauerman. Genetic characterization of chicken anemia virus from commercial broiler chickens in Alabama. Avian Dis. 45:373-388. 2001.
169. van Santen, V. L., B. Kaltenboeck, K. S. Joiner, K. S. Macklin, and R. A. Norton. Real-time quantitative PCR-based serum neutralization test for detection and titration of neutralizing antibodies to chicken anemia virus. J. Virol. Meth. 115:123-135. 2004.
170. van Santen, V. L., H. Toro, and F. J. Hoerr .Biological characteristics of chicken anemia virus regenerated from clinical specimen by PCR. Avian Dis. 51:66-77. 2007.
171. Vaziry, A., A. Silim, C. Bleau, D. Frenette, and L. Lamontagne. Chicken infectious anaemia vaccinal strain persists in the spleen and thymus of young chicks and induces thymic lymphoid cell disorders. Avian Pathol. 40:377-385. 2011.
172. Vielitz, E., and H. Landgraf. Anaemia-dermatitis of broilers: Field observations on its occurrence, transmission and prevention. Avian Pathol. 17:113-120. 1988.
173. von Bülow, V., B. Fuchs, E. Vielitz, and H. Landgraf. [Early mortality syndrome in chickens following double infection with Marek's disease virus and chicken anemia agent]. Zentralbl. Veterinarmed. B. 30:742-750. 1983.
174. von Bülow, V., B. Fuchs, and M. Bertram. Untersuchungen über den Erreger der infektiösen Anämie bei Hühnerküken (CAA) in vitro: Vermehrung, Titration, Serumneutralisationstest in indirekter Immunfluoreszentest. Zentralbl. Veterinarmed. B. 32:679-693. 1985.
175. von Bülow, V., R. Rudolph, and B. Fuchs. Folgen der Doppelinfektion von Küken mit Adenovirus oder Reovirus und dem Erreger der aviären infektiösen Anämie (CAA). Zentralbl. Veterinarmed. B. 33:717-726. 1986.
176. von Bülow, V., R. Rudolph, and B. Fuchs. Erhöhte Pathogenität des Erregers der aviären infektiösen Anämia bei Hühnerküken (CAA) bei simultaner Infektion mit Virus der Marekschen Krankheit (MDV), Bursitisvirus (IBDV) oder Reticuloendotheliosevirus (REV). J. Vet. Med. B. 33:93-116. 1986.
177. von Bülow, V., and Witt, M. Propagation of chicken anaemia agent in chicken embryos. Journal of Veterinary Medicine, B (Infectious Diseases, Immunology, Food Hygiene, Veterinary Public Health) 33:664-669. 1986.
178. von Bülow, V. Unsatisfactory sensitivity and specificity of indirect immunofluorescence tests for the presence or absence of antibodies to chicken anaemia agent (CAA) in sera of SPF and broiler breeder chickens. Zentralbl. Veterinarmed. B. 35:594-600. 1988.
179. von Weikel, J., P. Dorn, H. Spiess, and E. Wessling. Ein Beitrag zur Diagnostik und Epidemiologie der infektiösen Anaemia (CAA) beim Broiler. Berl. Münch. Tierärztl. Wschr. 99:119-121. 1986.
180. Witter, R. L., I. M. Gimeno, A. R. Pandiri, and A. M. Fadly. Tumor Diagnosis Manual: The Differential Diagnosis of Lymphoid and Myeloid Tumors in the Chicken. Amercian Association of Avian Pathologists, Jacksonville, FL. 2010.
181. Yuasa, N., T. Taniguchi, and I. Yoshida. Isolation and some characteristics of an agent inducing anemia in chicks. Avian Dis. 23:366-385. 1979.
182. Yuasa, N., T. Noguchi, K. Furuta, and I. Yoshida. Maternal antibody and its effect on the susceptibility of chicks to chicken anemia agent. Avian Dis. 24:197-201. 1980.
183. Yuasa, N., T. Taniguchi, T. Noguchi, and I. Yoshida Effect of infectious bursal disease virus infection on incidence of anemia by chicken anemia agent. Avian Dis. 24:202-209. 1980.
184. Yuasa, N. Propagation and infectivity titration of the Gifu-1 strain of chicken anemia agent in a cell line (MDCC-MSB1) derived from Marek's disease lymphoma. Natl. Inst. Anim. Health Q. (Jpn.) 23:13-20. 1983.
185. Yuasa, N., T. Taniguchi, M. Goda, M. Shibatani, T. Imada, and H. Hihara. Isolation of chicken anemia agent with MDCC-MSB1 cells from chickens in the field. Natl. Inst. Anim. Health Q. (Jpn.) 23:75-77. 1983.

186. Yuasa, N., T. Taniguchi, T. Imada, and H. Hihara. Distribution of chicken anemia agent (CAA) and detection of neutralizing antibody in chicks experimentally inoculated with CAA. Natl Inst. Anim. Health Q. (Jpn.) 23:78-81. 1983.
187. Yuasa, N., and I. Yoshida. Experimental egg transmission of chicken anemia agent. Natl. Inst. Anim. Health Q. (Jpn.) 23:99-100. 1983.
188. Yuasa, N., K. Imai, and H. Tezuka. Survey of antibody against chicken anaemia agent (CAA) by an indirect immunofluorescent antibody technique in breeder flocks in Japan. Avian Pathol. 14:521-530. 1985.
189. Yuasa, N., and K. Imai. Pathogenicity and antigenicity of eleven isolates of chicken anaemia agent (CAA). Avian Pathol. 15:639-645. 1986.
190. Yuasa, N., K. Imai, K. Watanabe, F. Saito, M. Abe, and K. Komi. Aetiological examination of an outbreak of haemorrhagic syndrome in a broiler flock in Japan. Avian Pathol. 16:521-526. 1987.
191. Yuasa, N., K. Imai, and K. Nakamura. Pathogenicity of chicken anaemia agent in bursectomized chickens. Avian Pathol. 17:363-369. 1988.
192. Yuasa, N. Effect of chemicals on the infectivity of chicken anaemia virus. Avian Pathol. 21:315-319. 1992.
193. Zhang, X., Q. Xie, J. Ji, S. Chang, J. Liu, F. Chen, J. Ma, and Y. Bee. Complete genome sequence analysis of a recent chicken anemia virus isolate and comparison with a chicken anemia virus isolate from human fecal samples in China. J. Virol. 86:10896-10897. 2012.

CHAPTER 5

VIRUS-INDUCED IMMUNOSUPPRESSION: MAREK'S DISEASE VIRUS INFECTION AND ASSOCIATED SYNDROMES

Isabel M. Gimeno and Arun R. Pandiri

Introduction

Marek's disease (MD) is a highly contagious lymphoproliferative disease of chickens caused by an alphaherpesvirus of the Genera *Mardivirus* [58] known as Marek's disease virus (MDV). [23-24] MD is one of the major concerns for the poultry industry as it can lead to tremendous economic losses in the absence of proper control methods. Even using adequate control methods, in 1984, it was estimated that mortality and condemnation losses associated with MD were at $169 million in the United States and $943 million worldwide. [90] MD has been successfully controlled by vaccination since 1969. [25] The great efficacy of MD vaccines, however, has negative consequences. The use of MD vaccines has been accompanied by an increase in virulence of MDV. [118] Emergent MDV strains not only are able to break protection conferred by currently available vaccines but also have increased neurovirulence [45] and immunosuppressive potential. [19]

MDV-induced lymphomas (commonly known as MD) are by far the best studied outcome of MDV infection. However, in addition to lymphomas, MDV is able to induce a variety of non-neoplastic diseases/syndromes encompassing nervous system (neurological syndromes), lymphoid organs (lymphodegenerative syndrome), and circulatory system (arteriosclerosis). Furthermore, MDV can induce immunosuppression (MDV-IS) that seems to be a consequence of both neoplastic and non-neoplastic processes. The economical impact of the MDV-induced non-neoplastic syndromes is difficult to assess but might be more relevant than initially estimated; especially MDV-IS. MDV has a complex interaction with the immune system and can induce immunosuppression by different mechanisms, some of which are poorly understood. Because of its complexity, MDV-IS has not been properly studied and it is difficult to monitor under field conditions. In the opinion of the authors, MDV-IS has long been neglected by the poultry industry and the research community. An effort will be made in this chapter to emphasize this aspect of the disease.

The goal of this chapter is to aid poultry veterinarians and diagnosticians in understanding the various manifestation of MDV infection, the repercussions of different syndromes under field conditions, and the methods of detection and control.

Etiology

MDV is an alpha-herpesvirus in the genus *Mardivirus* and subfamily *Alphaherpesvirinae* (http://ncbi.nlm.nih.gov/ICTVdb/ICTVdB). Genus *Mardivirus* includes three species viz. *Gallid herpesvirus* 2 (formerly MDV serotype 1), *Gallid herpesvirus* 3 (formerly MDV serotype 2), and *Meleagrid herpesvirus* 1 (formerly MDV serotype 3). *Gallid herpesvirus* 2 (serotype 1) are oncogenic viruses of chickens. *Gallid herpesvirus* 3 (serotype 2) are non-oncogenic viruses of chickens. *Meleagrid herpesvirus* 1 (serotype 3) are non-oncogenic viruses of turkeys and are commonly known as turkey herpesvirus or HVT. In this chapter, the term MDV will indicate serotype 1 MDV since virulence is unique for this serotype. Related herpesviruses of serotypes 2 and 3 will be indicated by the corresponding serotype.

Based on their virulence, serotype 1 MDV can be further classified into pathotypes. [118] To date, four pathotypes have been described: mild (m), virulent (v), very virulent (vv), and very virulent plus (vv+). Biologically, the newly emergent more virulent MDVs differ clearly from less virulent MDVs. They are able to break vaccine immunity and this is the criteria for the gold standard pathotyping system [120]; they are more neurovirulent [45]; they have a expanded host range [48]; and they seem to be more immunosuppressive. [19] The association between pathotype and MDV-IS ability will be further discussed in the last section of this chapter. Molecularly, however, there are minor differences between vMDV, vvMDV, and vv+MDV [103] and at this point it has not been possible to establish a pathotyping system based on molecular features.

The causes of MDV evolution are not well elucidated. It is speculated that the changes in poultry production systems during 1950s may have been a major trigger for the initial changes in MDV (from mMDV to vMDV). After the first shift in virulence of MDV, all subsequent waves of evolution of virulence were linked to the introduction of different generations of vaccines. [118] The observation that viruses from each successive wave acquired the ability to overcome the immunity induced by the previously generation of vaccines, strongly suggests that the evolution is primarily aimed at avoiding/overcoming the vaccine-induced response. The fact that none of the current MD vaccines induces sterilizing immunity, prevents reinfection or superinfection, or prevents challenge viruses from being shed, could be a major triggering factor for the evolution of MDV.

MDV has unique features that differentiate it from other alpha-herpesviruses (reviewed in ref. 99). It is a cell associated virus with lymphotropic properties similar to those of gammaherpesvirus. It establishes latency in lymphocytes. Furthermore, it carries an oncogene (*meq*) and is able to transform latently infected lymphocytes and form lymphomas. However, its molecular structure and genomic organization are similar to alphaherpesvirus [12], thus its classification into this group of viruses. Details on the genomic structure of MDV are beyond the scope of this chapter and readers are encouraged to peruse other sources. [99]

MDV can establish three different kinds of interaction with the host cells: productive infection, latent infection and transforming infection (Table 1).

- Productive infection implies replication of viral DNA, synthesis of viral protein, and in some cases, production of viral particles. Based on the production of viral particles, there are two kinds of productive infections: fully productive infection and restrictive productive infection.
  - Fully productive infection results in the development of large numbers of enveloped, fully infectious virus. This kind of infection only occurs in the feather follicle epithelium (FFE) and it is of major importance in the epidemiology of the disease, as it is the main, if not the only, source of infectious MDV particles. [17]
  - By contrast, in restrictive productive infection, nonenveloped and noninfectious viruses are formed. This type of infection occurs in vitro in cell culture and in vivo in lymphocytes and macrophages.
- Latent infection is defined as the presence of viral genome with no or limited production of viral antigens or infectious virus. [76]
- Transforming infection only occurs in cells infected with serotype 1, since other serotypes have no oncogenic potential. Activated T cells, mainly of phenotype $CD4^+$ $CD8^-$, are the target cells for transformation.

Epidemiology

Chickens are the natural host for MDV, but quails, turkeys and pheasants are also susceptible to virus infection and disease. [99] It is suspected that more virulent MDVs have increased ability to induce disease in turkeys than less virulent MDVs. This chapter will address the clinical and pathological manifestation of MD in chickens. A more detailed description of MD in other species can be found in other reviews. [54,99]

Table 1. MDV-host cell interactions.

TYPE OF INFECTION		CELL TYPES		INFECTIOUS VIRIONS	VIRAL DNA LOAD	ANTIGEN EXPRESSION
Cytolytic or productive	Partially productive	In vitro	CEF, DEF, CKC	No	Very high	• High • All antigens
		In vitro	B cells, T cells, macrophages	No	Very high	• High • All antigens
	Fully productive	In vivo	Feather follicle epithelium	Yes	Very high	• High • All antigens
Latency		In vivo	• T cells mainly • B cells, non-myelinating Schwann cells	No	Very low	• Low to none • Only *meq*
		In vitro	Quail cell line (QT35)	No	Very low	• Low to none • Only *meq*
Transformation		In vivo	$CD4^+CD8^-$ T cells mainly	No	Medium to high	• Low to none • Only *meq*
		In vitro	$CD4^+CD8^-$ T lymphoblastic lines mainly	No	Medium to high	• Low to none • Only *meq*

CEF: chicken embryo fibroblasts; DEF: duck embryo fibroblasts; CKC: chicken kidney cells.

MDV infection is transmitted by the airborne route. Transmission of the infection occurs readily between chickens by direct or indirect contact. Epithelial cells in the keratinizing layer of the FFE support fully productive infection and these cells serve as a source of infection to other chickens. The virus is generally associated with desquamated, keratinized FFE cells which are shed along with molted feathers and as dander. Virus shedding begins about 2 weeks post infection (wpi) [63], with maximal shedding occurring between 3-5 wpi. [121] Once the infection is introduced into a chicken flock, regardless of vaccination status, infection spreads quickly from chicken to chicken. Replication of the virus in the feather follicle can be detected by the presence of nuclear inclusion bodies in the infected cells or by evaluation of the expression of MDV antigens (Fig. 1). Vertical transmission of MDV has not been reported.

MDV is ubiquitous and MDV infection in most cases does not result in MD. Vaccination does not prevent superinfection and this might be a major factor in the evolution of MDV towards greater virulence. Vaccinated chickens become a perfect ecosystem in which a variety of MDVs replicate and those better fit MDVs survive the immune response and spread in the flock. Chickens that are adequately protected by vaccination or are genetically resistant do not develop MD after MDV infection. The lack of correlation between infection and disease is a major hurdle in the diagnosis of MD.

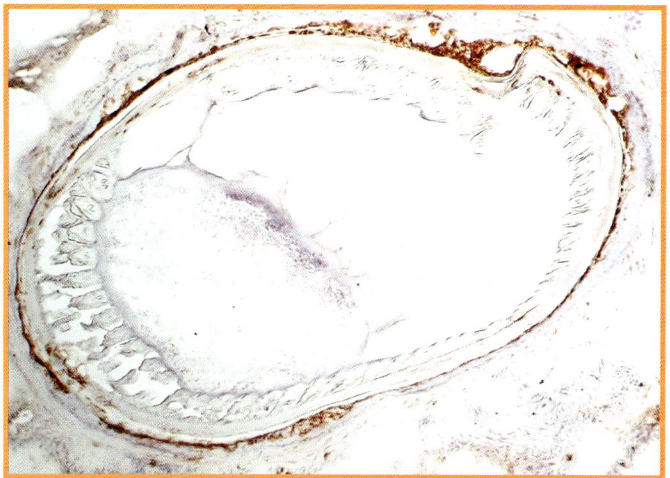

Fig. 1 | Expression of MDV pp38 protein (brown stain) in the feather follicle epithelium detected by immunohistochemistry (diaminobenzidine with hematoxylin counterstain).

Pathogenesis

The pathogenesis of MD is a very complex process and a detailed discussion is beyond the scope of this chapter. Further details can be found in numerous review papers. [20,99] In this chapter, only those events of the pathogenesis that are relevant for the development of the different MDV-induced syndromes and for diagnosis will be reviewed.

The pathogenesis of MDV differs in chickens that have maternal antibodies against MDV (MAb) and those lacking MAb. It also differs between chickens that are genetically susceptible or resistant to the disease and between vaccinated and unvaccinated chickens. In this section, events occurring after infection of susceptible chickens lacking MAb and not vaccinated against MD are described. Differences in the pathogenesis in chickens bearing MAb, resistant against MD or vaccinated against MD are presented in Table 2.

The natural route of MDV infection is via respiratory tract following inhalation of infectious virus in desquamated FFE and in dust from a contaminated environment. The role of the lung in MD pathogenesis is not clear and it is presumed that phagocytes in the lung pick up the virus and carry it to lymphoid organs such as the bursa of Fabricius, thymus, and spleen. At this early point in the infection, there is no associated pathology in the lung but viral antigen has been detected in pulmonary parenchymal cells [2,87,89] and B lymphocytes. [3]

MDV reaches the lymphoid organs within 24-36 hours after intratracheal inoculation. In unvaccinated chickens lacking MAb, a productive cytolytic infection is established in the lymphoid organs between 3-6 days post infection (dpi). The initial target cells for the cytolytic infection are B lymphocytes. [101] This productive infection leads to necrosis and inflammation of the lymphoid organs resulting in a condition referred to as lymphodegenerative syndromes. Lymphodegenerative syndromes are associated with a transient immunosuppression (Fig. 2) (discussed in the latter sections of this chapter).

The necrosis of B lymphocytes in the lymphoid organs elicits an inflammatory response and the recruitment of numerous inflammatory cells, especially macrophages, T and B lymphocytes and some heterophils. The activation of T lymphocytes is of particular relevance in the pathogenesis of MDV as resting T lymphocytes are refractory to MDV infection. Activated T lymphocytes can also support productive infection but in most cases infection becomes latent after T lymphocytes are infected. The switch from cytolytic infection to latency occurs rapidly and by 7-8 days evidence of cytolytic infection in the lymphoid organs is minimal. Latent infection, however, can be detected by this time not only in lymphoid organs but also in peripheral blood lymphocytes (PBL) and in the feather pulp. [9,49]

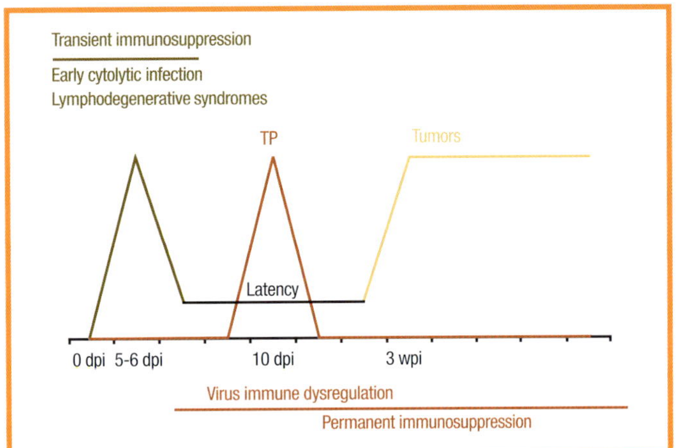

Fig. 2 | Marek's disease virus induced immunosuppression (MDV-IS) in the context of MDV pathogenesis. MDV can induce a transient immunosuppression associated with the early replication and cytolytic infection in the lymphoid organs. This MDV-IS only occurs in chickens not vaccinated against MD and lacking maternal antibodies against MDV. In addition, MDV can induce a permanent immunosuppression associated with immune dysregulation occurring during the stages of latency and transformation. Permanent MDV-IS occurs in chickens regardless of the maternal antibody status. Recent studies indicated that it can occur also in MD vaccinated chickens that are otherwise well protected against MD. dpi: days post inoculation; wpi: weeks post inoculation; TP: transient paralysis.

Latently infected PBL are the disseminators of MDV to other tissues in the chicken. As early as 6 dpi, MDV can be detected in the eye, brain and peripheral nerves.[43,82] Depending on the virulence of the virus and the genetic resistance of the chickens, MDV can reactivate in some of the lymphocytes infiltrating the brain and induce an acute inflammatory response. The consequence of this inflammatory response in the brain is the development of vasculitis and vasogenic edema, responsible for eliciting the clinical signs of transient paralysis (TP).[1,43,60,107,108] In some cases, inflammatory lesions in the brain (perivascular cuffing, gliosis) are not associated with the development of TP. Early inflammatory lesions in the peripheral nerves (neuritis) are not associated with any clinical manifestation. Early inflammatory lesions in the eye can be detected as early as 6 dpi and they can progress in distribution and severity and cause panophthalmitis with complete destruction of the retina.[82]

A second wave of cytolytic infection (secondary cytolytic infection) is detected in most epithelial tissues by the end of the 2nd wpi. Because of its relevance in transmission, productive infection of the FFE is particularly important. Replication of MDV in the FFE occurs in genetically resistant as well as susceptible birds regardless of the virulence of the MDV strain. It also occurs in vaccinated chickens regardless of the level of protection that vaccines confer against a particular challenge. MDV most likely is transferred to the FFE by infected lymphocytes within lymphoid aggregates that develop in the perifollicular dermis as early as 7 dpi. The lymphoid aggregates can develop into either necrotic areas consisting of FFE cells and degenerating lymphocytes (dermatitis) or into cutaneous tumors (skin leukosis). The secondary cytolytic infection is also associated with a permanent immunosuppression (Fig. 2) (discussed in the latter sections of this chapter).

Vascular changes within major blood vessels have been detected as early as 15 dpi although evident lesions of vascular sclerosis occur much later in the course of MDV infection.[38,80] MDV antigens have been demonstrated in smooth muscle cells of affected arteries as early as 1 month after inoculation. Also, vascular lesions were found to be latently infected with MDV.[37] The exact pathogenesis of arteriosclerosis is unknown but it is thought that MDV induces necrosis of the smooth muscle cells and this, together with the known alterations in lipid metabolism, might play a role in the development of arteriosclerosis.[20] Arteriosclerosis only occurs in unvaccinated chickens lacking MAb.

Latently infected T lymphocytes can be transformed leading to the development of lymphomas. Transformation can occur within the lymphocytes infiltrating any tissue. Therefore, MDV-induced lymphomas can be detected in nerves, brain, skin, and any viscera. Clinical manifestation of MDV induced lymphomas depends on the location and extension of the tumors. For the purpose of this chapter MD is referred to as MDV-induced lymphomas. Other MDV-induced syndromes will be referred by their respective syndrome names.

MDV-induced syndromes

MDV is able to induce a variety of syndromes that are divided into two categories: non-neoplastic and neoplastic. In addition, MDV can induce immunosuppression that might have both a non-neoplastic and a neoplastic component. Details of each syndrome and tools for their respective diagnosis and control are described below.

Non-neoplastic syndromes

Transient paralysis (TP)

Field relevance: TP only occurs in unvaccinated chickens without MAb. In field conditions, TP was described in young pullets (8-18 weeks-old) prior to the widespread use of vaccines.[21,64,125] In countries where vaccination of broilers is not a common practice, TP can be a problem in these chickens (30-40 days-old).[55]

Table 2. Pathogenesis of Marek's disease virus infection.

DPI	LOCATION		PATHOLOGICAL EVENTS	SUSCEPTIBLE WITHOUT MAb	SUSCEPTIBLE WITH MAb	GENETICALLY RESISTANT/PROTECTED BY VACCINATION
0-1	Lung		None	Yes	Yes	Yes
3-6	Lymphoid organs		• Lymphodegenerative syndromes • Lymphoid organ atrophy	Yes	No	No
> 7	Blood (viremia)		None	Yes	Yes	Yes
> 7	Various tissues	Brain	• Vasculitis, edema • Transient paralysis	Yes	No or delayed	No or reduced
		Nerves	• Neuritis • No clinical signs	Yes	Yes	Yes
		Eye	• Panophtalmitis • Blindness	Yes	No or delayed	No or reduced
		FFE	• Necrosis • Full productive infection (shedding)	Yes	Yes	Yes
		Other tissues	• Necrosis, inflammation • No clinical signs	Yes	Yes	Yes
> 21	Various tissues		• Neoplasia • Lymphoma development	Yes	Yes	No or reduced
> 15	Blood vessels		Arteriosclerosis	Yes	No	No

DPI: days post inoculation; **MAb:** Maternal antibodies against Marek's disease virus; **FFE:** feather follicle epithelium.

Clinical signs: TP occurs 8 to 12 days following infection with an oncogenic MDV [21,64,125] and it is characterized by a flaccid paralysis that initially affects neck muscles and later tends to become generalized (Figs. 3a-b). The onset of TP is very abrupt and most chickens with TP recover completely within 24 to 48 hours. An acute form of TP occurs after infection with highly virulent MDV (vv and vv+ MDV). [119] In acute TP, chickens die within 24 to 48 hours.

Gross lesions: TP is not associated with any gross lesions. However, most of the chickens suffering TP have atrophy of the bursa of Fabricius and thymus because of concomitant lymphodegenerative syndromes.

Histopathology: vasogenic edema and vasculitis are responsible for the establishment of TP (Fig. 3c). Other brain lesions such as perivascular cuffing, lymphocytosis and gliosis may be detected after recovery from TP or in infected but clinically normal chickens, and therefore these lesions cannot be associated with TP. [42,108]

Diagnosis: diagnosis of TP can be made in most cases by the characteristic clinical signs (sudden onset of flaccid neck paralysis that become generalized and in a short time chickens either recover or die) and by epidemiological information (unvaccinated and lacking MAb). Evaluation of the microscopic lesions in the brain can confirm the existence of vasculitis and edema in the brain. Detection of MDV DNA in the brain is not an adequate method of diagnosis for TP as it can also be detected in infected chickens without TP. [119] TP has to be differentiated from other diseases producing paralysis (e.g. botulism, peripheral neuropathy) or brain lesions (e.g. Newcastle disease, avian influenza, west Nile virus, encephalomalacia, encephalomyelitis, toxoplasmosis, bacterial encephalitis). Criteria for differential diagnosis of TP have been reviewed elsewhere. [54]

Control: vaccination with any of the currently available MD vaccines protects against the development of TP.

Lymphodegenerative syndromes

Field relevance: lymphodegenerative syndromes only occur in unvaccinated chickens lacking MAb. Therefore, the relevance of these syndromes in the field is minimal.

Clinical signs: no clinical signs are normally associated with this syndrome.

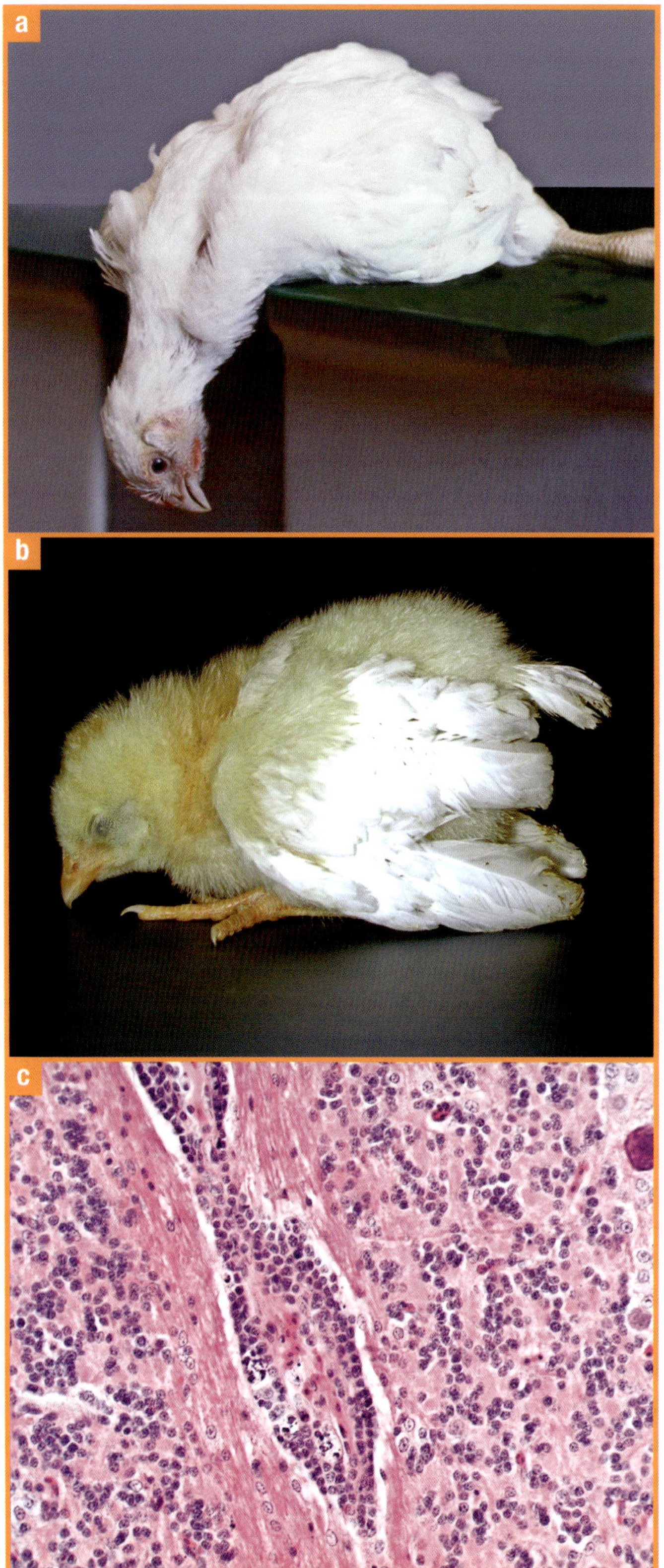

Fig. 3 Transient paralysis (TP). (a) Chicken showing flaccid neck paralysis that is characteristic of TP. (b) Chicken showing depression and limb paralysis. Please note that this chicken (10 days old) still maintains baby feathers due to delayed maturation secondary to viral infection; (c) Cerebellum: vasculitis and perivascular edema are characteristic of TP.

Gross lesions: bursa of Fabricius and thymus are atrophic and yellowish as early as 6-8 dpi (Fig. 4a). The spleen is enlarged and in many cases marbled at 4-6 dpi. After infection with highly virulent MDV (vv and vv+ MDV), necrotic foci can be observed mainly in the spleen at about 7-10 dpi. [114] Necrosis in lymphoid organs is more evident when 1-day-old susceptible chickens are inoculated with a highly virulent MDV.

Histopathology: the productive infection in lymphoid organs reaches a peak at 5-6 dpi and it is accompanied by cytolysis of lymphocytes and other cells, hyperplasia of reticular cells, accumulation of macrophages and infiltration by granulocytes. In the thymus, the cytolytic infection and hyperplasia of reticular cells occur mainly in the medulla, and the cortex is markedly atrophied (Fig. 5a). Similar changes occur in the bursa, with destruction of the normal architecture (Fig. 5b). When atrophy of the bursa and thymus is not reversible, connective tissue replaces the parenchyma and the lumen is lined by unfolded/undulating epithelium (Figs. 4b-c).

Immunohistochemistry: early cytolytic infection in lymphoid organs is characterized by the production of abundant viral antigen (both early and late viral antigens), as can be detected by a variety of techniques. Most of the antigens in the bursa and thymus can be detected in the medulla where necrosis is evident (Figs. 5c-d). In severe cases, viral antigens can be detected in both medulla and cortex (Figs. 5e-f).

Diagnosis: lymphodegenerative syndromes do not occur in chickens vaccinated against MD or in chickens bearing MAb. Therefore, it is a highly uncommon scenario under field conditions. In unvaccinated chickens, MDV could induce lymphoid organ atrophy once MAb levels decrease (around 3 weeks of age). In those cases, diagnosis of lymphodegenerative syndromes is very difficult and a variety of other diseases of infectious (infectious bursal disease, chicken infectious anemia, etc.) and non-infectious (aflatoxins, stress) etiology have to be included in the differential diagnosis as all of them could induce necrosis and atrophy of the lymphoid organs. Detection of MDV antigens in the lymphoid organs has very little diagnostic value because it is transient (5-6 dpi) and occurs before the lymphoid organ atrophy is apparent.

Control: vaccination with any of the currently available MD vaccines protects against the development of lymphodegenerative syndromes.

Early inflammatory lesions in other tissues

Field relevance: MDV induces inflammatory and degenerative lesions in various organs that are not accompanied by the de-

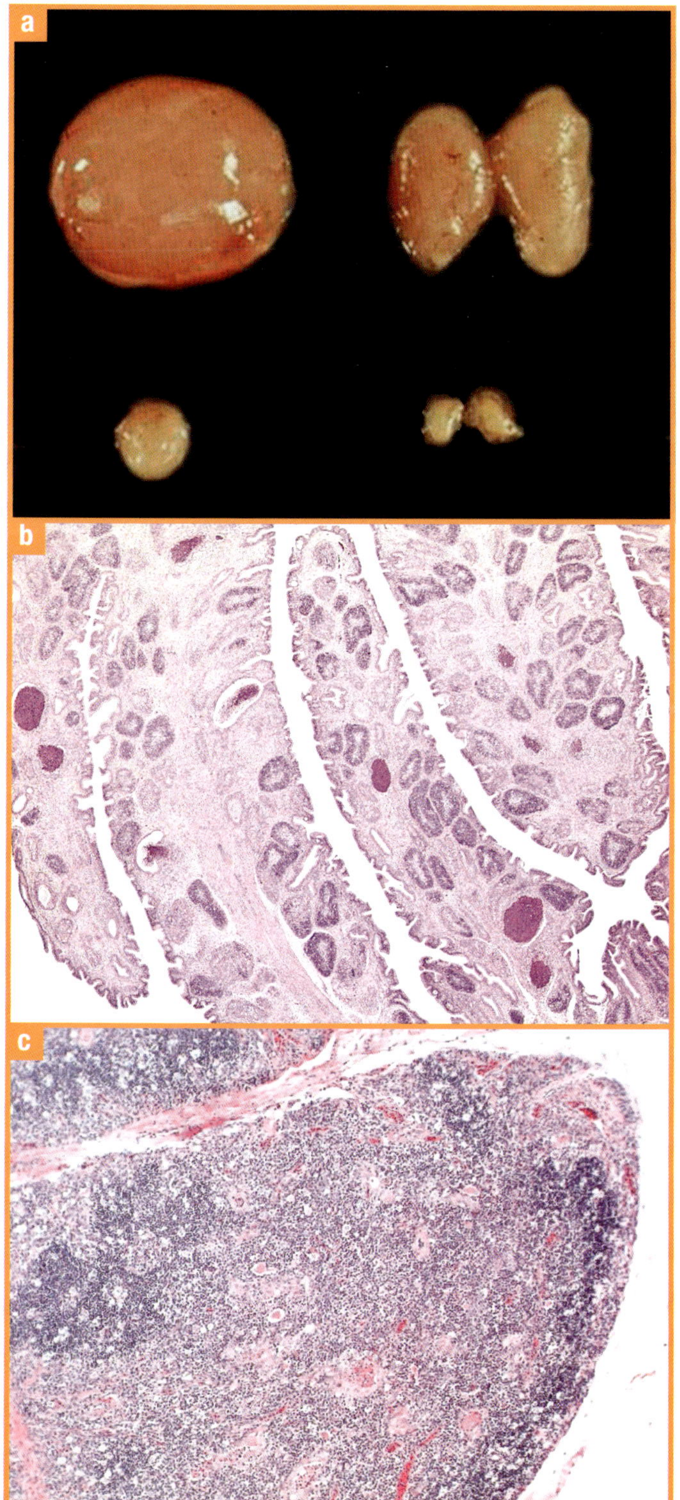

Fig. 4 Lymphoid organ atrophy associated with MDV infection. (a) The bursa of Fabricius (left) and two thymic lobes (right) in the upper row are from healthy uninfected chickens. Severely atrophied bursa of Fabricius and two thymic lobes of chickens 10 days after inoculation with very virulent plus (vv+) MDV strain 648A can be observed in the low row. (b) Photomicrograph of a severely atrophied bursa of Fabricius (hematoxylin and eosin stain). (c) Photomicrograph of a severely atrophied thymic lobe (hematoxylin and eosin stain).

velopment of clinical signs and that may or may not develop into neoplastic lesions (Figs. 6a-d). It is important to differentiate between those inflammatory lesions (indication of MDV infection) and neoplastic lesions (indication of MD).

Clinical signs: none.

Gross lesions: none.

Histopathology: inflammatory infiltrates in the nerves (Fig. 6a) can occur very early after MDV infection (7-8 dpi) and is of particular relevance due to the confusions in diagnosis. Mild inflammatory lesions in the nerves can be induced by all three MDV serotypes and they can regress without inducing clinical signs. It is important that these inflammatory lesions do not get confused with lymphomas in nerves. This is also true for the presence of mononuclear perivascular cuffing in the brain that is not associated with vasculitis and edema (Fig. 6b). Those lesions are common in chickens infected with MDV but are not related to any disease.

Early lesions in skin are not normally associated with clinical signs or gross lesions such as enlarged feather follicles and in general have to be identified by microscopic analysis. They are important as they seem to be necessary for the infection of the FFE and therefore for the transmission of the infection. Early pathological changes in the skin include dermatitis (perifollicular and follicular) as well as degeneration in the FFE due to the replication of MDV.

Diagnosis: the relevance of these inflammatory lesions is presented in the differential diagnosis with tumors induced by MDV.

Control: inflammatory lesions are a common finding in chickens infected with MDV regardless of their health status. MDV is ubiquitous and except those flocks maintained under specific pathogen free (SPF) conditions, commercial flocks will invariably be infected with MDV and chickens will have MDV-induced inflammatory lesions, with or without MD. The presence of MDV-induced inflammatory lesions alone does not support a diagnosis of MD but just of MDV infection. Furthermore, MDV-induced inflammatory lesions in chickens with tumors due to other etiologies might complicate the diagnosis and in these cases additional tests will be required for confirming the diagnosis.

Panophthalmitis and ocular disease

Field relevance: the relevance of ocular lesions in the field is unknown. Increased ocular lesions have been associated with outbreaks induced by highly virulent MDV (vv and vv+ MDV).[39,104] Vaccination does not always result in protection against ocular lesions.[82] The progression in the severity of the ocular lesions undoubtedly will result in blindness. However, the economic

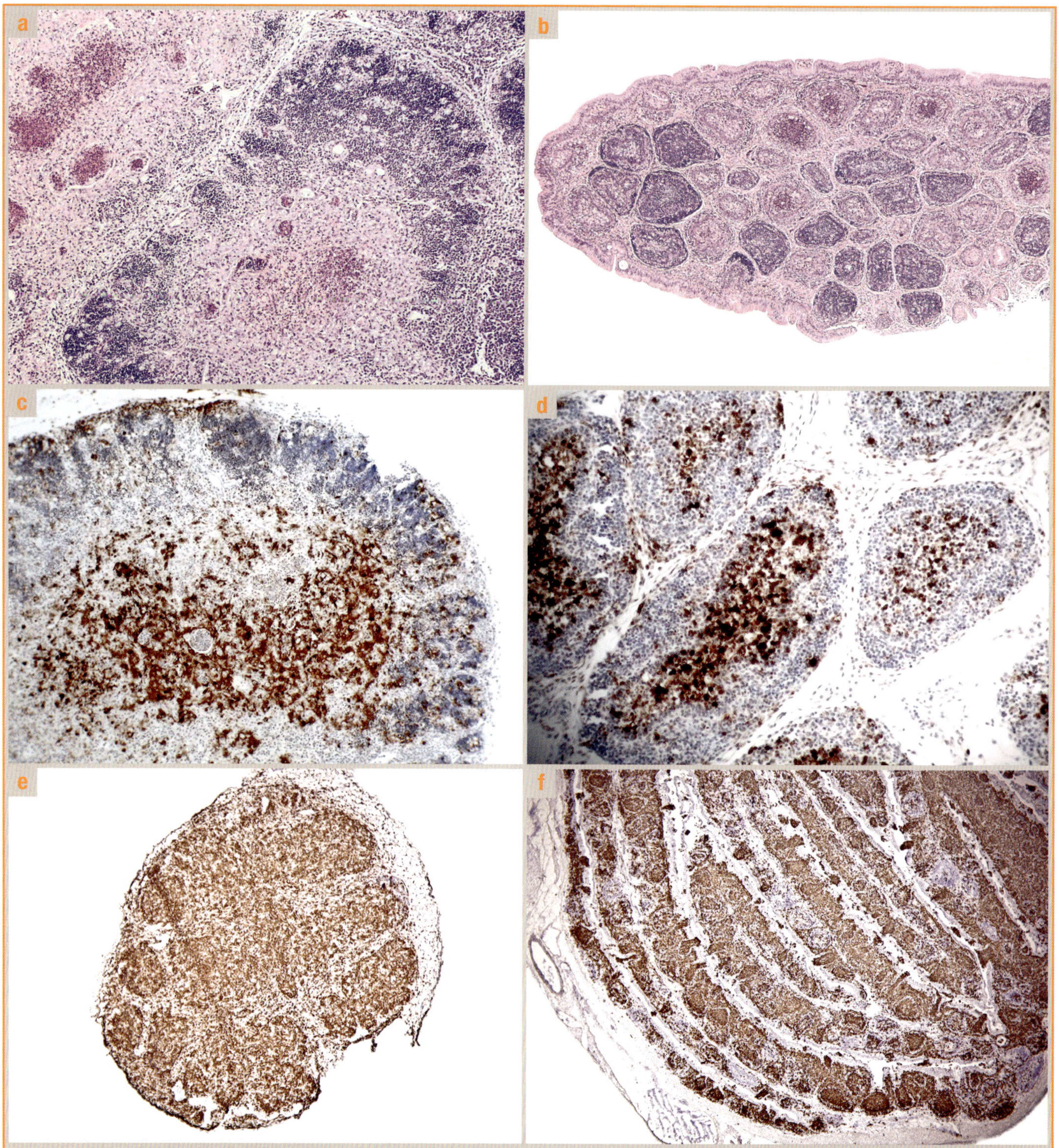

Fig. 5 Lymphodegenerative syndromes. (a) Photomicrograph of thymus showing severe necrosis and depletion of lymphocytes in the cortex and medulla (hematoxylin and eosin stain). (b) Photomicrograph of the bursa of Fabricius showing severe multifocal necrosis of the bursal follicles and marked depletion of lymphocytes (hematoxylin and eosin stain). (c) Photomicrograph demonstrating MDV pp38 antigen expression (brown stain) by immunohistochemistry in the thymus of a chicken, please note viral antigen expression is limited to the thymic medulla (diaminobenzidine with hematoxylin counterstain). (d) Photomicrograph demonstrating MDV pp38 antigen expression (brown stain) by immunohistochemistry in the bursa of Fabricius of a chicken, please note viral antigen expression is limited to the medulla within the bursal follicles (diaminobenzidine with hematoxylin counterstain). (e) Photomicrograph demonstrating MDV pp38 antigen expression (brown stain) by immunohistochemistry in the thymus in a chicken, please note viral antigen expression is expressed in both the cortex and medulla of the thymic lobes (diaminobenzidine with hematoxylin counterstain). (f) Photomicrograph demonstrating MDV pp38 antigen expression (brown stain) by immunohistochemistry within the bursa of Fabricius in a chicken, please note viral antigen expression is expressed diffusely within all the follicles encompassing the cortex and medulla (diaminobenzidine with hematoxylin counterstain). Severity of viral antigen expression indicates high viral replication and is related to subsequent lymphoid organ atrophy.

consequences of blindness in commercial poultry have not been evaluated.

Clinical signs: birds with ocular involvement may show evidence of blindness. [39,83,104] The blindness can be unilateral or bilateral. Recognition of clinical blindness requires careful observation and it is usually overlooked in the field.

Gross lesions: gross ocular changes, including loss of pigmentation in the iris ("grey eye") and irregularity of the pupil, are caused by mononuclear infiltration within the iris. Cataracts, conjunctivitis, occasionally with multifocal hemorrhages and corneal edema have also been observed [39] (Fig. 7).

Histopathology: MDV-induced lesions in the eye can be classified as early lesions (6 to 11 days post inoculation, dpi) and late lesions (26 to 56 dpi) based on the location and severity of the lesions. [82] The early lesions involve iris, ciliary body and choroid layer and are characterized by endothelial cell hypertrophy, vasculitis, and infiltration of lymphocytes, plasma cells, macrophages, and heterophils (Figs. 8a-b). Late lesions consist of severe lymphohistiocytic uveitis, keratitis, pectenitis, vitreitis, retinitis, and segmental to diffuse retinal necrosis (Figs. 8c-d).

Immunohistochemistry: expression of MDV antigen pp38 can be detected in the cells infiltrating choroid layer at 11 dpi; and in the retina, uveal tract and corneal epithelium during later stages of infection. [82] No expression of oncoprotein *meq* has been detected, which rules out that infiltrated cells were transformed.

Diagnosis: ocular lesions are normally associated with other lesions induced by MDV and aid in the diagnosis. The finding of ocular lesions without the presence of other symptoms in flocks affected by MDV is unlikely. Gross and histopathological evaluation of the eye together with the history of the flock and other lesions will help in the diagnosis.

Control: vaccination protects partially against the development of ocular lesions. Pandiri et al. [82] demonstrated that vaccination with HVT protected against the early lesions but did not protect against the late lesions when chickens were challenged with a vv+ strain 648A. On the other hand, vaccination with CVI988 protected against both types of ocular lesions.

Arteriosclerosis

Field relevance: arteriosclerosis only occurs in unvaccinated chickens lacking MAb. Therefore, the relevance of these lesions in the field is minimal. Moreover, lesions develop very slowly and they might not be apparent during the short life span of commercial poultry.

Clinical signs: no clinical signs are normally associated with these lesions.

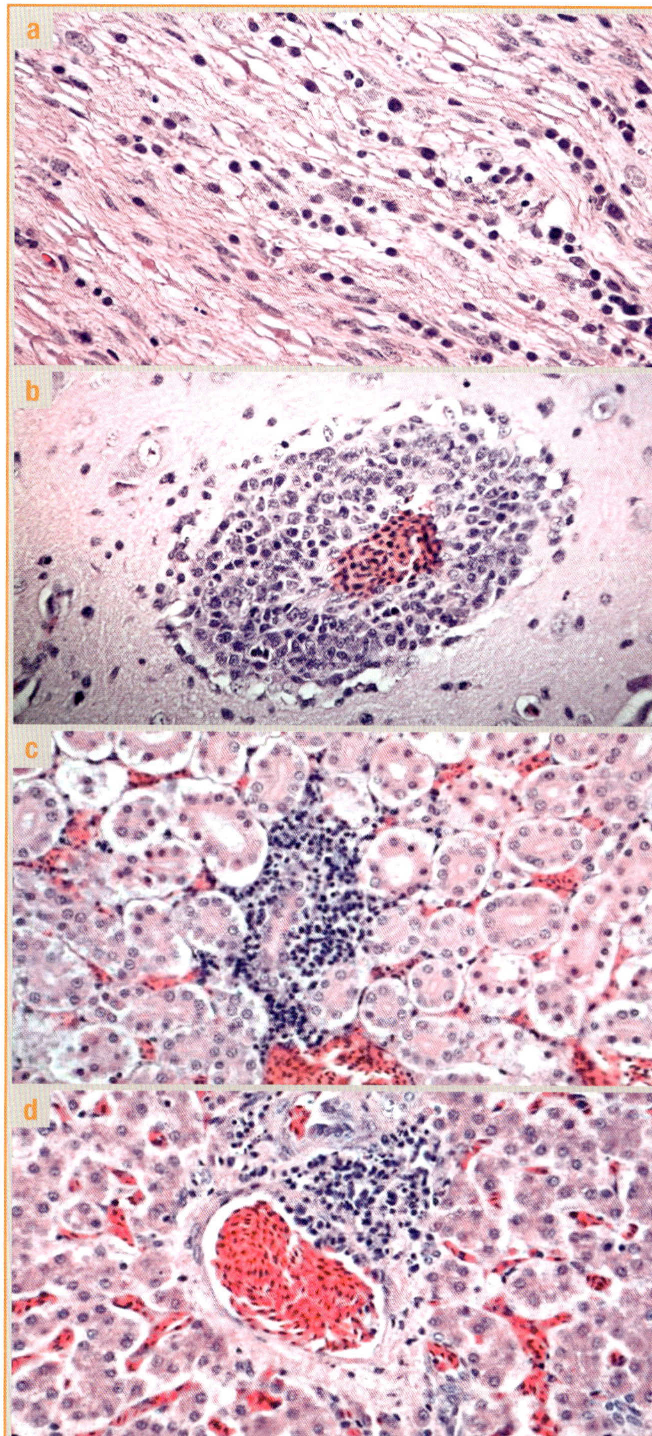

Fig. 6 Photomicrographs demonstrating inflammatory lesions induced by MDV in various tissues that are not associated with Marek's disease. (a) Inflammatory lesions in the sciatic nerve 8 days after inoculation with very virulent (vv) MDV strain Md5. (b) Perivascular cuffing in the brain of a chicken 10 days after inoculation with v MDV strain GA that was not associated with transient paralysis. (c) Inflammatory lesions in the kidney of a 21-day-old chicken vaccinated with CVI988 at one day of age and challenge with vv MDV strain Md5 at 5 days of age. (d) Inflammatory lesions in the liver from a 21-day-old chicken vaccinated with CVI988 at day of age and challenged with vv MDV strain Md5 at 5 days of age. All sections are stained with hematoxylin and eosin. None of the chickens that had the above lesions had tumors.

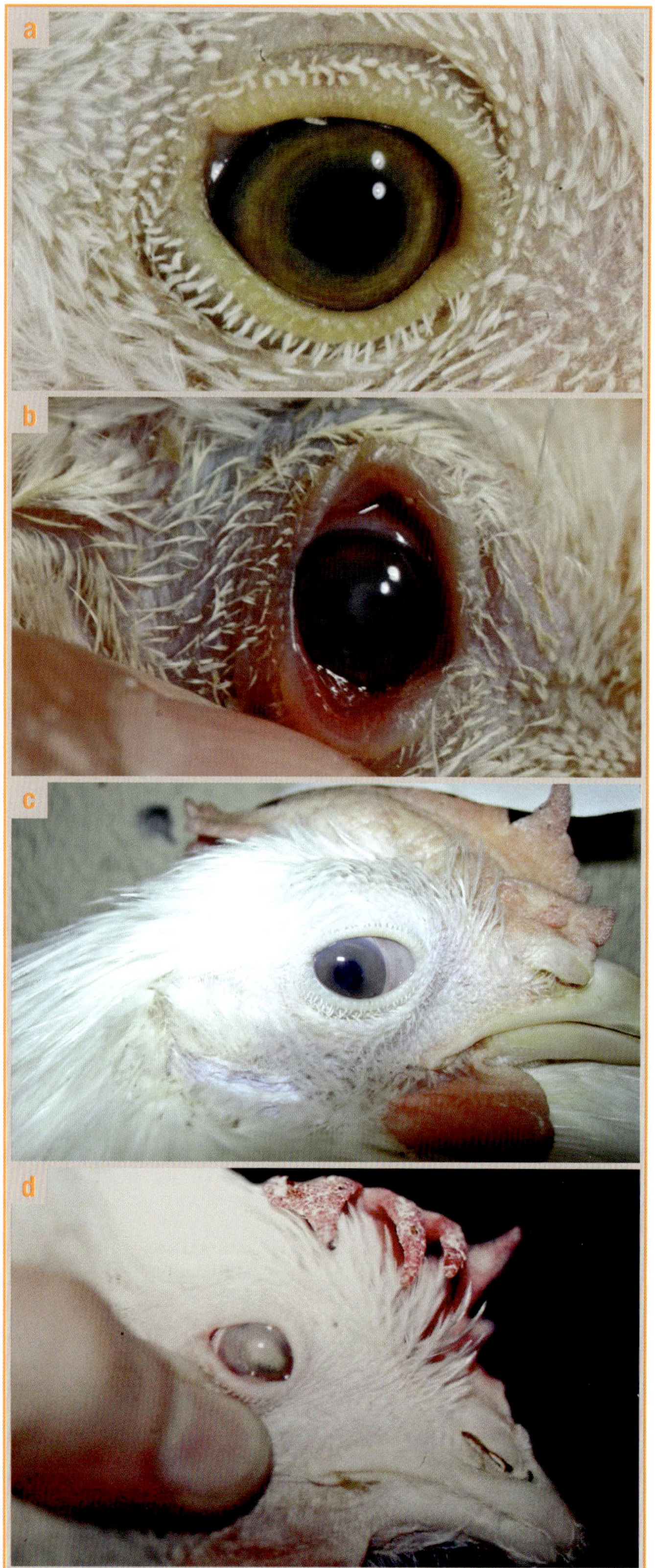

Fig. 7 MDV-induced ocular lesions. (a) Normal chicken eye. (b) Iris with pale white areas and irregular pupil, also note the marked conjunctivitis. (c) Exophthalmia accompanied by a protruding nictitating membrane, also note the pupil is irregular and the iris is diffusely grey. (d) Diffuse corneal opacity and cataract.

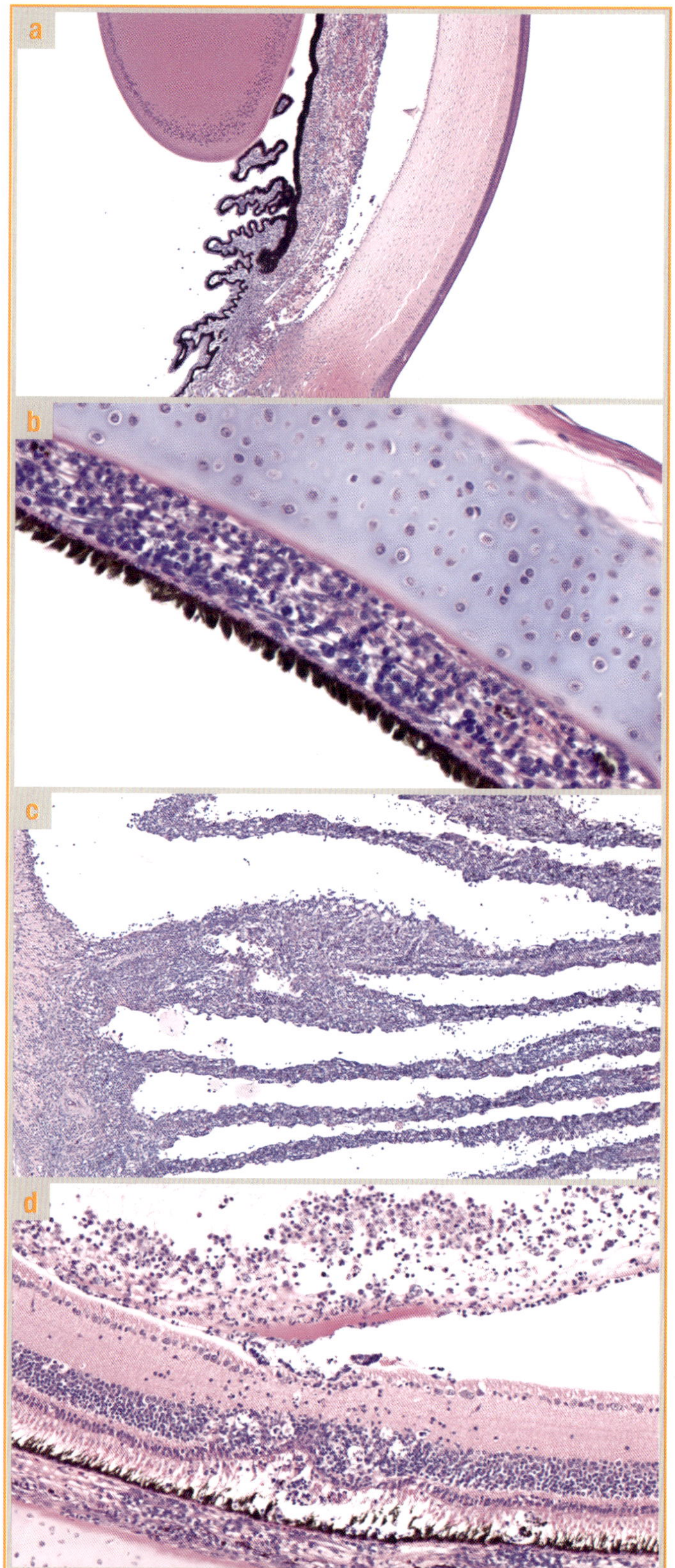

Fig. 8 Photomicrographs of MDV-induced eye lesions. (a-b) Early lesions: infiltration of lymphocytes within the iris (a) and choroid layer (b) 11 days following inoculation with vv+ MDV 648A. (c-d) Late lesions: infiltration of macrophages and lymphocytes in the pecten (c) and in the vitreous and retina (d); also note the retinal detachment in figure d. All sections are stained with hematoxylin and eosin.

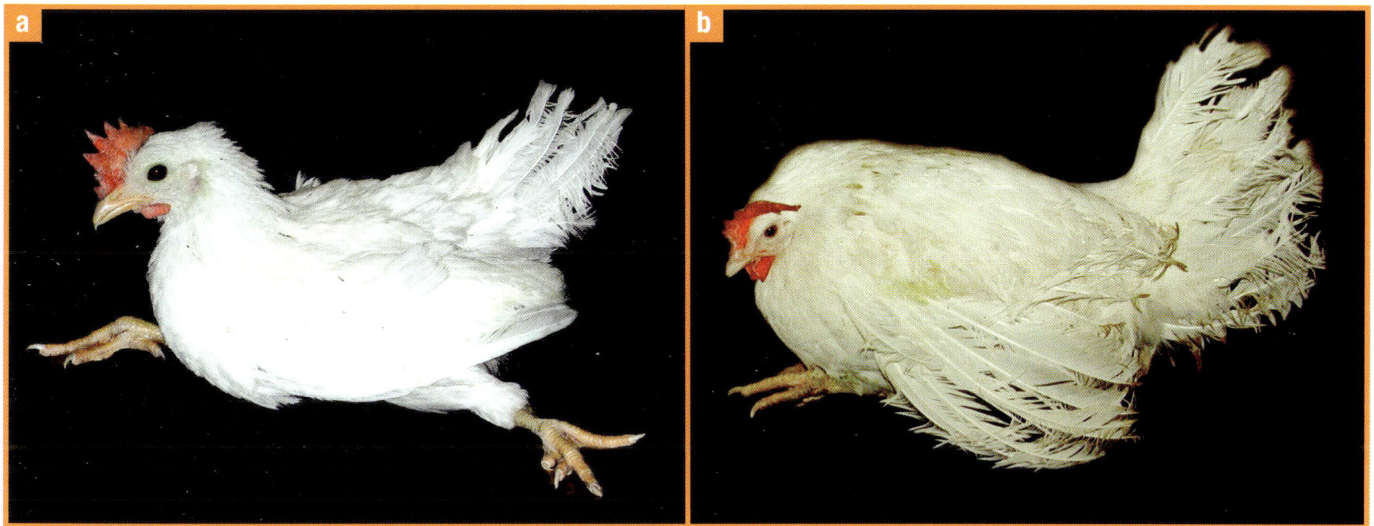

Fig. 9 | Neurological clinical signs in chickens with Marek's disease. (a) Chicken with paralysis of the legs. (b) Chicken with paralysis of the wings.

Gross lesions: gross lesions are not apparent and are commonly missed during necropsy. However, enlargement of the major arteries can be noted with careful evaluation. [36]

Histopathology: infiltrates of lymphocytes, macrophages and cholesterol deposits within the tunica intima and media as well as hyperplasia of the tunica muscularis are the most common lesions induced by MDV in the arteries.

Immunohistochemistry: MDV antigens have been detected by immunofluorescence in the tunica media of affected arteries as early as 1 month after infection. [36]

Diagnosis: the diagnosis of MDV-induced arteriosclerosis is uncommon because it only occurs in unvaccinated chickens lacking MAb. In addition, lesions are not apparent until very late in the pathogenesis of the disease and life span of commercial poultry is usually short.

Control: vaccination with any of the currently available MD vaccines protects against the development of arteriosclerosis.

Neoplastic syndromes (tumors)

Field relevance

The development of tumors is the MDV-induced syndrome of most relevance in the field and it is normally named MD. The rest of the syndromes associated with MDV infection are normally referred to by the name of the induced syndrome. MD is by far one of the most relevant diseases of poultry and a major threat for the poultry industry in absence of proper control methods. The incidence of MD differs between countries and the current global situation has been recently reported. [34]

Clinical signs

Symptoms associated with the development of MDV-induced lymphomas vary according to the location of the tumors and very few are specific for MD. Stunting, depression, lethargy, paleness and diarrhea are nonspecific clinical signs that may be observed, especially when the course of the disease is prolonged. Neurological clinical signs are common and depend on the involvement of the peripheral nerves as well as the brain (Figs. 9a-b). Torticollis and tremors are characteristic of the persistent neurological disease due to the neoplastic infiltration in the central nervous system. [42] Asymmetric progressive paralysis that evolves to complete spastic paralysis of one or more of the extremities is the most characteristic sign of peripheral nerve dysfunction (brachial and/or sciatic nerve involvement). Involvement of the vagus nerve usually is associated with crop paralysis and gasping.

Gross lesions

The gross changes commonly present in MD are enlargement of peripheral nerves and spinal ganglia, and lymphoma formation in various organs and tissues. Skin lesions are also observed and they are more common in meat-type chickens than in egg-type chickens. In a more detailed description:

- Visceral organs (Figs. 10-11): lymphomas may occur in virtually any organ. The distribution of the tumor in an organ can be diffuse, nodular, or both. When diffuse, viscera appear enlarged, sometimes to several times the normal size, and with grey to white discoloration. When nodular, lymphomas appear as one or several white to grey firm nodules with smooth surface.

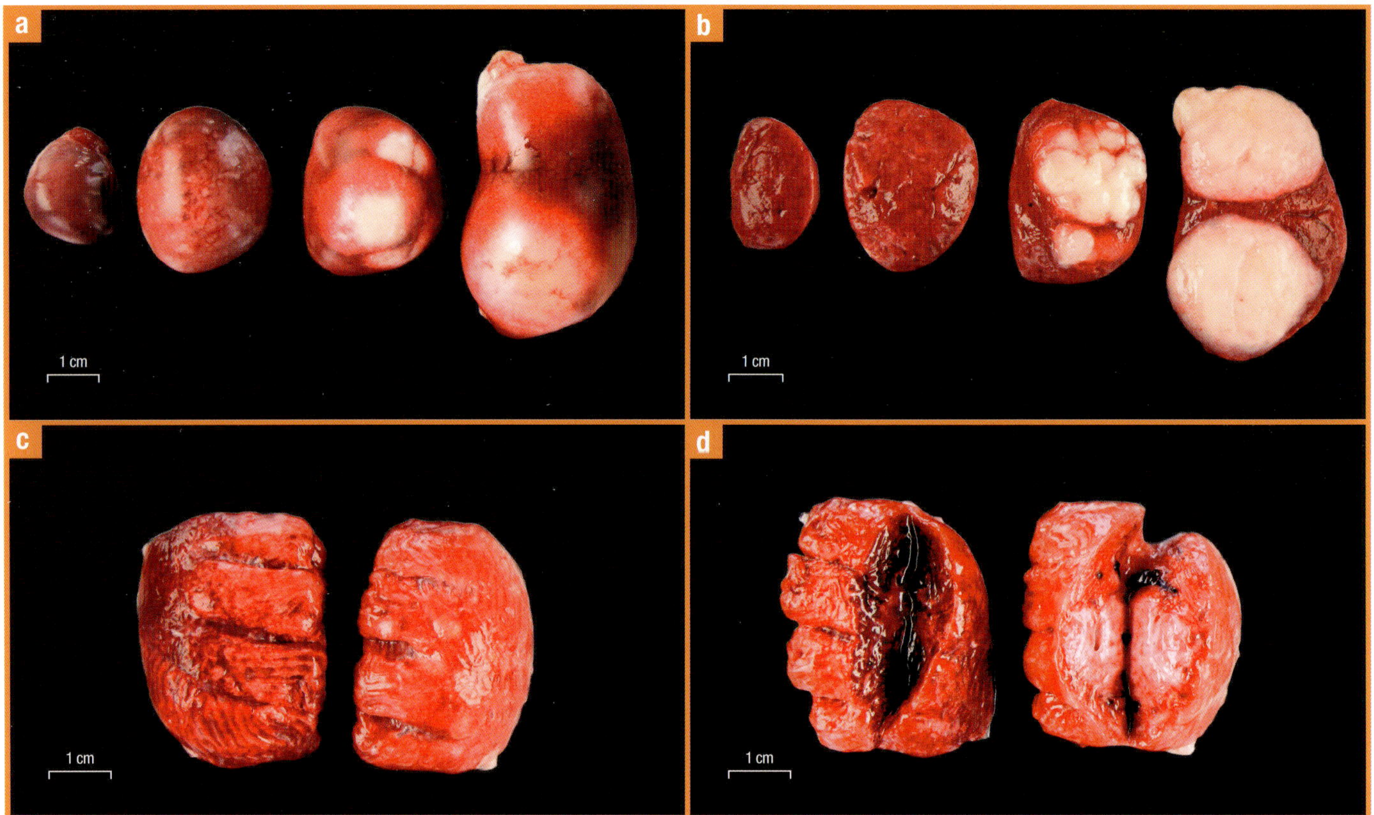

Fig. 10 | MDV-induced tumors in spleen and lung. (a-b) From left to right: normal spleen, enlarged spleen with diffuse infiltration, enlarged spleen with multifocal nodular lymphomas, and the severely enlarged spleen with markedly enlarged lymphomas that appear more obvious on cut surface (b). (c-d) The left lung is from a healthy uninfected chicken and the right lung shows a nodular tumor, which is more obvious by palpation or on the cut surface (d).

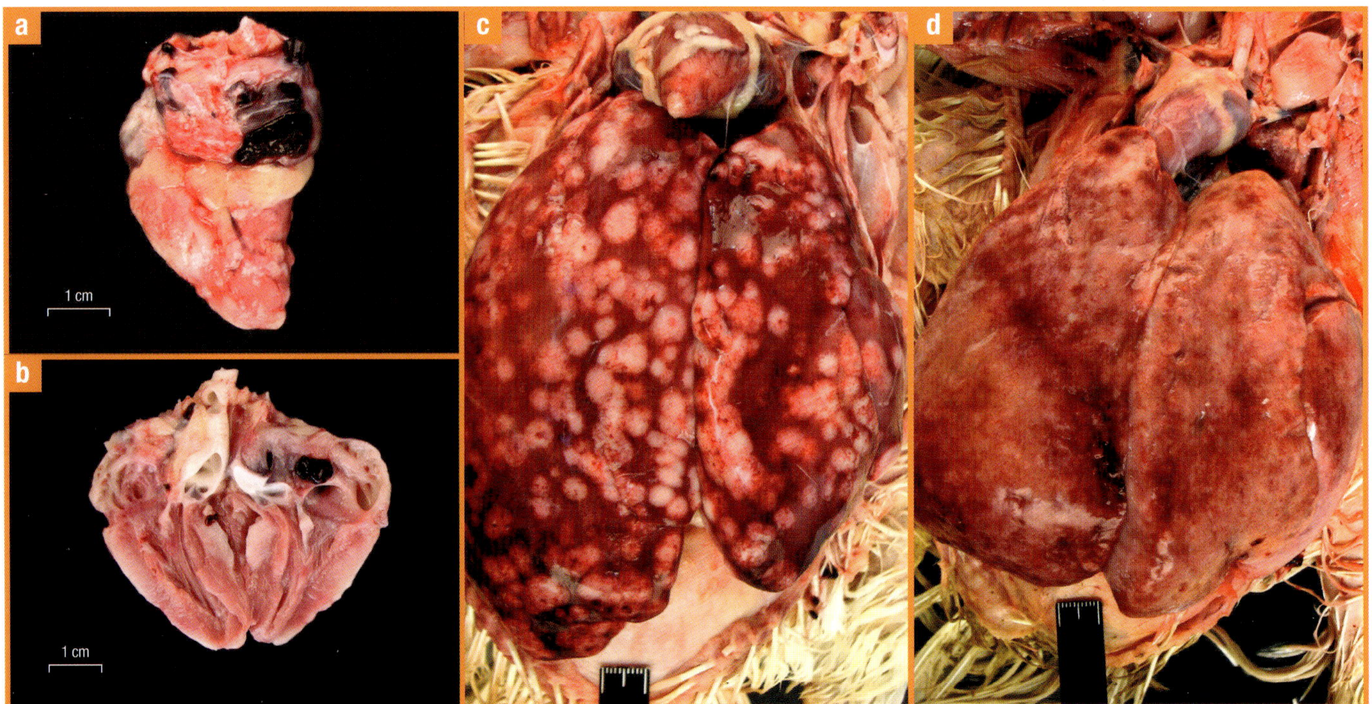

Fig. 11 | MDV-induced tumors in heart and liver. (a-b) Numerous multifocal lymphoma nodules in the heart. On cut surface, the extent of the myocardial invasion by the lymphoma may be observed. (c-d) Lymphomas in the liver with nodular multifocal distribution (c) or diffuse distribution (d).

- Integument (Fig. 12): skin lymphomas are mainly associated with feather follicles and they are more evident in dressed carcasses, although they can also be present in non-feathered areas such as comb, wattles, and shanks. Initial lesions do not seem to be neoplastic and are characterized by severe cutaneous erythema (Fig. 12a). These lesions progress to neoplasia and few or several follicles become enlarged (Fig. 12b). In severe cases, lesions from several follicles coalesce and form gross nodules (Figs. 12c-d). Initially, there are whitish nodules but in some cases they are ulcerated with brown crust formation. Comb and wattles can be also affected. Lesions in the skin of the shanks start with reddish discoloration (Alabama Red Leg) and tend to progress into skin tumors with ulcerated crusts.
- Peripheral nerves (Fig. 13): the enlargement of the peripheral nerves is one of the main lesions associated with MD and it has important diagnostic value as it allows the differentiation between MD and lymphoid leukosis. Although visceral tumors

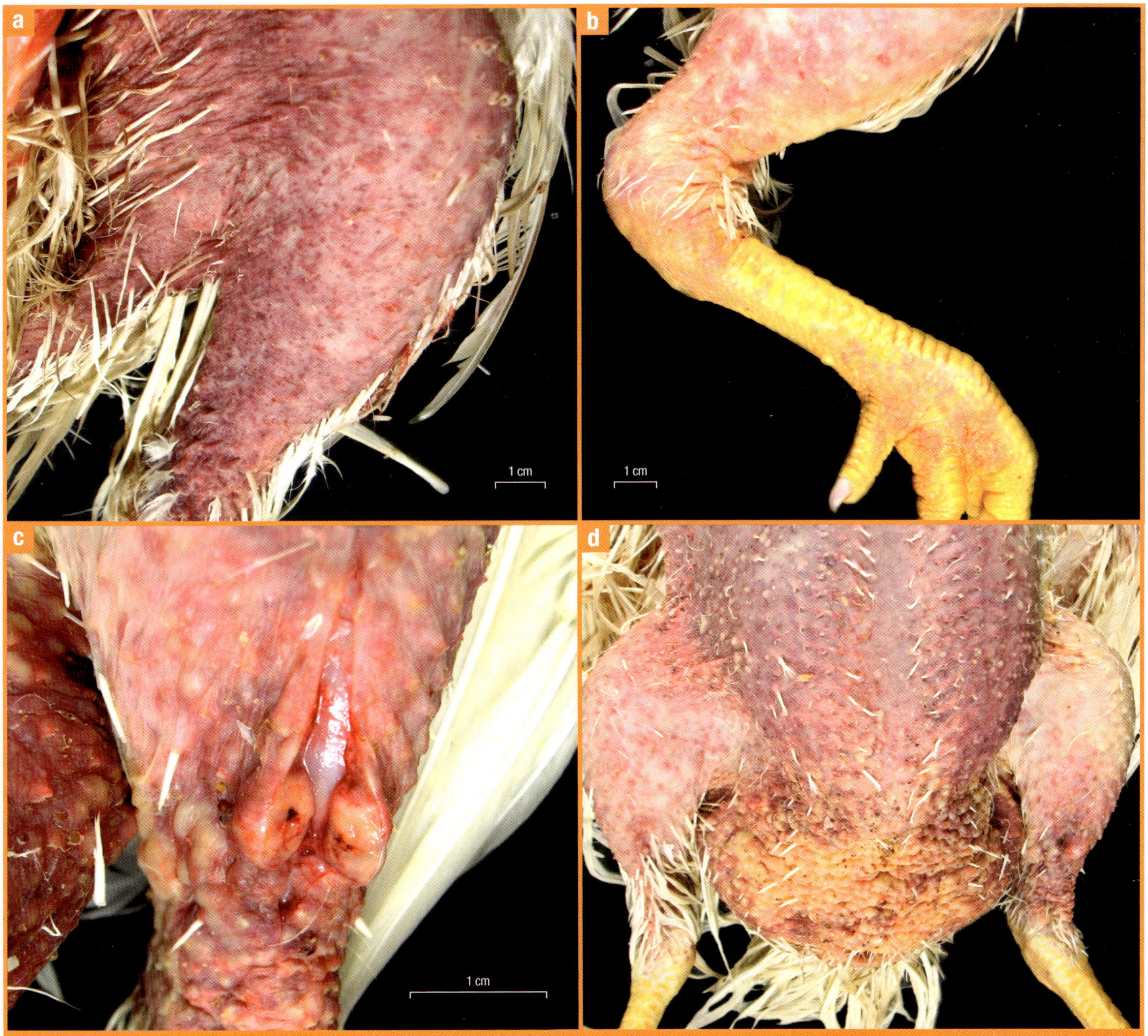

Fig. 12 | MDV-induced cutaneous lesions. (a) Severe, diffuse cutaneous erythema in the thigh of a chicken. (b) Early cutaneous lymphomas in the leg and shank, small nodules can be appreciated in both feathered and unfeathered skin. (c) Variably sized cutaneous lymphoma nodules in the leg of a chicken. (d) Generalized and extensive nodular cutaneous lymphomas in a chicken carcass.

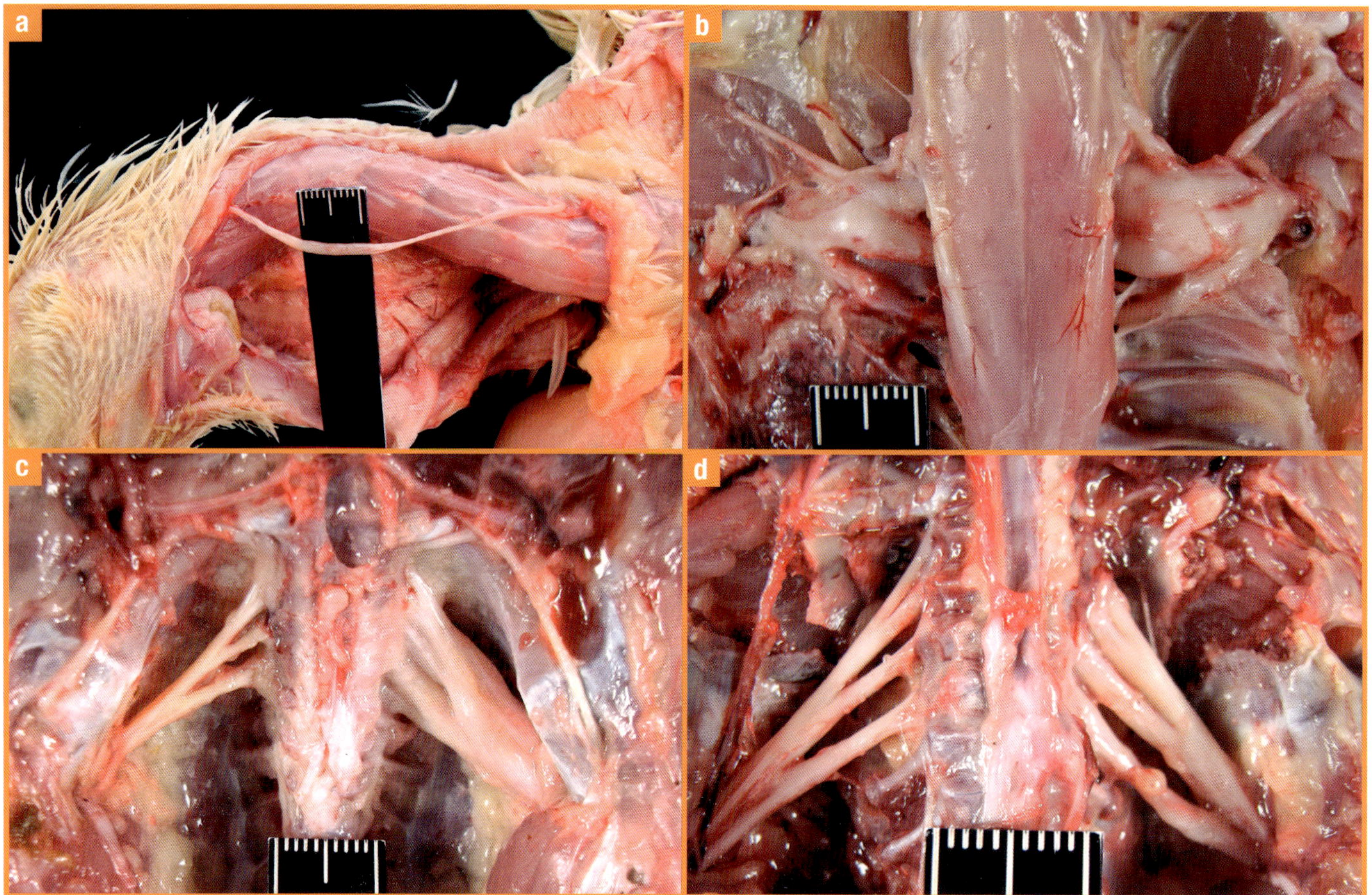

Fig. 13 | MDV-induced lymphomas in peripheral nerves. (a) Marked enlargement of the vagus nerve. (b) Marked bilateral enlargement of brachial plexi. (c) Severe unilateral enlargement of a sciatic plexus. (d) The bilateral sciatic plexi are variably enlarged but the sciatic nerve branches on the right are more severely affected.

can occur in the absence of gross nerve lesions, if nerves are affected the MD diagnosis is very much simplified. Any nerve or ganglia can be affected. Nerve enlargement can be uniform along its length (Figs. 13a-c) or it might be segmental and nodular (Fig. 13d). Lesions can be unilateral or bilateral. Affected nerves or affected areas of the nerves are usually up to 2-5 times the normal thickness. In severe cases, the enlarged nerves lose their normal glistening cross-striations, have a grey to yellow discoloration, and sometimes are edematous and/or hemorrhagic.

- Histopathology (Fig. 14): regardless of the location, lymphomas induced by MDV have the same microscopic characteristics. Therefore, a general description will be made followed by specific characteristics of the lymphomas in different tissues. MD lymphomas can be focal, well demarcated from the normal parenchyma of the viscera or they can infiltrate diffusely and destroy the normal parenchyma. MD lymphomas consist of a mixture of small and medium sized lymphocytes, lymphoblasts, and macrophages. [86] Plasma cells are rarely present. The lymphoid tumor cells are pleomorphic, with abundant cytoplasm, and fairly large atypical nuclei with prominent nucleoli (Fig. 14a). Because of the inflammatory component in MD lymphomas, it is particularly difficult to differentiate initial stages of the lymphoma from normal lymphoreactive areas or from severe inflammatory lesions induced by MDV.

Peripheral nerve lesions have been classified as two types (A and B). [84] Type A is characterized by a marked infiltration of neoplastic lymphoid cells that destroy the structure of the nerve (Fig. 14b). Microscopic characteristics of the lymphomas in nerves are the same as those describe in other tissues. Type B lesions are inflammatory in nature and are characterized by infiltration of plasma cells, edema and variable degree of demyelination (Figs. 14c-d). The pathogenesis of B type lesions is poorly understood but chronological studies showed that they occur late in the pathogenesis of MD and probably are secondary to the immune response against type A lesions. [66]

Immunohistochemistry

Although experimentally MDV is able to transform cells of a variety of types, under natural conditions most of the neoplastic transformed cells are considered to be $CD4^+$ (Fig. 15a) $CD8^-$ (Fig. 15b) T lymphocytes expressing the antigens MATSA and AV37 (Fig. 15c), the latter being analogous to the human CD30 antigen.[14,92] Expression of MDV antigens is quite restrictive in transformed T lymphocytes. Sporadically, a few cells in the tumors express early antigens such as pp38 and ribonucleotide reductase. The expression of these antigens is inconsistent and varies greatly from tumor to tumor. It is now considered that cells expressing those early antigens might be undergoing a reactivation of the infection.[99] The oncogene *meq*, however, is consistently highly expressed in lymphomas as well as in lymphoblastic cell lines (Fig. 15d).

Diagnosis

The diagnosis of lymphomas is fundamentally different from the diagnosis of many other diseases of chickens and presents numerous challenges to the diagnostician. The first thing to keep in mind is that the presence of MDV does not imply disease since MDV is ubiquitous and most infected chickens do not develop MD. It is also important to consider that there are other viruses that can induce lymphomas in poultry, such as avian leukosis virus (ALV) and reticuloendotheliosis virus (REV). Although organ and tissue tropisms differ, there is no truly pathognomonic lesion for any of the lymphomas induced by these viruses. Finally, there are other syndromes of non-infectious etiology, such as peripheral neuropathy that can induce lesions in the peripheral nerves that are very similar to MDV-induced type B lesions.[7,122] A simplified review of the diagnostic criteria is presented in Table 3. A manual on the differential diagnosis of poultry tumor diseases has been recently published[122] and readers are encouraged to read it for further details.

The diagnosis of MD is a multi-step process. The tentative diagnosis can be achieved on the farm by the evaluation of epidemiology, clinical signs, and pathology. Confirmation of the diagnosis in the laboratory may be done by histopathology, immunohistochemistry, and real-time PCR. Table 3 summarizes the main differential diagnoses to consider and the necessary tests to confirm a diagnosis.

Table 3. Differential diagnosis of viral tumor diseases in poultry.

GROSS LESIONS	AGE (WEEKS)	DIFFERENTIAL DIAGNOSIS	TEST TO CONFIRM DIAGNOSIS	
			AID IN THE DIAGNOSIS	CONFIRM DIAGNOSIS
Enlarged nerves	< 14	• Marek's disease • Peripheral neuropathy	Histopathology	Real-time PCR
	> 14	• Marek's disease • Peripheral neuropathy • Reticuloendotheliosis (neuritis)	Histopathology	Real-time PCR
Tumors in viscera + enlarged nerves	< 14	Marek's disease	Not necessary in most cases*	Not necessary in most cases*
	> 14	• Marek's disease • REV-induced tumors	• Histopathology • Immunohistochemistry	Real-time PCR
Tumors in viscera	< 14	• Marek's disease • Acutely transforming retrovirus	• Histopathology • Immunohistochemistry	Real-time PCR
	> 14	• Marek's disease • ALV-induced tumors • REV-induced tumors	• Histopathology • Immunohistochemistry	Real-time PCR
Tumors in the bursa of Fabricius	> 14	• Marek's disease • ALV-induced tumors • REV-induced tumors	• Histopathology • Immunohistochemistry	Real-time PCR

* The only exception to this would be the rare cases in which there are tumors and enlarged nerves (neuritis) induced by REV.

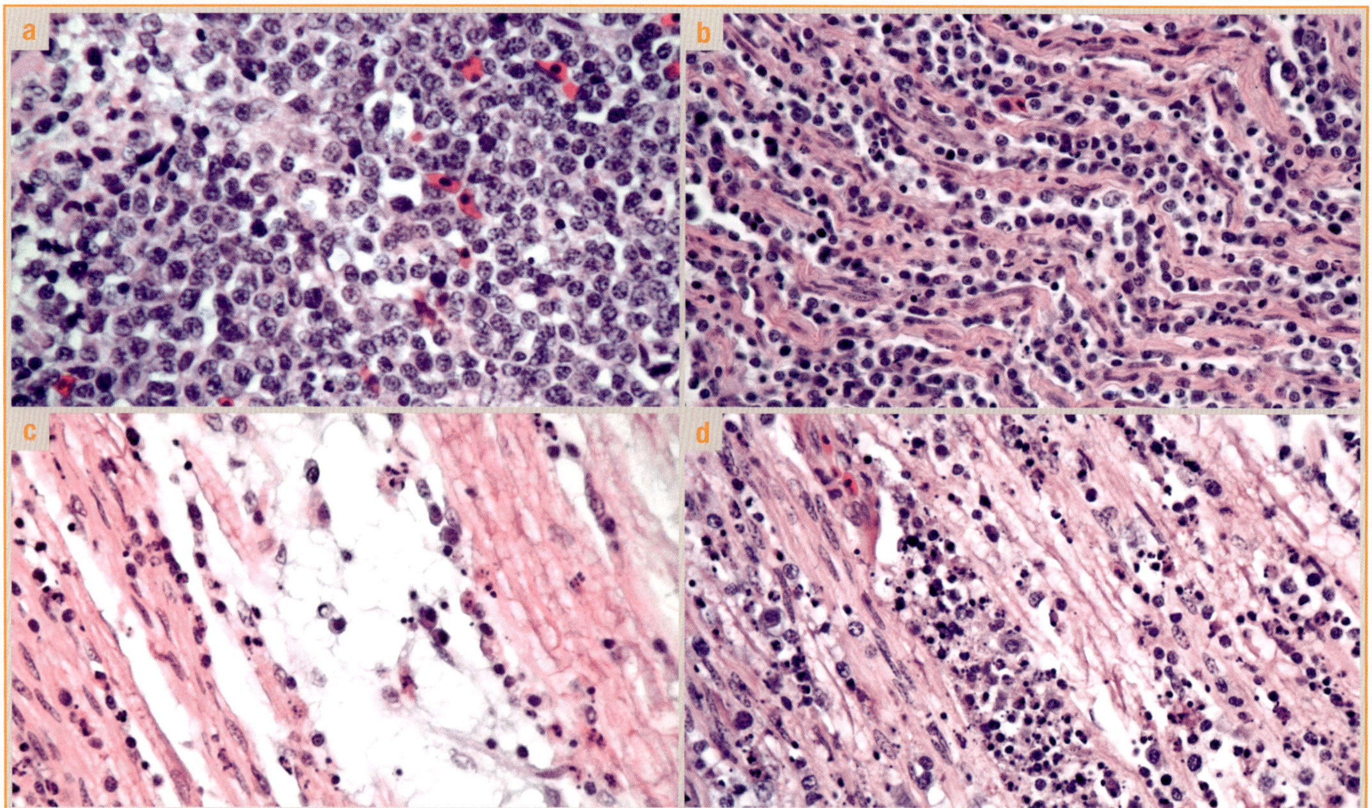

Fig. 14 Photomicrographs of MD lymphomas. (a) Lymphoma in the lung of a chicken, note that the neoplastic lymphocytes are heterogenous and pleomorphic with large vesicular nuclei. (b) Type A lesions in a nerve are characterized by a high density of neoplastic lymphocytes that infiltrate and separate the intervening nerve fibers. (c) Type B lesions in a nerve are characterized by chronic inflammatory cells like macrophages, lymphocytes and plasma cells accompanied by edema separating the nerve fibers. (d) Type B lesions in a peripheral nerve showing inflammatory cell infiltrates composed of macrophages, lymphocytes and heterophils that are often pycnotic and show karyolysis. These inflammatory lesions should not be confused with type A lesions that are neoplastic.

Tentative diagnosis

Age: both, REV and ALV, require longer to transform lymphocytes than MDV. Therefore, if a chicken younger than 14 weeks develop lymphomas, MDV is the most likely etiology. However, MDV is able to induce tumors in older chickens (> 14 weeks), thus limiting the value of this criterion.

Clinical signs: retroviruses do not induce specific clinical signs. Chickens with retrovirus-induced tumors will develop non-specific clinical signs such as depression, lethargy, ruffled feathers, etc. MDV can affect brain and peripheral nerves and if tumors develop in those tissues, chickens will develop neurological clinical signs (paralysis, ataxia, tremors, torticollis, etc.). However, if MDV-induced lymphomas do not affect the nervous system, clinical signs will be non-specific, just like those induced by retroviruses.

Gross pathology: involvement of the peripheral nerves is normally associated with MDV-induced lymphomas. If peripheral nerve enlargement is present, MDV is the most likely cause of the tumors. However, this assumption has two limitations. Peripheral neuropathy (PN) is a non-neoplastic syndrome that induces enlargement of peripheral nerves just like MD. [7,122] In the absence of visceral tumors and if only nerve lesions are present, further diagnostic tests are needed to differentiate between MD and PN. If there are both nerve and visceral tumors, then PN may be ruled out. However, REV can induce visceral lymphomas and cause neuritis that could be easily confused with MD. In this case, further diagnostic tests are needed (Table 3).

Detection of bursal tumors is a common feature in tumors induced by retroviruses (both ALV and REV). However, they are not present in all chickens with retrovirus-induced tumors. Also, MDV can induce bursal tumors that will look grossly identical to those induced by retroviruses.

Laboratory diagnosis

Histopathology: fresh samples of tumors and peripheral nerves from recently euthanized sick chickens should be collected and fixed in 10 % neutral buffered formalin for 24-48 hours. The criteria evaluated by pathologists include distribution of lesions and morphology of the tumor cells:

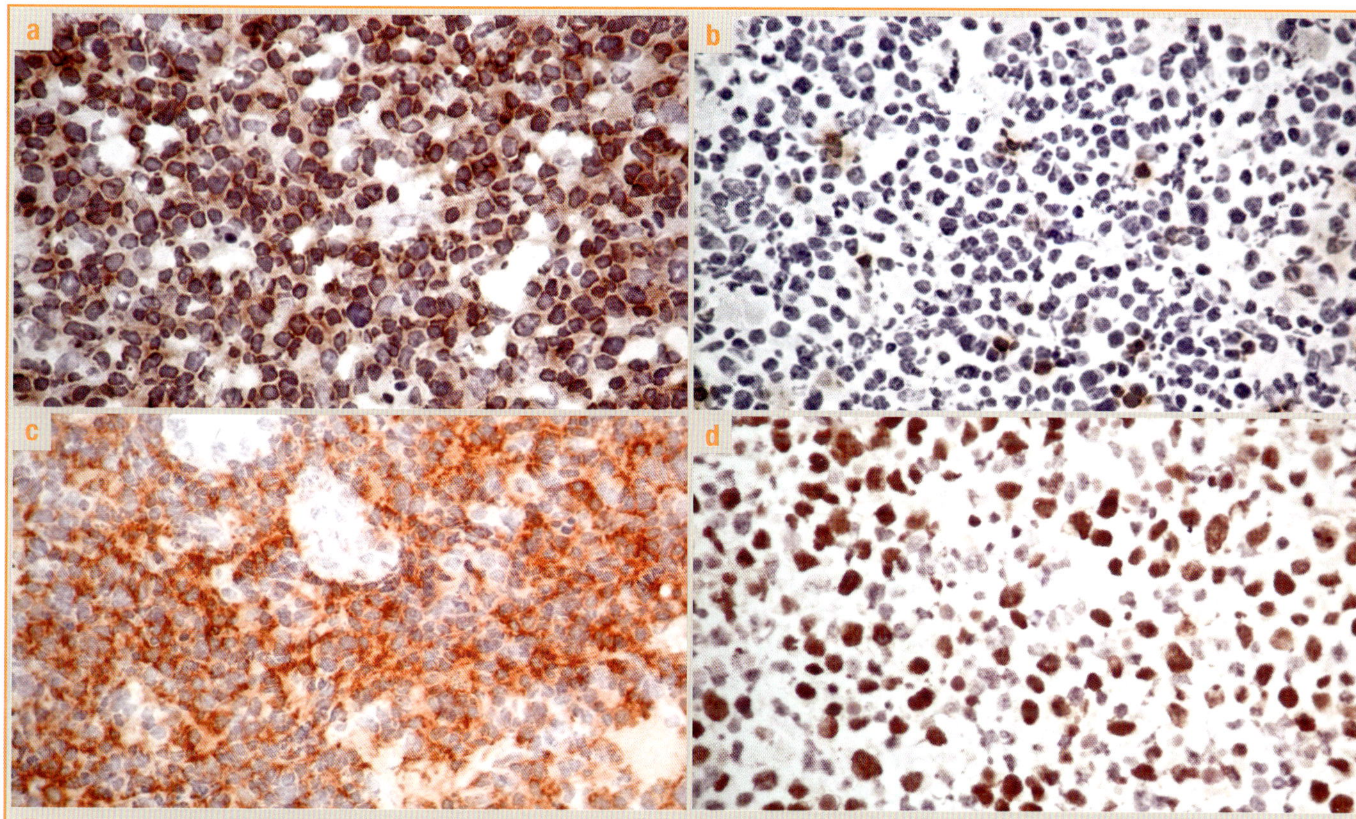

Fig. 15 Immunophenotype of MDV-induced lymphoma. (a) CD4 antigen expression in a MD lymphoma demonstrated by immunohistochemistry (brown stain), note that almost all the cells present in the tumor are strongly positive. (b) CD8 antigen expression in a MD lymphoma demonstrated by immunohistochemistry (brown stain), note that few scattered cells are positive. (c) CD30 antigen expression in a MD lymphoma demonstrated by immunohistochemistry (brown stain), note that almost all the cells present in the tumor are strongly positive. (d) Viral oncogene *meq* antigen expression in a MD lymphoma demonstrated by immunohistochemistry (brown stain), note that almost all the cells present in the tumor have strongly intranuclear staining.

- Lymphomas in visceral organs accompanied by lymphomas in nerves. These lesions are characteristic of MD and diagnosis can be confirmed by histopathology. However, it is important to confirm that nerve lesions are indeed neoplastic (type A) and not inflammatory. Inflammatory lesions in the nerves are an indication of MDV infection but not of MD.
- Lymphomas in nerves only. In this case, the diagnosis of MD may be made by histopathology if the lesions are type A. If lesions are type B, it is necessary to differentiate between MD and PN, due to overlapping morphologic features, using other methods such as real-time PCR or immunohistochemistry.
- Lymphomas in viscera only. Those lesions could be due to retrovirus or to MDV and further tests are needed to confirm the etiology.
- Lymphomas in the bursa. This lesion can be very helpful in the diagnosis by histopathology. Retrovirus-induced tumors in the bursa are intrafollicular lymphomas, whereas MDV-induced tumors in the bursa are interfollicular lymphomas.
- Morphology of tumor cells may also aid in the diagnosis if fresh samples are collected from euthanized chickens and properly fixed in 10 % neutral buffered formalin for 24-48 hours. ALV-induced lymphomas are formed by homogenous population of lymphoblasts while MDV-induced lymphomas are formed by a heterogeneous population of lymphoid cells of various sizes and macrophages. REV-induced lymphomas are normally identical to those induced by ALV, but sometimes they can be very similar to those induced by MDV.

One of the major challenges in the diagnosis of MD by histopathology is the differentiation between MDV-induced inflammatory lesions and MDV-induced lymphomas. First, MDV is the etiology for both of these lesions. Also, inflammatory lesions can progress to the development of neoplastic lesions but this is not always the case. Finally, lymphomas are composed of a mixture of pleomorphic neoplastic and inflammatory cells. Furthermore, even MDV vaccines (e.g. HVT) can induce inflammatory lesions.[113] Interpretation of borderline inflammatory/neoplastic lesions has to be done carefully based on other concurrent evidence of the disease (e.g. clinical signs, gross lymphomas, etc.). In many cases, further diagnostic tests are necessary to differentiate between lymphoid inflammation and MDV-induced lymphomas.

Immunohistochemistry: characterization of the phenotype of tumor cells by immunohistochemistry can be very useful in the differential diagnosis of poultry tumor diseases. MD tumors are composed of neoplastic T lymphocytes, and ALV-induced lymphomas are composed of neoplastic B lymphocytes. REV tumors are generally composed of B lymphocytes but sometimes they can also be of T lymphocytic origin. The major drawback of phenotypic characterization of tumor cells is that most commercially available antibodies against chicken antigens do not work very well in formalin fixed and paraffin embedded samples and tumor samples have to be snap frozen in liquid nitrogen to retain the antigenicity.

Detection of the oncogene *meq* in tumor cells by immunohistochemistry is more specific than identification of the immunephenotype of the tumor cell population. [46] MDV-induced tumor cells express high levels of the oncoprotein *meq* but this is absent in retrovirus-induced tumors or in PN lesions. The limitation of this technique, however, is that antibodies against the oncoprotein *meq* are not commercially available.

Expression of other immuno-markers such as MATSA and AV37 is high in MD tumors. [46] However, they are not specific to MD lymphomas since they can also be present in other lymphoid tumors and even in inflammatory lesions. [46,94] Therefore, its use in diagnostics is limited.

Real-time PCR: quantification of the MDV DNA by real-time PCR is highly useful for confirmation of MD tumors, since tumor tissues contain 100-fold higher levels of MDV DNA than latently infected tissues. [46] The same assay can be used for early diagnosis of MD as early as 3 weeks of age. [47] Quantification can be done by using a standard curve (absolute quantification) or by the Ct method (relative quantification). [46] However, the Ct method is recommended as it is easier to standardize in different laboratories and it does not require the use of a standard curve. Diagnosis of MD can be done using samples from tumors, blood, and feather pulp. [29] Samples can be stored frozen at -70 °C or they can be collected in FTA® cards. [28] The latter option has several advantages for storage and shipping.

Control

MD control is based on three criteria: good biosecurity, selection for genetic resistance and vaccination. Biosecurity and genetic resistance are currently used as important adjuncts to vaccination rather than as primary control strategies. The focus of this chapter will be mainly on vaccines and vaccination protocols. Reviews on MD vaccines and control procedures are available for further details. [11,48,96]

Genetics

The relevance of genetic resistance in the control of MD was observed several decades ago. [26] Indeed, it was the first method used to control the disease. Primary breeder companies frequently include MD resistance as one of the criteria for selection. The strategies to select for MD resistance have been reviewed [8] and include mainly mass selection (i.e. breeding from survivors) and family selection utilizing pedigreed offspring as breeders. There are two groups of genes in the chicken that influence MD resistance: major histocompatibility complex (MHC) genes and non-MHC genes. The relevance of MHC-genes in MD resistance has been amply demonstrated. [8] Particularly remarkable is the influence of B haplotype on the efficacy of MD vaccines and this influence depends on the serotype of the vaccine. [4-6]

Several non-MHC genes may also be involved in genetic resistance against MD. For example, line 6 and line 7 chickens differ markedly in MD susceptibility, but both lines are homozygous for the MHC B^2 allele. [30] Numerous studies have identified and mapped several quantitative trait loci (QTL) that may be linked to genetic resistance against MD. [13,112,123] The rapid technological advances in the complete genome sequencing of the chicken and SNP analysis (Single Nucleotide Polymorphisms) of various genetic lines with different susceptibilities to MD will aid in the identification of specific genes associated with resistance to MD.

Biosecurity

Taking the example of specific-pathogen-free flocks, MD may be eradicated from a farm if ideal conditions of biosecurity are followed. Unfortunately, the use of filtered air and positive pressure housing is not economically feasible for the poultry industry. However, a proper biosecurity plan will be of great help to control MD. There are two critical points in any MD biosecurity plan:

- Reduce initial levels of MDV on the farm by preventing entry of MDV into the building.
- Avoid contamination of the environment by preventing MDV from leaving the building.

Measures to reduce initial levels (all in-all out systems, single age buildings, etc.) of MDV have been widely emphasized although not always practiced. Measures to avoid contamination of the environment, however, are not always well recognized and there are two issues that deserve more attention: air management and disposal of chicken carcasses and manure. Biofilters designed to remove odors from air emanating from livestock facilities might be a solution to decrease the level of MDV contamination in the air exiting poultry farms. [105] Carcasses are usually burned or buried but disposal of manure does not normally receive the attention it requires. Composting has been shown to be a satisfactory alternative procedure for discarding both carcasses and manure. [105]

Vaccination

Vaccination protocols

Type of vaccines: modified live vaccines are the keystone for protecting against MD. There is a large selection of licensed MD vaccines representing three MDV serotypes. In general, the three types of formulations in ascending order of efficacy are: HVT alone, HVT plus a serotype 2 strain, and CVI988 serotype 1 strain (Rispens) with or without viruses of serotypes 2 and 3. A decade ago, a novel serotype 1 MDV vaccine (strain BH16) was introduced in Australia and it seemed to confer at least as much protection as CVI988. [61,62] Recently, several recombinant vaccines using HVT as a vector have become available and they are widely used alone (mainly in broiler chickens) or in combination with vaccines of serotypes 1 and 2. In addition, recombinant vaccines using serotype 1 strains (either as a vector expressing genes of other viruses or by deleting partially or completely the oncogene *meq*) have been developed and are still under experimental evaluation. [31,72,75,126]

MD vaccines are highly cell associated viruses. They are produced in chicken embryo cells, stored in liquid nitrogen, and administered as viable cell suspensions. HVT, but not serotype 1 and 2 MDV, can be produced as a cell-free suspension and stored in a lyophilized state. However, the cell-associated form of HVT vaccine has been most widely used because it is more efficacious than cell-free virus in the presence of MAb.

Vaccine administration: early immunity is essential since most chicks face challenge from MDV within the first few days of being introduced into their brooding pens. Therefore, MD vaccines are administered to chicks at hatch by subcutaneous or intramuscular inoculation, or in ovo at embryonic days 18 (via amniotic) or 19 (intraembryonic route). [100] Cell-associated vaccines are very labile. Only viable infected cells are capable of transmitting the vaccine virus, so handling is of crucial importance for a vaccine to retain its efficacy. [56] Failures in the cold chain (MD vaccines should be stored in liquid nitrogen and maintained under refrigeration), improper thawing conditions, and reconstitution in inadequate diluents can severely reduce vaccine titers. Other factors, such as mixing with antibiotics [27,35], joint administration with other vaccines [91], or long delays in vaccination after reconstitution can also decrease vaccine titers. Finally, dilution of vaccines to reduce vaccination costs is a common practice worldwide, especially in the broiler chicken industry. The negative effects of administering suboptimal doses of vaccine have been recently reported. [49] Besides of suboptimal vaccine dose, there are other factors that influence the efficacy of vaccines such as an early challenge with MDV before the vaccine-induced immunity has been elicited; decreased immune competence of the chicken by either infectious or non-infectious causes; and presence of highly virulent MDVs (Fig. 16).

There are three strategies (protective synergism, revaccination, and the use of adjuvants) that are commonly used to augment vaccine efficacy:

- Protective synergism: it is the basis for the bivalent vaccines developed in the 1980s. Combination of the SB-1 strain (serotype 2) and the FC126 strain (serotype 3, HVT) provides better protection than either of the vaccines alone. [95,115] Synergism is strongly serotype specific and is especially evident in the combination of serotypes 2 and 3. [116] No protective synergism has been reported in the combination of serotype 1 with serotypes 2 or 3. The mechanisms involved in the protective synergism are poorly understood and represent an overlooked but important area for future research.
- Revaccination: the practice of administering a second dose of MD vaccine at a later time (revaccination) has been used in commercial poultry for many years. Recent studies demonstrated that the benefit of double vaccination can be achieved by using a less efficacious first vaccine followed by a more efficacious second vaccine. [50] In ovo vaccination followed by a second vaccination at day of age seems to be the most beneficial protocol. [50] An early and strong activation of T lymphocytes following the in ovo vaccination seem to be, at least partially, responsible for the benefits of double vaccination. [52]
- Use of adjuvants: MD vaccines are administered in embryo or in one-day old chicks. The use of immunomodulators, such as cytokines, and adjuvants along with MD vaccines could enhance the innate immune response and induce an earlier maturation of the immune system of the chicken. Acemannan, a polysaccharide, has been licensed as an adjuvant of MD vaccines in the USA since 1992, but it is not widely used. Several studies have been conducted to include cytokines as adjuvants in MD vaccines to enhance the cellular immune response. [33,109] This area of research will continue in the future and may be a solution to increase the protection conferred by the current generation of vaccines.

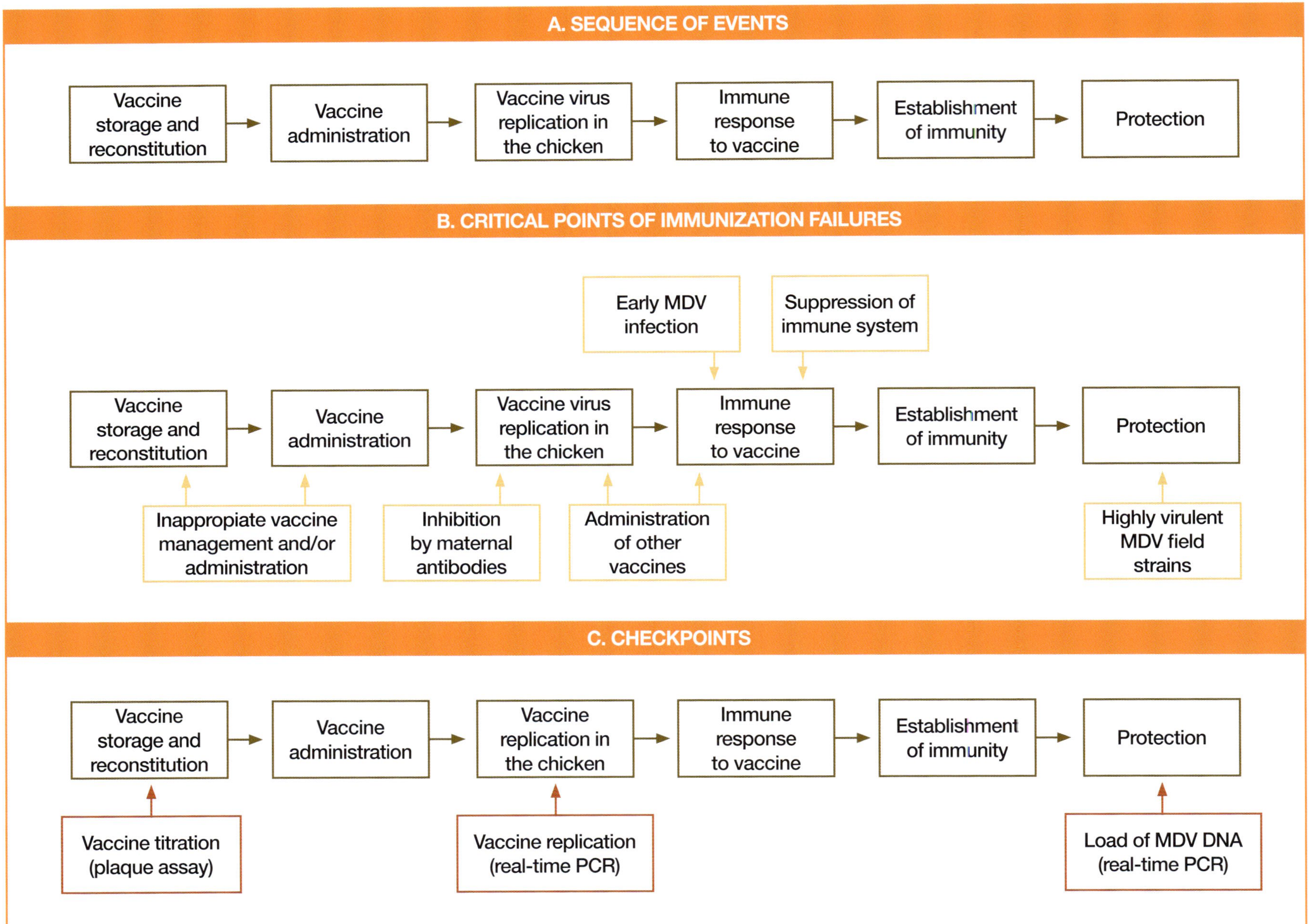

Fig. 16 | Critical points in immunization failures and checkpoints. (A) The expected outcome of MD vaccination is the establishment of immunity and protection against MD. The necessary steps for this process to be successful include proper vaccine storage, reconstitution and administration; adequate replication of the vaccine virus in the chickens; development of a proper immune responses; and the establishment of immunity. (B) Various factors (in yellow) can negatively affect the sequence of events necessary to achieve proper protection following MD vaccination. (C) In the event of an immunization failure, there are three checkpoints that can be monitored: vaccine titers, vaccine replication in the chicken and load of MDV DNA (early diagnosis).

Monitoring vaccination and protection

Because of the cell-associated nature of MD vaccines, they are labile and failures in vaccination may occur. In case of immunization failures, there are three aspects that can be monitored: vaccine titers by plaque assay, replication of the vaccine virus in the chickens by real-time PCR, and load of MDV DNA by real-time PCR for an early diagnosis (Fig. 16). Titration of vaccines by plaque assay should be conducted directly from the vaccine vial and after reconstitution in the diluent. When titration is not feasible, an alternative is possible to count live cells using a vital dye such as trypan blue. It is important to consider that counting live cells do not provide information about the vaccine titers. However, it can give a rough idea on how the vaccine has been handled.

Monitoring replication of the vaccine virus in the chicken can ensure that vaccination was correctly administered and there were no other factors inhibiting replication of the vaccines in the chicken. The evaluation of MD vaccine virus replication in chickens has traditionally been done by plaque assay. [22] Recently, specific primers for each MD serotype have been designed, and real-time PCR has slowly overtaken the traditional plaque assay. It has been recently demonstrated that feather pulp is an adequate sample to monitor MD vaccination for vaccines of all three serotypes. [9,29] The spleen can also be used, but this requires the euthanasia of the chickens. The use of blood is not advisable due to high number of false negative results, specially, for serotype 3 vaccines. [29] Samples can be collected fresh and stored frozen at -70 °C until processed, or on FTA® cards. [28] The latter has the advantage of easy storage and shipping. It is recommended to sample chickens between 1 and 3 weeks of age to monitor vaccine administration and replication. After 3 weeks of age, the levels of MD vaccine virus reach a plateau even if very low dose of vaccine was administered. [10,49]

Early diagnosis of MD can be done as early as 3 weeks of age by measuring MDV DNA load in blood or feather pulp. [47] This assay can be used to determine if a flock is properly protected against MD. High levels of MDV DNA are prognostic and indicate the possible development of tumors. Most chickens in a flock that is properly protected should have low levels of MDV DNA (latency levels) instead of high levels (tumor levels).

MDV immunosuppression (MDV-IS)

Field relevance

The immunosuppressive nature of MDV is well known (review in ref. 98). However, the relevance of MDV-IS in the field is greatly underestimated, mainly due to its complexity. MDV by itself can negatively affect the immune responses against a variety of diseases and vaccine efficacy (review in ref. 98). Immunosuppression is even more severe if MDV is concurrently present with other immunosuppressive agents such as chicken infectious anemia virus. [73,98] Due to a lack of adequate means to detect MDV-IS and the complexity in the field situation, there are no satisfactory methods to monitor and control it. Recently, it was demonstrated that MD vaccination cannot adequately protect against MDV-IS. [53] In this section, we will review the current knowledge on MDV-IS and focus on areas that warrant further research.

Pathogenesis of MDV-IS

MDV induces a transient immunosuppression associated with early viral replication (cytolytic infection) in the lymphoid organs, and a permanent immunosuppression associated with the secondary cytolytic infection and the development of lymphomas (Fig. 2).

The transient MDV-IS is induced by viruses of all three serotypes and therefore it is not related to the ability of the virus to induce tumors. Two mechanisms have been associated with transient MDV-IS: destruction of B and T lymphocytes due to the initial replication of the viruses in the lymphoid organs, and due to the presence of suppressor macrophages capable of inhibiting replication of lymphocytes in vitro.

The destruction of B and T lymphocytes due to the initial replication of viruses in lymphoid organs is most likely caused by apoptosis. [77,78] The resulting lymphoid atrophy of the bursa of Fabricius and thymus is easy to diagnose by gross inspection or by histopathology. Destruction of lymphoid cells depends greatly on the viral replication rates and it is influenced by MD vaccination status, levels of MAb, and genetic susceptibility against MDV (Table 1). In susceptible chickens that lack MAb and are not vaccinated against MD, vv and vv+ MDV pathotypes replicate more and for a longer period than v or m MDV pathotypes [19,124], and tend to induce severe lymphoid organ atrophy. This is also the case for the experimental serotype 1 MDV vaccines lacking oncogene *meq* [69,72,102], or for MDV strains with REV LTR (long terminal repeat) inserted in their genomes. [51,65,106,117] On the other hand, vaccines of serotypes 2 and 3, or attenuated serotype 1 MDV CVI988 replicate at low rate in the lymphoid organs and they induce minor lesions in the bursa. [40] In chickens that are vaccinated against MD or bearing MAb, early replication in the lymphoid organs is greatly decreased and no lymphoid organ atrophy can be appreciated. [85] Since most chickens in the poultry industry have MAb and are vaccinated against MD, it is highly unlikely that this early immunosuppressive mechanism has any impact under field conditions.

In vitro mitogen stimulation of lymphocytes is often impaired early after infection during the cytolytic phase (days 3-6). [67,88,97] This early immunosuppression is induced not only by serotype 1 MDV, but also by serotype 2 SB-1 strain and HVT, and contributes to the transient MDV-IS. [41] The impaired response is caused by the induction of suppressor macrophages, and the removal of these cells restores the responsiveness of lymphocytes to mitogen stimulation. [67] MDV-induced suppressor macrophages are able to suppress mitogen stimulation in normal lymphocytes. [68] The role of suppressor macrophages in chickens bearing MAb or in chickens that are vaccinated against MDV is unknown.

The permanent MDV-IS, that occurs later in the pathogenesis, is only induced by oncogenic viruses, and occurs regardless of the MAb status of the chickens. [53] We have recently demonstrated that it occurs even in chickens vaccinated against MD that were otherwise protected against the development of lymphomas. [53] The permanent MDV-IS is very complex and difficult to study. It is not related to lymphoid organ atrophy and commonly remains undetected. Permanent MDV-IS is very likely underestimated and might have an economical impact that is arguably as important as MDV-induced tumors. It has been demonstrated that several mechanisms may contribute to permanent MDV-IS.

Development of lymphomas seems to be correlated with permanent MDV-IS [93,111], although the exact role of lymphomas on immunosuppression is poorly understood. It has been speculated that immunosuppression induced by neoplastic cells might lead to increased severity of the secondary cytolytic infection, and therefore reduce the number of B and T lymphocytes. [99] MD tumor cells express various antigens that can interfere with the immune responses, such as chicken fetal antigen that interferes with natural killer cell activity [81], and CD30 antigen that may switch the immune responses toward a Th2 bias. [16,98] On the other hand, MD tumor cells can down-regulate the CD28 antigen, a co-stimulatory molecule for T-cell activation, and this could be a mechanism for immune evasion by the tumors. [15] Li et al. [70] demonstrated that deletion of *meq* decreases the ability of MDV to suppress the humoral immune responses against avian influenza and Newcastle disease following vaccination against those viruses. Deletion of oncogene *meq* also seems to reduce the ability of the vv+ MDV strain 648A to interfere with the protection conferred by infectious laryngotracheitis vaccines (Gimeno et al., unpublished). Recently, Matsuyama-Kato et al. [74] demonstrated that the chicken PD-1/PD-L1 (programmed death-1/programmed death-ligand 1) pathway has immunoinhibitory functions and they reported that tumor cells transformed by MDV express high levels of PD-1 and PD-L1.

Further studies on MDV-IS

In the opinion of the authors, MDV-IS research should focus on the permanent MDV-IS. A better understanding on the mechanisms behind MDV-IS will lead to development of proper diagnostic and control tools that will aid the poultry industry.

There have been several limitations to study permanent MDV-IS:

- Lack of a proper laboratory model.
- Complexity of MDV-IS mechanisms.
- Limited reagents to evaluate immune responses in chickens.
- Limited knowledge on the role of several molecules on the chicken immune system.

Extensive recent advances in research on the chicken's immune system (reviewed in ref. 32) and the development of new immunological reagents will aid in overcoming some of these limitations.

We have recently developed a model to evaluate permanent MDV-IS indirectly by assessing the negative effect on the immune responses against infectious laryngotracheitis vaccines. [53] We have named this model as the MDV-IS LT model and it has proved to be very useful to evaluate permanent MDV-IS. We are currently using this model to evaluate some of the mechanisms involved in MDV-IS, to evaluate factors that affect the severity of the immunosuppression, to evaluate diagnostic criteria, and to test different control methods.

A major keystone in the research of MDV-IS is the relationship between virulence, lymphomas, and immunosuppression. More virulent strains have the ability to overcome vaccine-immune responses and cause tumors in resistant chickens. On the other hand, it seems that more virulent MDVs are also more immunosuppressive. At this point, it is unknown if being more immunosuppressive is critical for the virus to overcome the immune response and induce more tumors. And finally, it could be that the more virulent viruses are more oncogenic and the lymphomas are responsible for inducing greater immunosuppression. Further studies to elucidate the relationship between virulence, lymphomas and immunosuppression are warranted.

Other mechanisms, unrelated to tumors, have been associated with permanent MDV-IS. MDV can dysregulate several aspects of the immune responses. It has been demonstrated that MDV down-regulates MHC-I [43,57], dysregulates MHC-II either by up-regulation [18,79] or down-regulation [71,110], and increases nitric oxide (NO) that could lead to NO-induced apoptosis of lymphocytes and immunosuppression. [59] Pathotype seems to have an effect on the ability of MDV to dysregulate the immune responses. Infection with vv+ MDV strains has been shown to produce higher levels of nitric oxide (NO) in vivo than infections with v MDV strains. [59] In addition, severe down-regulation of MHC-I occurs in chickens inoculated with the 648A strain after 10 passages in cell culture (vv+ MDV), but not with GA strain (v MDV) [43] or with the strain 648A attenuated at 40 passages in cell culture. [44]

Diagnosis of MDV-IS

The only part of MDV-IS that can be measured is the lymphoid organ atrophy associated with the early replication of the virus in the lymphoid organs. As mentioned above, this early MDV-IS is greatly reduced in commercial chickens because they bear MAb and are commonly vaccinated against MD. Therefore, the histopathological evaluation of the lymphoid organs to diagnose MDV-IS has little use. Under laboratory conditions, in vitro assays such as mitogen stimulation assays, antibody responses to antigens, cytotoxic T lymphocyte assays, natural killer assays, and specific antigen proliferation assays have been used to demonstrate MDV-IS. Unfortunately, it will be very difficult to standardize these techniques for routine diagnosis under field conditions, and at present there are no adequate methods to detect the permanent MDV-IS.

Control of MDV-IS

Transient MDV-IS is easily controlled by vaccination against MDV. Control of permanent MDV-IS is more complex and it might not be achieved successfully by the current generation of vaccines. [53]

References

1. Abdul-Careem, M.F., B.D. Hunter, A.J. Sarson, A. Mayameei, H. Zhou, and S. Sharif. Marek's disease virus-induced transient paralysis is associated with cytokine gene expression in the nervous system. Viral Immunol. 19:167-176. 2006.
2. Adldinger, H.K., and B.W. Calnek. Pathogenesis of Marek's disease: Early distribution of virus and viral antigens in infected chickens. J.Natl.Cancer Inst. 50:1287-1298. 1973.
3. Baaten, B.J., K.A. Staines, L.P. Smith, H. Skinner, T.F. Davison, and C. Butter. Early replication in pulmonary B cells after infection with Marek's disease herpesvirus by the respiratory route. Viral Immunol. 22:431-444. 2009.
4. Bacon, L.D., and R.L. Witter. Influence of turkey herpesvirus vaccination on the B-haplotype effect on Marek's disease resistance in 15.B-congenic chickens. Avian Dis. 36:378-385. 1992.
5. Bacon, L.D., and R.L. Witter. B haplotype influence on the relative efficacy of Marek's disease vaccines in commercial chickens. Poult.Sci. 73:481-487. 1994.
6. Bacon, L.D., and R.L. Witter. Serotype specificity of B-haplotype influence on the relative efficacy of Marek's disease vaccines. Avian Dis. 38:65-71. 1994.
7. Bacon, L.D., R.L. Witter, and R.F. Silva. Characterization and experimental reproduction of peripheral neuropathy in White Leghorn chickens. Avian Pathol. 30:487-499. 2001.
8. Bacon, L.D., H.D. Hunt, and H.H. Cheng. Genetic resistance to Marek's disease. In: Current Topics in Microbiology and Immunology. K. Hirai, ed. Springer-Verlag, Berlin. pp 121-142. 2001.
9. Baigent, S.J., L.J. Petherbridge, K. Howes, L.P. Smith, R.J. Currie, and V.K. Nair. Absolute quantitation of Marek's disease virus genome copy number in chicken feather and lymphocyte samples using real-time PCR. J. Virol. Methods 123:53-64. 2005.
10. Baigent, S.J., L.P. Smith, R.J. Currie, and V.K. Nair. Correlation of Marek's disease herpesvirus vaccine virus genome load in feather tips with protection, using an experimental challenge model. Avian Pathol. 36:467-474. 2007.
11. Bublot, M., and J.M. Sharma. Vaccination against Marek's disease. In: Marek's disease, an evolving problem. F. Davison and V.K. Nair, eds. Elsevier Academic Press, London. pp 168-185. 2004.
12. Buckmaster, A.E., S.D. Scott, M.J. Sanderson, M.E.G. Boursnell, L.J.N. Ross, and M.M. Binns. Gene sequence and mapping data from Marek's disease virus and herpesvirus of turkeys: implications for herpesvirus classification. J.Gen. Virol. 69:2033-2042. 1988.
13. Bumstead, N. Genomic mapping of resistance to Marek's disease. Avian Path. 27:S78-S81. 1998.
14. Burgess, S.C., P. Kaiser, and T.F. Davison. A monoclonal antibody that recognizes the chicken homologue of CD30, a tumor antigen in Marek's disease. Current Progress in Avian Immunology. 2001.
15. Burgess, S.C., and T.F. Davison. Identification of the neoplastically transformed cells in Marek's disease herpesvirus-induced lymphomas: Recognition by the monoclonal antibody AV37. J. Virol. 76:7277-7292. 2002.
16. Burgess, S.C., J.R. Young, B.J. Baaten, L. Hunt, L.N. Ross, M.S. Parcells, P.M. Kumar, C.A. Tregaskes, L.F. Lee, and T.F. Davison. Marek's disease is a natural model for lymphomas overexpressing Hodgkin's disease antigen (CD30). Proc Natl Acad Sci U S A. 101:13879-13884. 2004.
17. Calnek, B.W., A.M. Alexander, and D.E. Kahn. Feather follicle epithelium: a source of enveloped and infectious cell-free herpesvirus from Marek's disease. Avian Dis. 14:219-233. 1970.
18. Calnek, B.W., K.A. Schat, L.J.N. Ross, W.R. Shek, and C.L.H. Chen. Further characterization of Marek's disease virus infected lymphocytes. I. In vivo infection. Intl. J. Cancer 33:389-398. 1984.
19. Calnek, B.W., R.W. Harris, C. Buscaglia, K.A. Schat, and B. Lucio. Relationship between the immunosuppressive potential and the pathotype of Marek's disease virus isolates. Avian Dis. 42:124-132. 1998.
20. Calnek, B.W. Pathogenesis of Marek's disease virus infection. In: Current Topics in Microbiology and Immunology. K. Hirai, ed. Springer-Verlag, Berlin. pp 25-56. 2001.
21. Cho, B.R., S.G. Kenzy, and W.J. Mathey. Histologic and microbiologic studies of chickens with transient paralysis. Avian Dis. 14:587-598. 1970.
22. Cho, B.R. A simple in vitro differentiation between turkey herpesvirus and Marek's disease virus. Avian Dis. 25:839-846. 1981.
23. Churchill, A.E. Herpes-type virus isolated in cell culture from tumors of chickens with Marek's disease. I. Studies in cell culture. J.Natl.Cancer Inst. 41:939-950. 1968.
24. Churchill, A.E., and P.M. Biggs. Herpes-type virus isolated in cell culture from tumors of chickens with Marek's disease. II. Studies in vivo. J.Natl.Cancer Inst. 41:951-956. 1968.
25. Churchill, A.E., L.N. Payne, and R.C. Chubb. Immunization against Marek's disease using a live attenuated virus. Nature 221:744-747. 1969.
26. Cole, R.K. Studies on genetic resistance to Marek's disease. Avian Dis. 12:9-28. 1968.
27. Colwell, W.M., D.G. Simmons, J.R. Harris, T.G. Fulp, J.H. Carrozza, and T.A. Maag. Influence of some physical factors on survival of Marek's disease vaccine virus. Avian Dis. 19:781-790. 1975.
28. Cortes, A.L., E.R. Montiel, and I.M. Gimeno. Validation of Marek's disease diagnosis and monitoring of Marek's

disease vaccines from samples collected in FTA cards. Avian Dis 53:510-516. 2009.

29. Cortes, A.L., E.R. Montiel, S. Lemiere, and I.M. Gimeno. Comparison of blood and feather pulp samples for the diagnosis of Marek's disease and for monitoring Marek's Disease vaccination by real time PCR Avian Dis. 55:302-310. 2011.
30. Crittenden, L.B., R.L. Muhm, and B.R. Burmester. Genetic control of the susceptibility to the avian leukosis complex. 2. Marek's disease. Poult.Sci. 51:261-267. 1972.
31. Cui, X., L.F. Lee, H.D. Hunt, W.M. Reed, B. Lupiani, and S.M. Reddy. A Marek's disease virus vIL-8 deletion mutant has attenuated virulence and confers protection against challenge with a very virulent plus strain. Avian Dis. 49:199-206. 2005.
32. Davison, F., B. Kaspers, and K.A. Schat Avian Immunology, 1st ed. Elsevier, London. 2008.
33. Djeraba, A., E. Musset, J.W. Lowenthal, D.B. Boyle, A.M. Chausse, M. Peloille, and P. Quere. Protective effect of avian myelomonocytic growth factor in infection with Marek's disease virus. J. Virol. 76:1062-1070. 2002.
34. Dunn, J., and I.M. Gimeno. Current status of Marek's disease in the United States and worldwide based on a questionnaire survey. Avian Dis. in press. 2013.
35. Eidson, C.S., R.K. Page, and S.H. Kleven. In vivo and in vitro studies on the effect of gentamicin sulfate on the efficacy of the turkey herpesvirus vaccine. Poult.Sci. 57:1519-1525. 1978.
36. Fabricant, C.G., J. Fabricant, and C.R. Minick. Herpesvirus-induced atherosclerosis in chickens. Fed.Proc. 42:2476-2479. 1983.
37. Fabricant, C.G. Atherosclerosis: The consequence of infection with a herpesvirus. Adv.Vet.Sci.Comp.Sci. 30:39-66. 1985.
38. Fabricant, C.G., and J. Fabricant. Atherosclerosis induced by infection with Marek's disease herpesvirus in chickens. American Heart J. 138:S465-S468. 1999.
39. Ficken, M.D., M.P. Nasisse, G.D. Boggan, J.S. Guy, D.P. Wages, R.L. Witter, J.K. Rosenberger, and R.M. Nordgren. Marek's disease virus isolates with unusual tropism and virulence for ocular tissues: clinical findings, challenge studies and pathological features. Avian Pathol. 20:461-474. 1991.
40. Fletcher, O.J., C.S. Eidson, and S.H. Kleven. Bursal lesions in chickens inoculated with Marek's disease vaccines. Avian Dis. 16:153-162. 1972.
41. Friedman, A., E. Shalem-Meilin, and E.D. Heller. Marek's disease vaccines cause temporary B-lymphocyte dysfunction and reduced resistance to infection in chicks. Avian Pathol. 21:621-631. 1992.
42. Gimeno, I.M., R.L. Witter, and W.M. Reed. Four distinct neurologic syndromes in Marek's disease: Effect of viral strain and pathotype. Avian Dis. 43:721-737. 1999.
43. Gimeno, I.M., R.L. Witter, H.D. Hunt, L.F. Lee, S.M. Reddy, and U. Neumann. Marek's disease virus infection in the brain: virus replication, cellular infiltration and major histocompatibility complex antigen expression. Vet. Path. 38:491-503. 2001.
44. Gimeno, I.M., R.L. Witter, H.D. Hunt, S.M. Reddy, and U. Neumann. Differential attenuation of the induction by Marek's disease virus of transient paralysis and persistent neurological disease: a model for pathogenesis studies. Avian Pathol. 30:397-409. 2001.
45. Gimeno, I.M., R.L. Witter, and U. Neumann. Neuropathotyping: a new system to classify Marek's disease virus. Avian Dis. 46:909-918. 2002.
46. Gimeno, I.M., R.L. Witter, A.M. Fadly, and R.F. Silva. Novel criteria for the diagnosis of Marek's disease virus-induced lymphomas. Avian Path. 34:332-340. 2005.
47. Gimeno, I.M., A.L. Cortes, and R.F. Silva. Load of Challenge Marek's Disease Virus DNA in Blood as a Criterion for Early Diagnosis of Marek's Disease Tumors. Avian Dis 52:203-208. 2008.
48. Gimeno, I.M. Marek's disease vaccines: a solution for today but a worry for tomorrow? Vaccine 26 Suppl 3:C31-41. 2008.
49. Gimeno, I.M., A.L. Cortes, E.R. Montiel, S. Lemiere, and A.R. Pandiri. Effect of diluting Marek's disease vaccines on the outcomes of Marek's disease virus infection when challenge with highly virulent Marek's disease viruses. Avian Dis.55:302-10. 2011.
50. Gimeno, I.M., R.L. Witter, A.L. Cortes, S.M. Reddy, and A.R. Pandiri. Standardization of a model to study revaccination against Marek's disease under laboratory conditions. Avian Pathol. 41:59-68. 2011.
51. Gimeno, I.M., R.L. Witter, A.L. Cortes, and W.M. Reed. Replication ability of three highly protective Marek's disease vaccines: implications in lymphoid organ atrophy and protection. Avian Pathol. 40:573-579. 2011.
52. Gimeno, I.M., A.L. Cortes, R.L. Witter, and A.R. Pandiri. Optimization of the protocols for double vaccination against Marek's disease using commercially available vaccines: evaluation of protection, vaccine replication, and activation of T cells. Avian Dis. 56:295-305. 2012.
53. Gimeno, I.M., N.M. Faiz, E.R. Montiel, A.L. Cortes, M. West, and J.S. Guy. Immunosuppression induced by Marek's disease virus: is it affecting the efficacy of infectious laryngotracheitis vaccines? In: 9th International Meeting on Marek's disease and avian Herpesviruses. Berlin. p 35. 2012.
54. Gimeno, I.M., A. Miles, and R.L. Witter. Marek's disease. In: AAAP slides study sets. AAAP, ed. AAAP. 2003.
55. Gimeno, I.M., M. Pizarro, and P. Villegas. Histopathological study of the flaccid paralysis syndrome in Spanish broiler flocks and its relationship with transient paralysis Marek's disease virus induced. In: Current Research on Marek's Disease. R.F. Silva, H.H. Cheng, P.M. Coussens, L.F. Lee and L.F. Velicer, eds. American Association of Avian Pathologists, Inc., Kennett Square, Pennsylvania. pp 98-103. 1996.

56. Halvorson, D.A., and D.O. Mitchell. Loss of cell-associated Marek's disease vaccine titer during thawing, reconstitution and use. Avian Dis. 23:848-853. 1979.
57. Hunt, H.D., B. Lupiani, M.M. Miller, I.M. Gimeno, L.F. Lee, and M.S. Parcells. Marek's disease virus down regulates surface expression of MHV (B complex) class I (BF) glycoproteins during active but not latent infection of chicken cells. Virology 282:198-205. 2001.
58. ICTVdB-Management. 00.031.1.03 Mardivirus. In: C. Buchen-Osmond ICTVdB- The universal virus database, version 4. Columbia University, New York, USA. 2006.
59. Jarosinski, K.W., R. Yunis, P.H. O'Connell, C.J. Markowski-Grimsrud, and K.A. Schat. Incluence of genetic resistance of the chicken and virulence of Marek's disease virus (MDV) on nitirc oxide responses after MDV infection. Avian Dis. 46:636-649. 2002.
60. Jarosinski, K.W., B.L. Njaa, P.H. O'Connell, and K.A. Schat. Pro-inflammatory responses in chicken spleen and brain tissues after infection with very virulent plus Marek's disease virus. Vir. Immunol. 18:148-161. 2005.
61. Karpathy, R.C., G.A. Firth, and G.A. Tannock. Derivation, safety and efficacy of a Marek's disease vaccine developed from an Australian isolate of very virulent Marek's disease virus. Aust. Vet.J. 80:39-44. 2002.
62. Karpathy, R.C., G.A. Firth, and G.A. Tannock. Field evaluations of safety and efficacy of an Australian Marek's disease vaccine. Aust.Vet.J. 81:222-225. 2003.
63. Kenzy, S.G., and P.M. Biggs. Excretion of the Marek's disease agent by infected chickens. Vet.Rec. 80:565-568. 1967.
64. Kenzy, S.G., B.R. Cho, and Y. Kim. Oncogenic Marek's disease herpesvirus in avian encephalitis (temporary paralysis). J.Natl. Cancer Inst. 51:977-982. 1973.
65. Kim, T., J. Mays, A. Fadly, and R.F. Silva. Artificially inserting a reticuloendotheliosis virus long terminal repeat into a bacterial artificial chromosome clone of Marek's disease virus (MDV) alters expression of nearby MDV genes. Virus Genes. 2011.
66. Lawn, A.M., and L.N. Payne. Chronological study of the ultrastructural changes in the perpheral nerves in Marek's disease. In: Resistance and Immunity to Marek's Disease. P.M. Biggs, ed. Commission of the European Communities, Luxembourg. pp 133-143. 1980.
67. Lee, L.F., J.M. Sharma, K. Nazerian, and R.L. Witter. Suppression and enhancement of mitogen response in chickens infected with Marek's disease virus and the herpesvirus of turkeys. Infect.Immun. 21:474-479. 1978.
68. Lee, L.F., J.M. Sharma, K. Nazerian, and R.L. Witter. Suppression of mitogen-induced proliferation of normal spleen cells by macrophages from chickens inoculated with Marek's disease virus. J.Immunol. 120:1554-1559. 1978.
69. Lee, L.F., K.S. Kreager, J. Arango, A. Paraguassu, B. Beckman, H. Zhang, A. Fadly, B. Lupiani, and S.M. Reddy. Comparative evaluation of vaccine efficacy of recombinant Marek's disease virus vaccine lacking Meq oncogene in commercial chickens. Vaccine 28:1294-1299. 2010.
70. Li, Y., A. Sun, S. Su, P. Zhao, Z. Cui, and H. Zhu. Deletion of the Meq gene significantly decreases immunosuppression in chickens caused by pathogenic Marek's disease virus. Virol J 8:2. 2011.
71. Lian, L., L.J. Qu, J.X. Zheng, C.J. Liu, Y.P. Zhang, Y.M. Chen, G.Y. Xu, and N. Yang. Expression profiles of genes within a subregion of chicken major histocompatibility complex B in spleen after Marek's disease virus infection. Poult Sci 89:2123-2129. 2010.
72. Lupiani, B., L.F. Lee, X. Cui, I.M. Gimeno, A. Anderson, R.W. Morgan, R.F. Silva, R.L. Witter, H.J. Kung, and S.M. Reddy. Marek's disease virus-encoded Meq gene is involved in transformation of lymphocytes but is dispensable for replication. Proc Natl Acad Sci U S A 101:11815-11820. 2004.
73. Markowski-Grimsrud, C.J., and K.A. Schat. Infection with chicken anemia virus impairs the generation of pathogen-specific cytotoxic T lymphocytes. Immunology 109:283-294. 2003.
74. Matsuyama-Kato, A., S. Murata, M. Isezaki, R. Kano, S. Takasaki, O. Ichii, S. Konnai, and K. Ohashi. Molecular characterization of immunoinhibitory factors PD-1/PD-L1 in chickens infected with Marek's disease virus. Virol J 9:94. 2012.
75. Morgan, R.W., J. Kent, and A.S. Anderson. Marek's disease virus gC and meq mutants with dramatic reductions in tumour incidences and horizontal transmission. Avian Path. 27:S89-S89. 1998.
76. Morgan, R.W., Q. Xie, J.L. Cantello, A.M. Miles, E.L. Bernberg, J. Kent, and A. Anderson. Marek's disease virus latency. In: Current Topics in Microbiology and Immunology. K. Hirai, ed. Springer-Verlag, Berlin. pp 223-244. 2001.
77. Morimura, T., K. Ohashi, Y. Kon, M. Hattori, C. Sugimoto, and M. Onuma. Apoptosis and CD8-down-regulation in the thymus of chickens infected with Marek's disease virus - Brief report. Arch.Virol. 141:2243-2249. 1996.
78. 78. Morimura, T., K. Ohashi, Y. Kon, M. Hattori, C. Sugimoto, and M. Onuma. Apoptosis in peripheral $CD4^{+}T$ cells and thymocytes by Marek's disease virus-infection. Leukemia 11:206-208. 1997.
79. Niikura, M., T. Kim, H.D. Hunt, J. Burnside, R.W. Morgan, J.B. Dodgson, and H.H. Cheng. Marek's disease virus up-regulates major histocompatibility complex class II cell surface expression in infected cells. Virology 359:212-219. 2007.
80. Njenga, M.K., and C.A. Dangler. Endothelial MHC class II antigen expression and endarteritis associated with Marek's diseasevirus infection in chickens. Vet. Pathol. 32:403-411. 1995.

81. Ohashi, K., T. Mikami, H. Kodama, and H. Izawa. Suppression of NK activity of spleen cells by chicken fetal antigen present on Marek's disease lymphoblastoid cell line cells. Intl.J.Cancer 40:378-382. 1987.
82. Pandiri, A.K., A.L. Cortes, L.F. Lee, and I.M. Gimeno. Marek's disease virus infection in the eye: chronological study of the lesions, virus replication, and vaccine-induced protection. Avian Dis. 52:572-580. 2008.
83. Pappenheimer, A.M., L.C. Dunn, and V. Cone. Studies on fowl paralysis (neurolymphomatosis gallinarum). I. Clinical features and pathology. J. Exper. Med. 49:63-86. 1929.
84. Payne, L.N., and P.M. Biggs. Studies on Marek's disease. II. Pathogenesis. J.Natl.Cancer Inst. 39:281-302. 1967.
85. Payne, L.N., and M. Rennie. Pathogenesis of Marek's disease in chicks with and without maternal antibody. J. Natl. Cancer Inst. 51:1559-1573. 1973.
86. Payne, L.N. Pathology. In: Marek's disease. L.N. Payne, ed. Martinus Nijhoff, Boston. pp 43-75. 1985.
87. Phillips, P.A., and P.M. Biggs. Course of infection in tissue of susceptible chickens after exposure to strains of Marek's disease and turkey herpesvirus. J.Natl.Cancer Inst. 49:1367-1373. 1972.
88. Powell, P.C. In vitro stimulation of blood lymphocytes by phytohaemagglutinin during the development of Marek's disease. Avian Pathol. 9:471-475. 1980.
89. Purchase, H.G. Virus-specific immunofluorescent and precipitin antigens and cell-free virus in the tissues of birds infected with Marek's disease. Cancer Res. 30:1898-1908. 1970.
90. Purchase, H.G. Clinical disease and its economic impact. In: Marek's disease. L.N. Payne, ed. Martinus Nijhoff, Boston. pp 17-42. 1985.
91. Rosenberger, J.K. Reovirus interference with Marek's disease vaccination. In: Proceedings of the Western Poultry Disease Conference. pp 50-51. 1983.
92. Ross, L.J.N., G. O'Sullivan, C. Rothwell, G. Smith, S.C. Burgess, M. Rennie, L.F. Lee, and T.F. Davison. Marek's disease virus EcoRI-Q gene (meq) and a small RNA antisense to ICP4 are abundantly expressed in CD4+ cells and cells carrying a novel lymphoid marker, AV37, in Marek's disease lymphomas. J.Gen.Virol. 78:2191-2198. 1997.
93. Schat, K.A., R.D. Schultz, and B.W. Calnek. Marek's disease: Effect of virus pathogenicity and genetic susceptibility on response of peripheral blood lymphocytes to concanavalin-A. Proc.8th Intl.Symp.Comp.Res.Leuk.Rel.Dis.:46-46. 1977.
94. 94. Schat, K.A., and B.W. Calnek. Demonstration of Marek's disease tumor associated surface antigen in chickens infected with nonocogenic Marek's disease virus and herpesvirus of turkeys. J. Natl. Cancer Inst. 61:855-857. 1978.
95. 95. Schat, K.A., B.W. Calnek, and J. Fabricant. Characterization of two highly oncogenic strains of Marek's disease virus. Avian Pathol. 11:593-605. 1982.
96. Schat, K.A., and E. Baranowski. Animal vaccination and the evolution of viral pathogens. Rev. sci. tech. Off. int. Epiz. 26:327-338. 2007.
97. Schat, K.A., R.D. Schultz, and B.W. Calnek. Marek's disease: Effect of virus pathogenicity and genetic susceptibility on response of peripheral blood lymphocytes to concanavalin-A. In: Advances Comparative Leukosis Research. P. Bentvelzen, J. Hilgers and D.S. Yohn, eds. Elsevier, Amsterdam. pp 183-186. 1978.
98. Schat, K.A. Marek's disease immunosuppression. In: Marek's disease an evolving problem. F. Davison, Venugopal, N., ed. Elsevier, Compton. pp 142-155. 2004.
99. Schat, K.A., and V.K. Nair. Marek's disease. In: Diseases of Poultry, 12th ed. Y.M. Saif, A.M. Fadly, J.R. Glisson, L.R. McDougald, L.K. Nolan and D.E. Swayne, eds. Blackwell Publishing Professionals, Ames, Iowa. pp 449-514. 2008.
100. Sharma, J.M., and B.R. Burmester. Resistance to Marek's disease at hatching in chickens vaccinated as embryos with the turkey herpesvirus. Avian Dis. 26:134-149. 1982.
101. Shek, W.R., K.A. Schat, and B.W. Calnek. Characterization of non-oncogenic Marek's disease virus-infected and turkey herpesvirus infected lymphocytes. J.Gen.Virol. 63:333-341. 1982.
102. Silva, R.F., J.R. Dunn, H.H. Cheng, and M. Niikura. A MEQ-deleted Marek's disease virus cloned as a bacterial artificial chromosome is a highly efficacious vaccine. Avian Dis 54:862-869. 2010.
103. Spatz, S.J., and R.F. Silva. Polymorphisms in the repeat long regions of oncogenic and attenuated pathotypes of Marek's disease virus 1. Virus Genes 35:41-53. 2007.
104. Spencer, J.L., F. Gilka, J.S. Gavora, R.J. Hampson, and D.J. Caldwell. Studies with a Marek's disease virus that caused blindness and high mortality in vaccinated flocks. In: 4th International Symposium on Marek's Disease, 19th World's Poultry Congress. World's Poultry Science Association, Amsterdam. pp 199-202. 1992.
105. Spencer, J.L., and J. Guan. Public health implications related to spread of pathogens in manure from livestock and poultry operations. Methods Mol Biol 268:503-515. 2004.
106. Sun, A.J., X.Y. Xu, L. Petherbridge, Y.G. Zhao, V. Nair, and Z.Z. Cui. Functional evaluation of the role of reticuloendotheliosis virus long terminal repeat (LTR) integrated into the genome of a field strain of Marek's disease virus. Virology 397:270-276. 2010.
107. Swayne, D.E., O.J. Fletcher, and L.W. Schierman. Marek's disease virus-induced transient paralysis in chickens: Demonstration of vasogenic brain oedema by an immunohistochemical method. J.Comp.Pathol. 101:451-462. 1989.

108. Swayne, D.E., O.J. Fletcher, and L.W. Schierman. Marek's disease virus-induced transient paralysis in chickens. 1. Time course association between clinical signs and histological brain lesions. Avian Pathol. 18:385-396. 1989.
109. Tarpey, I., P.J. Davis, P.J.A. Sondermeijer, C. van Geffen, I. Verstegen, V.E. Schijns, J. Kolodsick, and R. Sundick. Expression of chicken interleukin-2 by turkey herpesvirus increases the immune response against Marek's disease virus but fails to increase protection against virulent challenge. Avian Pathol. 36:69-74. 2007.
110. Thanthrige-Don, N., L.R. Read, M.F. Abdul Careem, H. Mohammadi, A.I. Mallick, and S. Sharif. Marek's disease virus influences the expression of genes associated with IFN-gamma-inducible MHC class II expression. Viral Immunol 23:227-232. 2010.
111. Theis, G.A., R.A. McBride, and L.W. Schierman. Depression of in vitro responsiveness to phytohemagglutinin in spleen cells cultured from chickens with Marek's disease. J.Immunol. 115:848-853. 1975.
112. Vallejo, R.L., L.D. Bacon, H.-C. Liu, R.L. Witter, M.M. Groenen, J. Hillel, and H.H. Cheng. Genetic mapping of quantitative trait loci affecting susceptibility to Marek's disease virus induced tumors in F2 intercross chickens. Genetics 148:349-360. 1998.
113. Witter, R.L., J.M. Sharma, and L. Offenbecker. Turkey herpesvirus infection in chickens: induction of lymphoproliferative lesions and characterization of vaccinal immunity against Marek's disease. Avian Dis. 20:676-692. 1976.
114. Witter, R.L., J.M. Sharma, and A.M. Fadly. Pathogenicity of variant Marek's disease virus isolants in vaccinated and unvaccinated chickens. Avian Dis. 24:210-232. 1980.
115. Witter, R.L. Protection by attenuated and polyvalent vaccines against highly virulent strains of Marek's disease virus. Avian Pathol. 11:49-62. 1982.
116. Witter, R.L. Influence of serotype and virus strain on synergism between Marek's disease vaccine viruses. Avian Pathol. 21:601-614. 1992.
117. Witter, R.L., D. Li, D. Jones, L.F. Lee, and H.J. Kung. Retroviral insertional mutagenesis of a herpesvirus: A Marek's disease virus mutant attenuated for oncogenicity but not for immunosuppression or in vivo replication. Avian Dis. 41:407-421. 1997.
118. Witter, R.L. Increased virulence of Marek's disease virus field isolates. Avian Dis. 41:149-163. 1997.
119. Witter, R.L., I.M. Gimeno, W.M. Reed, and L.D. Bacon. An acute form of transient paralysis induced by highly virulent strains of Marek's disease virus. Avian Dis. 43:704-720. 1999.
120. Witter, R.L., B.W. Calnek, C. Buscaglia, I.M. Gimeno, and K.A. Schat. Classification of Marek's disease viruses according to pathotype: philosophy and methodology. Avian Patho 34:75-90. 2005.
121. Witter, R.L. Epidemiology of Marek's disease - a review. P.M. Biggs, G. de-The and L.N. Payne, eds. International Agency for Research on Cancer, Lyon. pp 111-122. 1972.
122. Witter, R.L., I.M. Gimeno, A.K. Pandiri, and A.M. Fadly Tumor Diagnosis Manual: The Differential Diagnosis of Lymphoid and Myeloid Tumors in the Chicken, First ed. The American Association of Avian Pathologists, Jacksonville, Florida 2010.
123. Xu, M., H. Zhang, L. Lee, H. Gao, S. Sharif, R.F. Silva, and M. Heidari. Gene expression profiling in rMd5- and rMd5deltameq-infected chickens. Avian Dis. 55:358-367. 2011.
124. Yunis, R., K.W. Jarosinski, and K.A. Schat. Association between rate of viral genome replication and virulence of Marek's disease herpesvirus strains. Virology:142-150. 2004.
125. Zander, D.V. Experiences with epidemic tremor control. In: Proceedings of the 8th Western Poultry Disease Conference. pp 18-23. 1959.
126. Zelnik, V., P. Tyers, G.D. Smith, C.L. Jiang, and L.J.N. Ross. Structure and properties of a herpesvirus of turkeys recombinant in which US1, US10 and SORF3 genes have been replaced by a lacZ expression cassette. J.Gen.Virol. 76:2903-2907. 1995.

CHAPTER 6

VIRUS-INDUCED IMMUNOSUPPRESSION: RETICULOENDOTHELIOSIS AND OTHER IMMUNOSUPPRESSIVE VIRUSES

Guillermo Zavala

Introduction

Induced immunosuppression has been well documented for a small group of avian lymphotropic viruses including those causing Marek's disease (MD), infectious bursal disease (IBD) and chicken infectious anemia (CIA).[39,112,114] Notably, all three disease agents have specific tropism for cells of the immune system and all are ubiquitous in the poultry house environment; thus, they invariably challenge chickens reared commercially almost anywhere in the world, regardless of the level of sanitation and the degree of pathogenicity of local strains. Uncontrolled infection with these viruses is incompatible with commercial production of chicken meat and eggs. Therefore, effective strategies for controlling MD, IBD and CIA have been developed and include the use of effective biosecurity, sanitation and immunizations that allow managing economically all three diseases in the field. Because MD, IBD and CIA viruses (MDV, IBDV and CIAV) are lymphotropic and all three are capable of inducing at least cytolysis and/or apoptosis, their effects on the immune system are readily noticeable and measurable. Other viruses that are not specifically lymphotropic do not induce a direct or a primary damage to the immune system, albeit some level of immunosuppression can occur during the course of infection. Newcastle disease virus (NDV) can induce transient lymphopenia shortly after infection[107,118,152], which likely translates into some level of immunosuppression. Most research regarding avian influenza (AI) in chickens does not involve studies on immunosuppression. However, the effects of avian influenza viruses (AIV) on the immune system have been studied in mammalian systems, demonstrating that such viruses replicate and cause lytic infections in lymphocytes, monocytes and macrophages[52,117], likely contributing to immunosuppression, in addition to the direct damage to respiratory cells in low pathogenic AIV infection, or to multiple tissues in highly pathogenic AIV infection. H9 AIV infection causes immunosuppression associated with lymphocytic depletion in ducks.[78] In chickens, AI viruses of various virulence levels can infect, replicate and deplete lymphoid cell aggregates in the Peyer's patches of the intestine, as well as in lymphoid organs such as the thymus, spleen and bursa of Fabricius.[126] The role of other viruses in immunosuppressive disease is even less direct and somewhat controversial. Avian reoviruses have been associated with some poorly defined forms of immunosuppression associated with lymphocytic depletion in primary lymphoid organs such as the bursa and thymus[68,78], with some reovirus strains specifically targeting T cells in the thymus.[116] Perhaps one of the most controversial virus-associated immunosuppressive conditions involves fowl adenovirus (FAdV) infection. In chickens, FAdV infects multiple epithelial cells but not cells of mesodermal origin, and in most cases there is some evidence of immunosuppression.[51] However, such immunosuppression is more widely accepted as being caused by one or more other viruses such as MDV[112], CIAV[114] and most commonly, IBDV.[39,108] Thus, FAdV-induced inclusion body hepatitis is likely the result of predisposing immunosuppression caused by another virus such as IBDV, or early infection with FAdV in the absence of homologous maternal antibodies. Avian poxviruses infect primarily epithelial cells.[135] However, it has been suggested circumstantially that fowl poxviruses may induce transient lymphopenia and possibly immunosuppression. Rather than direct immunosuppression caused by poxviruses, immune modulation to avoid immune responses has been documented and is known to be an immunoevasion mechanism for the virus to thrive in infected subjects.[113,136] However, in all likelihood most of the depressing effects on the immune system are probably associated with the presence of complete or near complete reticuloendotheliosis virus (REV) proviral sequences inserted into the genomes of fowl poxviruses and their transcribed gene products, which are responsible for disturbances in the immune system that include impaired leukocyte blastogenesis, impaired immune regulation through cytokine dysregulation, and decreased serological responses and immunity to ordinary pathogens.[157] REV is primarily an oncogenic virus but it also causes severe immunosuppression.[50] Among the oncogenic viruses MDV, REV and members of the avian leucosis/sarcoma complex (ALV or ALSV), MDV and REV are clearly the best examples of immunosuppressive oncogenic viruses since they have been distinctly documented as such.[7,15,16,41,50,69,112-114,138,139,145,157] Commercial flocks affected with oncogenic ALVs in the field appear immunosuppressed when the frequency of infection is high and if chickens are infected with viruses that cause a high incidence of clinical disease and mortality associated with tumors because affected flocks tend to express other types of infections. Some suggestion of immunosuppression has been reported in cases of infection with members of the avian leucosis/sarcoma group of retroviruses.[74] However, clear evidence of a putative immunosuppressive potential has not been demonstrated.

Reticuloendotheliosis virus is an oncogenic virus that also causes severe immunosuppression.

Etiology

MDV, CIAV and IBDV have been discussed on previous chapters as immunosuppressive agents. Other viruses causing some form of documented immunosuppression or immune dysfunction include NDV [107,118,152], AIV [52,78,117,126], avian reovirus [68,78,116], hemorrhagic enteritis virus [102] and REV.[7,15,41,42,50,113,145,157] This section concentrates on REV.

Reticuloendotheliosis (RE) is a lymphoproliferative and immunosuppressive condition caused by viruses in the REV group.[50] The representative strains of REV include:[12,42,157]

- REV-A, a non-defective replication-competent virus from turkeys and causing late onset lymphomas.
- REV-T (REV-A), a defective non-replicating virus from turkeys that requires REV-A or an equivalent virus as a helper virus.
- REV-T, carries a transduced cellular oncogene (v-*rel*) and causes acute death.
- CSV, chick syncytial virus.
- DIAV, duck infectious anemia virus.
- SNV, spleen necrosis virus.

Classification

REV is classified within the family *Retroviridae*, subfamily *Orthoretrovirinae*, genus *Gammaretrovirus*.[14] REV is a virus antigenically, morphologically and structurally unrelated to the ALV group of retroviruses[70], which are classified as *Alpharetroviruses*.[42]

Nucleic acids and chemical composition

Infectious virions are relatively spherical and have a diameter of approximately 100 nm.[7] Depending on the preparation of the specimen for electron microscopy, virions display projections approximately 10 nm in length.[50] The glycoprotein envelope of REV is composed of an outer surface (SU) protein and an inner transmembrane (TM) protein. The SU protein is essential for virus attachment and it also stimulates production of neutralizing antibody in non-tolerant birds.[8,157] TM is supported by the matrix (MA) protein, which in turn sits on the capsid (CA, or p30) protein. The nucleoprotein (NP) is in close contact with both the CA protein centrifugally and centripetally with the virus nucleic acid. As with other simple retroviruses, infectious virions also package a reverse transcriptase (RT) protein, a polymerase (RNA-dependent DNA polymerase), a protease (PRO) and an integrase (IN).

The genome of the reticuloendotheliosis virus contains three genes: *gag*, *pol*, and *env*.

The structure and replication of retroviruses has been reviewed extensively.[24,25,50] The non-defective proviral genome of the only American REV isolate sequenced in full has a length of approximately 8,300 bp and displays the canonical gene sequence of simple retroviruses such as ALV[7]; namely, the genome contains three essential genes designated *gag*, *pol*, and *env*. Such three genes are flanked by two identical long terminal repeats (LTR) in the integrated proviral DNA genome (see Virus replication), or by two distinct complementary terminal repeats in the RNA genome. As in other avian retroviruses, the *gag* gene encodes primarily structural proteins including the group specific antigen (CA, or *gs*, or *gsa*), the matrix protein (MA) and the nucleoprotein (NP). The *pol* gene encodes an RNA-dependent DNA polymerase also known as reverse transcriptase (RT), and an integrase (IN). The *env* gene encodes a polyprotein that is eventually post-translationally cleaved and glycosylated and results in two mature proteins, the surface (SU) and the transmembrane (TM) proteins.

In the integrated proviral DNA (see Virus replication), these three major genes (*gag, pol, env*) are flanked by long terminal repeats (LTR) containing the U3 region with essential regulatory elements, an R region with a strong stop sequence, and the U5 region with sequences critical for virus integration into the cellular genome. Defective strains of REV display a shorter genome with deletions in the *gag* and *env* genes[25], and may contain substitutions representing a transduced viral oncogene known as v-*rel*.[151] This oncogene is a homolog of a turkey proto-oncogene known as c-*rel*, believed to have been transduced during viral infection and replication in turkey cells.[151] The v-*rel* protein is only present in defective REVs and is responsible for the enhanced oncogenic characteristics of the defective T-strain of REV.[13] However, most REV-induced tumors are the result of insertional activation of the cellular proto-oncogene c-*myc*.[61,105,127]

THREE GENES COMPOSE THE REV GENOME

- *gag* gene encodes structural proteins (group specific antigen protein, matrix protein, and nucleoprotein).
- *pol* gene encodes a reverse transcriptase and an integrase.
- *env* gene encodes a polyprotein that results in the surface and the transmembrane proteins.

Virus replication

The replication cycle of REV is analog to the replication cycle of other avian retroviruses, and has been reviewed in detail.[24] Briefly, the SU protein of the envelope attaches to a specific yet unidentified cell receptor, followed by virus entry after translocation of the TM protein, as it occurs with other avian retroviruses. Once in the cytosol and in cytoplasmic vesicles, the regulatory elements in the LTR promote the initiation and enhancement of RNA transcription to synthesize cDNA that eventually integrates into the cellular chromosome in the form of double stranded proviral DNA. Integration is mediated by the viral integrase (IN) and occurs at random spots in the cellular chromosomes. After integration, a cellular polymerase (DNA-dependent RNA polymerase) is responsible for the synthesis of genomic and subgenomic RNA, which travel to the endoplasmic reticulum (ER). Translation of spliced subgenomic RNA in the ER results in the production of polyproteins that are post-translationally cleaved and processed in the Golgi apparatus. The envelope proteins are glycosylated and the viral membranes fuse with those of the Golgi. Mature proteins migrate to the cell membrane where all the components of infectious virus particles are assembled and the mature or maturing virions exit the cell by budding without causing cytolysis.

Epidemiology

Host range

REV has been detected in multiple avian species, domestic and wild, making it a non-species-specific avian retrovirus. Known susceptible species include chickens, domestic and wild turkeys, ducks, geese, Attwater's prairie chickens, greater prairie chickens, Chinese partridges, Hungarian partridges and Japanese quail to name a few.[7,8,17,18,26,29,37,41,54,59,66,75,76,81,110,111,134,147,149,157,160]

Although it has been suggested that REV is more closely related to mammalian retroviruses[70], repeated efforts to demonstrate susceptibility to REV in humans have failed[65-67], confirming that REV is not a public health threat.

Geographical distribution

RE has been reported primarily in countries with temperate climate, albeit the virus has been detected in cold latitudes as well. Natural cases of RE have been noted more frequently in North America[1,49,50,95,98,101,142,144,147,160], the Middle East[29,31,85] and Asia, specifically in China, where it appears to induce significant losses to the local poultry industry.[20,27,63,64,138,140,153] Seroprevalence in the South Eastern United States was last examined in 2003 (Zavala and Cheng, unpublished) (Fig. 1).

Transmission

Members of the ALV group of retroviruses and the REV can be transmitted congenitally via the egg; horizontally by close contact; or iatrogenically via contaminated injectable vaccines or by using contaminated needles. Therefore eradication methods are based on prevention or interruption of congenital and horizontal transmission.[35,38,40,44-46,99,100,106,109,122,123,158,159] In addition, REV can be transmitted via insects or after infection with large molecular DNA viruses such as MDV or fowl poxvirus into which REV proviral DNA may have been inserted.[8,27,32,50,60,124,125,141,150,149,153] Contaminated MDV and fowl poxvirus vaccines have been implicated in outbreaks of clinical RE in at least the United States, Japan, Australia and China.[4,15,48,49,62,69,79,130,131,141,156] Furthermore, vaccine and field strains of MDV or fowl poxvirus frequently contain REV proviral inserts representing fragments of the REV genome such as the LTR, or even almost complete or complete REV genomes.[28,53,60,86,121,129,139,146,155]

Transmission in commercial flocks

Transmission of REV in commercial flocks is not always possible to explain. In some natural outbreaks of RE in commercial turkeys a feasible explanation for the outbreak was never found[26], whereas in some other cases vaccine contamination was determined to be the source of infection.[15,48,49,69,79,104,141] In some areas of the Southern United States a large proportion of breeder and layer flocks display serological evidence of field infection after 40 weeks of age, albeit clinical disease, mortality or tumors attributable to REV infection are virtually never found in the field (Zavala, personal observation).

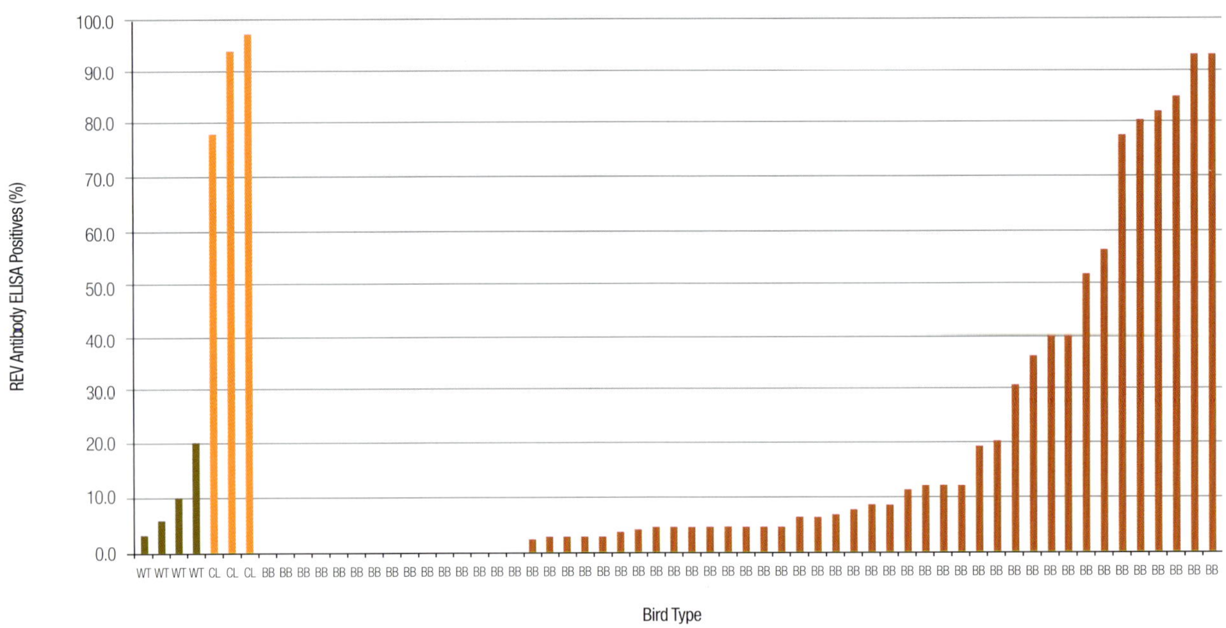

Fig. 1 | Seroprevalence of REV antibodies in wild turkeys (WT), commercial table egg layers (CL) and broiler breeders (BB) in the United States (2003). All groups of wild turkeys were juveniles, all layer and breeder flocks were sampled at random (50 hens per flock), and all ranged from 45 to 58 weeks of age.

Transmission in nature

Transmission of REV probably occurs most commonly as a result of exposure to REV mechanically transmitted by insects.[32,91,132,133] However, REV can be readily transmitted congenitally[149] or by close contact with infected birds, or exposure to contaminated faeces and environment.[50]

Pathogenesis

The timing of infection with REV is a critical determinant for the outcome of disease. One of the first indicators of infection is severe stunting and loss of uniformity (Fig. 2). Chickens or turkeys infected congenitally via the egg tend to become tolerant to infection and thus they do not develop a neutralizing immune response.[5,150] When infection occurs after a few days or weeks of age, persistent infection or viremia cannot be easily detected.[3,7,8] A robust seroconversion becomes evident as assessed by antibody enzyme-linked immunosorbent assay (ELISA) in chickens infected after a few weeks of age.[7] Adult meat-type grandparent hens infected after 50 weeks of age with the APC-566 strain of REV exhibited strong seroconversion within 12 days post-infection, and viremia lasted no more than 4 days after infection (Zavala and Barbosa, unpublished observation), confirming that when REV infection occurs during adult life (or after a few weeks of age) birds mount a robust immune response; viremia and shedding are interrupted, and clinical disease and mortality associated with REV infection do not occur.[3] However, turkeys exposed by contact may still develop lymphomas even when exposed after hatch.[83,84,96] Tolerant chickens or turkeys infected congenitally are likely to develop persistent viremia and virus shedding, clinical disease, neoplastic changes and eventually death.[5,149] REV is a lymphotropic retrovirus that most commonly causes slow lymphoid cell transformation.[42,50,49] The onset of detectable neoplasia frequently happens at or later than 16 weeks of age in commercial chickens infected with REV strains other than REV-T, albeit tumors may be detected earlier in some cases.[9,26,98,103,150] Tumors consist most commonly of B cell lymphomas, albeit T cell lymphomas have been reported experimentally and in natural outbreaks of REV infection.[26,50] In addition, an acute non-neoplastic syndrome with premature mortality and a runting disease syndrome have been described in young chickens.[92] In young susceptible birds, REV targets B cells in the bursa of Fabricius and other lymphoid organs. In slow onset lymphomas, multiple rounds of viremia and virus replication follow the initial infection until there is transformation of B cells, typically in the bursa of Fabricius. Transformed cells metastasize and invade multiple organs, including visceral organs and the gonads as well. Survivors that are able to reproduce for at least a few days or weeks will eventually produce infected progeny, thus extending infection to the following generation and serving as a source for horizontal transmission as well. Infection in young chickens or turkeys may result in immunosuppression regardless of the outcome of infection (see subsection on REV-induced immunosuppression).

REV infection resulting in B or T cell transformation is the outcome of insertional activation of a cellular proto-oncogene known as c-*myc*. [105,127] The strong promoter and enhancer sequences in the U3 region of the REV LTR drive the activation and transcription of c-*myc,* which in turn results in uncontrolled cell division and neoplasia. [105]

THE MOST IMPORTANT ITEMS ABOUT PATHOGENESIS OF REV

- REV infects susceptible birds congenitally, horizontally or iatrogenically.
- REV undergoes multiple rounds of persistent or intermittent viremia and virus shedding ensues in tolerant birds.
- REV induces transformation of B or T cells until slow onset B cell or T cell lymphomas develop followed by death.
- REV may induce severe immunosuppression at any time during the course of infection and disease.

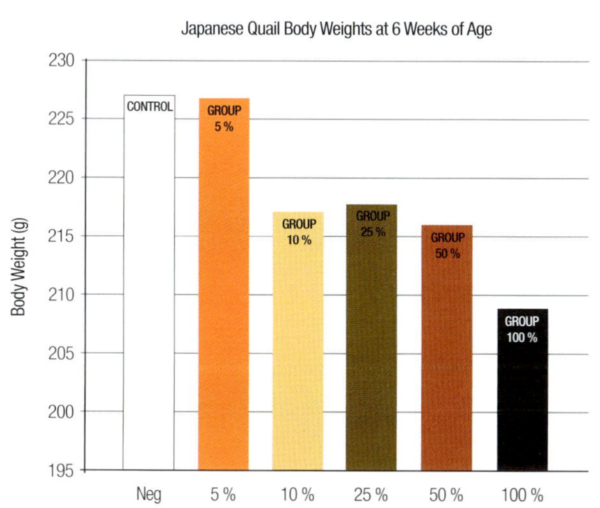

Fig. 2 Body weights of Japanese quail experimentally infected with the APC-566 strain of REV from Attwater's prairie chickens (*Tympanuchus cupido attwateri*). The white bar represents the mean 6-week-old body weight of uninfected quail; colored bars 5 % to 100 % represent mean body weights of quail infected as embryos where 5 %, 10 %, 25 %, 50 % or 100 % of the embryos received REV at 5 days of incubation and then grown to 6 weeks of age.

Clinical signs

The clinical signs induced after REV infections have been documented in various avian species. Japanese quail were stunted, unthrifty and developed tumors and mortality as early as 8 weeks of age after infection with the APC-566 REV isolate from wild birds of the United States. [8] Specific pathogen free (SPF) turkeys infected with the same isolate (APC-566) exhibited delayed growth, poor overall development and developed neoplasms by 13 weeks of age. [8] In a natural outbreak of RE in commercial turkeys clinical signs were noticed only after the processing plant reported increased condemnations due to tumors. [26] The RU-1 strain of REV induced stunting, neoplasms and mortality approaching 100 % in Peking ducks in a period of 6 months regardless of the age when the ducks were infected. [76] SPF chickens infected with an Australian isolate of REV displayed poor body development and increased mortality. [3] Chickens infected with REV either experimentally, naturally or accidentally through contaminated vaccines frequently develop stunting, feather abnormalities, anemia, leg paralysis and premature mortality associated with tumors. [4,15,49,69,79,156] Commercially raised Chinese partridges experienced a natural outbreak of RE showing wasting disease by 120 days of age. In that case, naturally dead birds displayed a collection of neoplasms in multiple internal organs. [20] Although not necessarily a clinical sign, proliferative cutaneous lesions around the eyes and beak commissures have been helpful in the clinical identification of REV-infected Attwater's and greater prairie chickens (*Tympanuchus cupido attwateri*). [160]

The clinical signs of REV appear mainly as poor overall growth, stunting, tumors and an increased mortality.

Pathology

Pathological changes induced by REV can be simply grouped into changes associated with non-neoplastic runting syndrome and changes associated with lymphoproliferative neoplasia, albeit other syndromes have been described such as "bursal lymphoma", "non-bursal lymphoma", and "acute reticulum cell neoplasia". [50]

Gross pathology

The first evidence of REV infection may be severe stunting [3,7,8] and the development of feather abnormalities, which have been described in chickens inoculated with the highly virulent REV-T strain [72], and after infection with REV isolated from contaminated MD vaccines. [62,156] Cutaneous lesions consisting of lymphocytic infiltrates in and around the feather follicles and the skin of the head are a frequent finding in Japanese quail, greater prairie chickens and Attwater's prairie chickens. [160] Such dermal infiltrates typically consist of mononuclear cells that appear to be more differentiated than the lymphoblastoid cells commonly found in visceral lymphomas, which would suggest possibly an inflammatory component rather than strictly a neoplastic change in the skin (Zavala, personal observation). Infiltrative peripheral nerve lesions with nerve thickening similar to lesions observed in MD have been observed in chickens inoculated experimentally. [148] Such infiltrations may be at least partially responsible for the leg paralysis reported in chickens infected with REV-contaminated MD vaccines. [69,156] An important feature of REV-induced pathology is atrophy of the thymus and bursa in young infected birds [4,26,92], prior to the enlargement of the bursa resulting from bursal lymphomas. Young Japanese quail developed severe thymus atrophy a few weeks post-infection with the REV APC-566 strain isolated from Attwater's prairie chickens. [7,8] An unusual form of severe proventriculitis has been reported in chickens infected with REV from contaminated MD vaccines. [62] Anemia has been associated with REV infection in some cases. [69]

Microscopic pathology

One of the most characteristic features associated with RE is the development of lymphomas [3,8,49,50,61,69,82,87,97,131,134,143,150,160], most of which are composed of cells bearing B cell markers [50], albeit in rare cases of RE in turkeys the predominant neoplastic cells displayed T cell surface markers rather than B cell markers. [26] The tumors in most REV-associated B cell lymphomas consist of solid sheets of large, undifferentiated, uniform lymphoblasts with a relatively large open nucleus and a prominent nucleolus. [93,94] Such cells display IgM on their surface and thus can easily be distinguished from other mononuclear cells. The neoplastic cells found in T cell lymphomas caused by REV in commercial turkeys were characterized as T helper cells on the basis of their cell surface markers ($CD3^+$, $CD4^+$ and $CD8^-$). [26] Such neoplastic cells may be found in multiple visceral organs. From the diagnostic standpoint it is important to determine whether there are detectable tumors in the bursa of Fabricius in order to support a possible diagnosis of RE. It is also important to be aware of the fact that in natural outbreaks of RE in chickens the tumor distribution and neoplastic cell morphology do not allow for differentiation from lymphoid leucosis and thus additional diagnostic approaches are necessary for proper differentiation and diagnosis. In general, gross and microscopic pathology are not diagnostic of RE. [43]

In natural outbreaks of RE, the tumor distribution and neoplastic cell morphology do not allow for differentiation from lymphoid leucosis.

Gross and microscopic pathology are not enough to accurately diagnose RE.

Immunosuppression

RE is a sporadic neoplastic disease that is also associated with significant immunosuppression [50,157], the severity of which depends at least on the type of virus involved and the age when birds acquire the infection. Some strains of REV are more virulent than others and tend to induce acute death before the infected birds develop lymphomas or before immunosuppression can be noticed clinically. [9,12,71,137] Early infection with REV is more likely to result in immune tolerance, immunosuppression, persistent viremia, virus shedding and development of neoplasia. [12,137,150] Immunosuppression is strongly influenced by the pre-REV-infection immune status and overall health of the bird or flock, and by concomitant insult by other immunosuppressive agents and non-infectious immunosuppressors.

In cases of RE where there is no intervention by any other factors, the possible outcomes of immunosuppression include: [157]

- Blood cell abnormalities.
- Impaired leukocyte blastogenesis.
- Disturbances in immune regulation.
- Decreased serological responses.
- Reduced immunity against ordinary avian pathogens.

Under field circumstances REV infection is likely to be complicated by the participation of a variety of disease agents, stress, environmental challenge, nutrition and the pressures of rapid growth or high egg production. Interactions between REV and other immunosuppressive viruses such as MDV, IBDV, CIAV, avian reovirus and hemorrhagic enteritis virus of turkeys are likely to occur in a commercial production environment.

Impairment of leukocyte blastogenesis

The ability to respond to T cell mitogens is an important indirect indication of the ability of an individual to confront neoplasia and a variety of viral and protozoal infections. Phytohemagglutinin A (PHA), concanavalin A (ConA) and lipopolysaccharide (LPS) are mitogens used to examine the proliferative competency of T cells after exposure to foreign antigens. Mitogenic stimulation of T cells can be studied by measuring the uptake of ^{3}H-thymidine in T cell cultures. Pokeweed mitogen (PWM) can also be used in a similar albeit less selective manner for studying less specific responses, since PWM can stimulate in vitro blastogenesis of both B and T cells. [115] Splenic cells and peripheral blood leukocytes obtained from birds infected with REV were unresponsive to blastogenic stimulation as early as 3 days post-infection with PHA. [12,115,137] Splenic cells and peripheral blood leukocytes (PBL) that become unable to divide retain their normal function and upon contact with naïve cells they render them also unable to multiply. [12,115,137] On this basis it has been proposed that the T cell suppression seen in REV-infected chickens probably results from the influence of suppressor cells in the spleen, is contact-mediated, and is cytostatic because the affected cells retain their function but lose their ability to multiply and consequently cytotoxic T cell proliferation is impaired. [19] This phenomenon is more likely to occur in immunotolerant chickens or turkeys because it is dependent on continuous exposure of splenocytes to REV, which is expected to happen in permanently viremic birds. However, this is not exclusive of birds infected young, since T cells of chickens infected between 4 and 6 weeks of age can still lose their ability to multiply and respond to mitogens like PHA, ConA and PWM. [137] In addition to suppressor splenocytes, thymus-dependent suppressor cells may interfere with the multiplication of splenocytes and PBLs. Treating cell culture supernatants with trypsin cancels the interference with blastogenic responses, suggesting a possible inhibitory protein factor or oligopeptide in this inhibitory role. These effects tend to be reduced after 10 weeks of age, which may reflect an age resistance factor or simply the onset of seroconversion and a diminishing virus exposure in the spleen. [115] The ability of REV to induce clinical disease and neoplasia does not disappear completely after 10 weeks of age. Instead, the time required for the onset of clinical signs and development of neoplasia is increased. In any event, responsiveness to PHA is maximally reduced when birds are infected congenitally or at a very young age and in that case T cell-related immunity is more severely affected. Impairment of cellular immunity in RE is further evidenced by delayed rejection of allogeneic skin grafts in REV-A-infected chickens [137], an effect that is controlled by the B locus, the chicken version of the MHC. It has been proposed that cellular immune competence may be compromised non-specifically in birds infected with REV-A. Surprisingly, neoplasia or immunosuppression did not develop in experiments done with chickens injected with low numbers of REV-transformed neoplastic cells. [137] This would suggest that birds that are not immunosuppressed should be capable of destroying transformed cells, and tumors may regress. However, a diminished cellular immune function renders the infected individual incapable of controlling effectively virus infection, its neoplastic consequences [157], and secondary or opportunistic infections and infestations.

Disturbances in immune regulation

REV is more closely related to some mammalian retroviruses morphologically, antigenically and genetically. [70] As such, REV shares with various mammalian retroviruses [Friend leukaemia virus (FLV), Moloney leukemia virus (MoLV), Rauscher leukemia virus (RLV), Mouse Mammary Tumor Virus (MMTV), human T cell leukemia virus types I and II (HTLV-I, HTLV-II), and Mason Pfizer Monkey virus (MPMV)] highly conserved immunosuppression-related interspecies amino acid sequences known as "immunosuppressive peptides" in their envelope gene. [23,56] The nucleotide sequences encoding the immunosuppressive peptide of REV have been identified in the transmembrane region of the envelope gene of REVs from multiple avian species, including the REV-A and APC-566 strains of REV, as well as multiple other isolates from Attwater's prairie chickens [7], greater prairies chickens, and commercial chickens of the United States and China (Zavala, unpublished). Immunosuppressive oligopeptides from mammalian retroviruses have been located in the TM region of the envelope gene, and several have been cloned, sequenced and expressed in the laboratory [22,55-58] (Fig. 3). The REV immunosuppressive oligopeptide is also located in the TM domain of *env*, contains only 17-18 amino acids and it has been implicated in dysregulation of type 1 and type 2 cytokines. [56] One of the viruses in which the immunosuppressive peptide has been most recently identified, the APC-566 strain, is oncogenic in

										10										20								
1	.	.	.	.	.	.	.	.	.	.	.	.	.	.	.	.	.										CKS-17.pro	Haraguchi, 1995
1	.	.	.	.	.	.	.	.	.	.	.	.	.	.	.	.	.	.									MN100021.pro	
1	L	Q	N	R	R	G	L	D	L	L	F	L	K	E	G	G	L	C	A	A	L	K	E	E	C	F	MoLV.pro	Haraguchi, 1997
1	.	.	.	.	.	.	.	.	.	.	.	.	.	.	.	.	.	.	.	.	.	.	.	.	.	.	AMCF.pro	
1	.	.	.	.	.	.	.	.	.	.	.	.	.	.	.	.	.	.	.	.	.	.	.	.	.	.	MMCF.pro	
1	.	.	.	.	.	.	.	.	.	.	.	.	.	.	.	.	.	.	.	.	.	.	.	.	.	.	AKV-murine end.pro	
1	.	.	.	.	.	.	.	.	.	.	.	.	.	.	.	.	.	.	.	.	.	.	.	.	.	.	FriendLV.pro	
1	.	.	.	.	.	.	.	.	.	.	.	.	.	.	.	.	.	.	.	.	.	.	.	.	.	.	GrossLV.pro	
1	.	.	.	.	.	.	.	.	.	.	.	.	Q	.	.	.	.	.	.	.	.	.	.	.	.	.	FeLV.pro	
1	A	.	.	.	.	.	.	.	.	.	.	W	E	Q	.	.	.	.	K	.	.	Q	.	Q	R	.	HTLV-I.pro	
1	A	.	.	.	.	.	.	.	.	.	.	W	E	Q	.	.	.	.	K	.	I	Q	.	Q	.	.	HTLV-II.pro	
1	.	.	.	.	.	.	.	.	.	.	T	A	E	Q	.	.	I	.	L	.	.	Q	.	K	.	.	MPMV.pro	
1	.	.	.	.	.	.	.	.	.	.	T	A	E	Q	.	.	I	.	L	.	.	Q	.	K	.	.	REV-A.pro	
1	.	.	.	.	.	.	.	.	.	.	T	A	E	Q	.	.	I	.	L	.	.	Q	.	K	.	.	SNV.pro - DQ003591	
1	.	.	.	.	.	.	.	.	.	.	T	A	E	Q	.	.	I	.	L	.	.	Q	.	K	.	.	REV 397 A.pro	
1	.	.	.	.	.	.	.	.	.	.	T	A	E	Q	.	.	I	.	L	.	.	Q	.	K	.	.	REV China.pro - nc006934	
1	.	.	.	.	.	.	.	.	.	.	T	A	E	Q	.	.	I	.	L	.	.	Q	.	K	.	.	apc-566.pro	
1	.	.	.	.	.	.	.	.	.	.	T	A	E	Q	.	.	I	.	L	.	.	Q	.	K	.	.	APC-793.pro	
1	.	.	.	.	.	.	.	.	.	.	T	A	E	Q	.	.	I	.	L	.	.	Q	.	K	.	.	APC-976.pro	
1	.	.	.	.	.	.	.	.	.	.	T	A	E	Q	.	.	I	.	L	.	.	Q	.	K	.	.	APC-1006.pro	
1	.	.	.	.	.	.	.	.	.	.	T	A	E	Q	.	.	I	.	L	.	.	Q	.	K	.	.	APC-1011.pro	
1	.	.	.	.	A	A	I	.	F	.	L	.	A	H	.	H	G	.	E	D	V	A	G	M	.	.	RSV.pro - Sonigo, 1986	

Fig. 3 | Amino acid alignment of the immunosuppressive peptide of REV and selected mammalian retroviruses. CKS-17 = Synthetic analog to the REV and mammalian immunosuppressive peptide; all viruses grouped under the Haraguchi references are of mammalian origin; SNV = spleen necrosis virus; all others are REV amino acid sequences. Dots represent identities to the Moloney leukaemia virus (MoLV) prototype immunosuppressive peptide; letters represent amino acid substitutions. Modified from: Barbosa et al., Virus Res. 124:68-77. 2007.

chickens, turkeys, Japanese quail and Attwater's prairies chickens and its immunosuppressive potential has been demonstrated in turkeys with compromised immune responses against at least NDV, IBDV and *Pasteurella multocida*.[7,8,160] Through studies with a synthetic peptide homologous to the immunosuppressive peptide of REV and known as CKS-17 it has been possible to document:[56]

- Inhibition of IL-2-dependent cell proliferation.
- Alloantigen-stimulated lymphocyte proliferation.
- Monocyte respiratory burst.
- Natural killer (NK) cell activity.
- Monocyte-dependent tumor destruction.
- Signal transduction mediated by IL-1.
- Delayed hypersensitivity reactions.
- LPS-induced mortality in mice.
- IgG synthesis stimulated by PWM.
- Activity of cytotoxic T cells.

CKS-17-treated cells experienced a burst of intracellular cAMP, which in turn creates a shift in cytokine balance by upregulating IL-10 and downregulating IL-2, IL-12 and TNF-α.[58] The overall result of these combined events is the suppression of cellular immunity.[58] One of the critical stimulant cytokines that CKS-17 (the homolog of the REV immunosuppressive peptide) inhibits is IL-2, a cytokine required for the proliferation of B and T lymphocytes. In addition, CKS-17 inhibits IL-12, which regulates T and NK cells and is also important in the development and differentiation of Th1 and Th2 cells; IFN-γ, which stimulates phagocytosis and killing by avian macrophages; and TNF-α, which is synthesized by macrophages and is responsible for stimulating systemic inflammation, $CD4^+$ lymphocytes, NK cells and neurons.

CKS-17, a synthetic peptide homologous to the immunosuppressive peptide of REV, inhibits IL-2, IL-12, IFN-γ, and TNF-α.

Type 2 cytokines that may be subject to dysregulation include IL-4, IL-5, IL-6, IL-10, and IL-13. Their functions are:

- IL-4 induces differentiation of naïve T helper cells from Th0 to Th2.
- IL-5 is a growth and differentiation factor for B cells and activation of eosinophils.
- IL-6 is a pro-inflammatory cytokine and plays an important role in tumor regression.
- IL-10 downregulates the expression of Th1 cytokines, MHC class II antigens and costimulatory molecules on macrophages.
- IL-13 is synthesized by activated Th2 cells and in conjunction with IL-4 intervenes in the maturation and differentiation of B cells. In addition, IL-13 upregulates CD23 and MHC class II expression and enhances the differentiation of B cells for production and release of IgE by B lymphocytes.

Taken as a whole, these events lead to severe dysregulation of cytokines and an overall suppression of cell mediated immunity, making the infected animal more prone to a variety of infections and infestations of viral, bacterial, fungal and parasitic nature, as well as to neoplasia in general.[157]

Immune responses to avian pathogens

Early infection with REV often leads to immunotolerance and lack of antibody responses against REV. On a flock basis there is production of detectable anti-REV antibodies regardless of the age of infection. Japanese quail, SPF turkeys and SPF chickens seroconverted against REV within 4 weeks post-infection, even when infection occurred within the first 3 days of age. Turkeys infected with the APC-566 strain of REV did seroconvert against REV and displayed evidence of immunosuppression, since the mean death time after *Pasteurella multocida* infection was shortened in REV-infected turkeys (Fig. 5). In addition, REV-positive turkeys produced lower ELISA antibody titers against vaccines containing inactivated IBDV and NDV (Fig. 4). The same turkeys developed feather abnormalities and lymphomas by 13 weeks of age, that is, some 12.5 weeks post-infection.[7] In a separate experiment, REV isolated from a contaminated MD vaccine induced decreased serological responses against REV, prolonged presence of NDV in respiratory tissues post-infection, increased severity of NDV-related clinical signs, and elevated mortality in

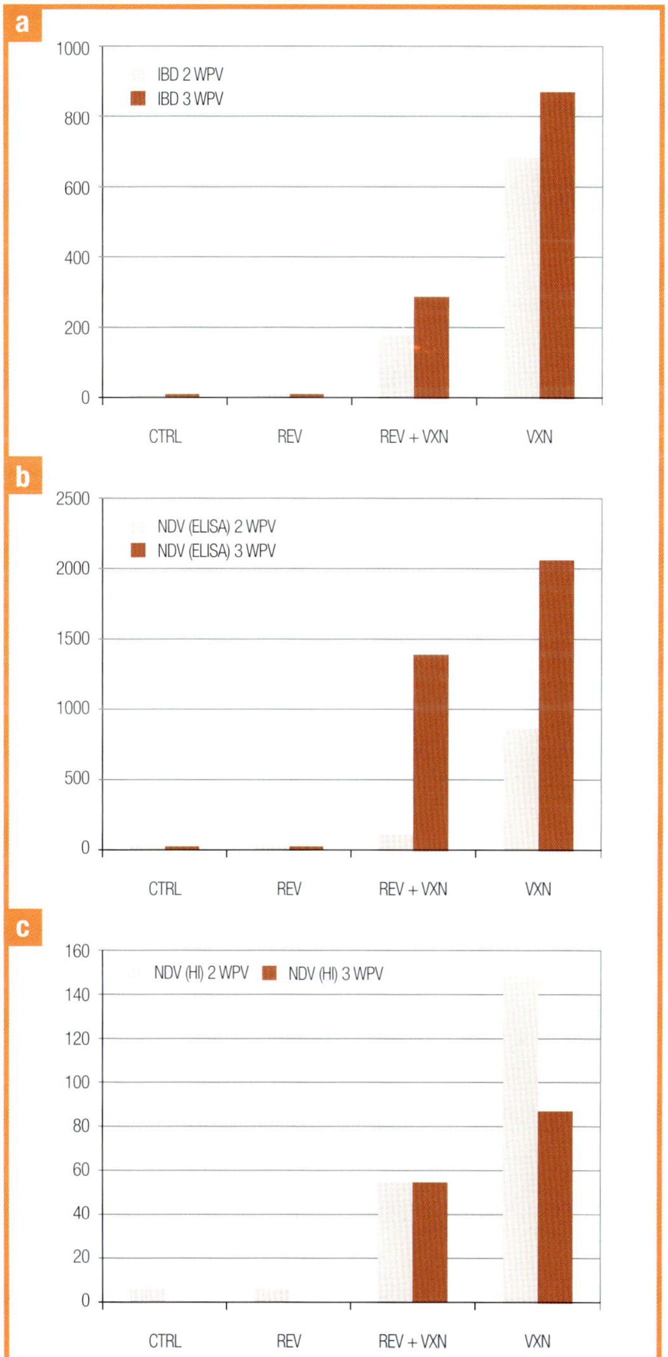

Fig. 4 | Serological responses in SPF turkeys infected with REV and vaccinated against either IBDV or NDV. Infected turkeys were challenged with the APC-566 strain of REV within the first 3 days of age and vaccinated against either IBDV or NDV at 4 weeks post-infection with REV. a) Infectious bursal disease (IBD) ELISA antibody titers at 2 weeks (light bars) and 3 weeks (dark bars) post-vaccination (WPV); b) Newcastle disease (NDV) ELISA antibody titers at 2 weeks (light bars) and 3 WPV (dark bars); c) Newcastle disease (NDV) hemoagglutination inhibition (HI) antibody titers at 2 weeks (light bars) and 3 WPV (dark bars). CTRL = Turkeys not infected with REV and not vaccinated against IBDV or NDV; REV = Turkeys infected with REV and not vaccinated against IBDV or NDV; REV + VXN = Turkeys infected with REV and vaccinated against IBDV or NDV; VXN = Turkeys not infected with REV and vaccinated against IBDV or NDV. Modified from: Barbosa et al., Virus Res. 124:68-77. 2007.

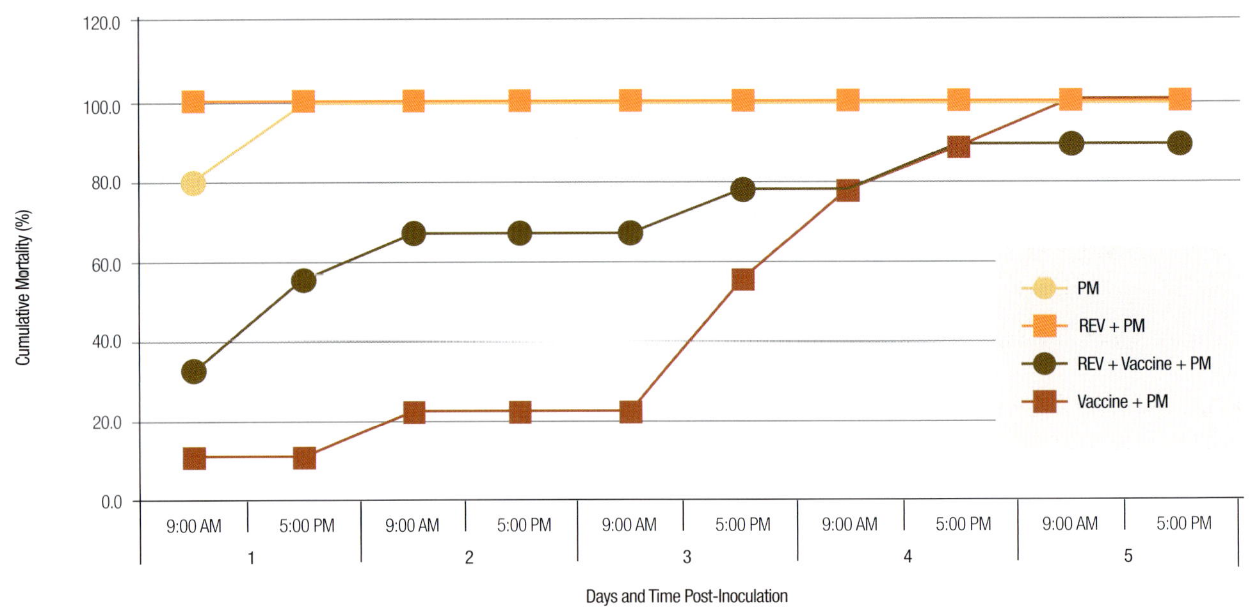

Fig. 5 Death time induced by *Pasteurella multocida* in REV-free and REV-infected SPF turkeys. Only relevant experimental groups are shown: PM = *P. multocida* only; REV+PM = *P. multocida* challenge + REV-infected; REV + Vaccine + PM = REV-infected + *P. multocida* bacterin + *P. multocida* challenge; Vaccine + PM = *P. multocida* bacterin + *P. multocida* challenge. The first turkeys to die after a virulent PM challenge were those infected with REV+PM in the absence of a bacterin; followed by turkeys challenged with PM without a bacterin; followed by vaccinated turkeys, infected with REV and challenged with PM; and finally turkeys vaccinated and challenged with PM without REV infection. Modified from: Barbosa et al., Virus Res. 124:68-77. 2007.

SPF chickens co-infected with REV and NDV, as opposed to chickens infected with NDV alone. [154]

Besides the reduction of immune competency against the bacterium *Pasteurella multocida*, decreased immune responses against other bacterial species such as *Salmonella typhimurium* (ST) have been documented. Deaths attributable to ST were higher in chickens co-infected with REV and ST than in chickens infected with ST alone. [88]

Increased severity of clinical signs, lesions, and mortality has been reported in chickens co-infected with infectious laryngotracheitis virus and REV and in birds co-infected with REV and fowl poxvirus. [50,90]

Experimental and natural infections with REV and ALV have been reported. [47] Co-infection with REV and ALV results in a higher frequency of ALV viremic chickens than in populations infected with ALV alone. In addition, chickens co-infected with REV and ALV responded less efficiently with sensitization against "symbolic" antigens such as sheep red blood cells (SRBC) and *Brucella abortus*. Furthermore, the strain used in such experiments, REV-T, induced a marked reduction of the bursa of

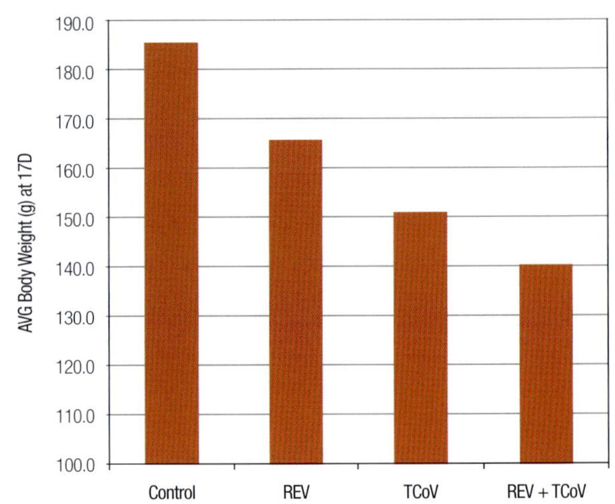

Fig. 6 Interactions between REV and a non-neoplastic, non-immunosuppressive virus (turkey coronavirus, TCoV). Dual infection with REV and TCoV resulted in enhanced depression at 17 days of age in experimentally-infected SPF turkeys.

Fabricius in commercial chickens.[47] Natural outbreaks with simultaneous infection with REV and ALV subgroup J (ALV-J) apparently facilitated vertical transmission of ALV-J and enhanced the expression of myelocytomas in commercial meat type and egg type chickens of China, including indigenous Chinese breeds.[27]

REV can interact with other immunosuppressive viruses such as MDV and CIAV, as has been shown experimentally and in natural outbreaks. REV-specific cytotoxic T cells are not responsive when chickens devoid of antibodies against CIAV are infected with CIAV at 9-17 days of age.[80] Immunity to MD vaccines is significantly reduced in chickens infected with REV.[145]

An additional and unusual form of viral interaction may occur from REV inserting fragments of its own genome or the complete REV genome into the genomes of large DNA viruses such as MDV and poxviruses, or simply by contamination of MD or fowl poxvirus vaccines, which may modify the virulence of MDV or poxviruses and the outcome of infection by any such viruses.[4,15,28,34,48,49,53,60,62,69,79,86,90,104,119-121,129-131,139,146]

Other forms of viral interactions exist and do not necessarily result in enhanced immunosuppression. In one experiment, a turkey strain designated as REV 397-A and isolated from a natural outbreak of RE in commercial turkeys was co-inoculated with turkey coronavirus (TCoV-TXp7), kindly provided by Dr. Mark Jackwood, University of Georgia. Turkeys co-infected with REV and turkey coronavirus expressed lower body weights than turkeys inoculated with either one of the viruses alone, suggesting that REV can interact in more ways than just immunosuppression (Fig. 6). Co-infection with TCoV and REV extended the period of detectable REV viremia and also the proportion of REV viremic turkeys in the experiment. Finally, the bursal microscopic lesions representing lymphocytic depletion were more severe in the turkeys that received both viruses instead of either one alone (Turner, Zavala, Barbosa and Cheng, unpublished).

REV infection can result in enhanced frequency and severity of lesions associated with *Eimeria tenella*[89], indicating that REV not only compromises responses against other viruses but to protozoa as well, which is expected since cellular immunity is clearly compromised.[21,22,55-58]

Economic effects

Other than in commercial chickens of China, clinical RE occurs only sporadically elsewhere in the world. Field infection in adult chickens and turkeys is evidenced by frequent seroconversion observed in commercial flocks, rarely with any evidence of clinical disease, mortality or virus shedding into fertile eggs. The exception has been occasional outbreaks associated with contaminated vaccines against MD or fowl poxvirus.[49,62,72,73] In those cases, economic losses have been rather dramatic and resulted from high mortality with tumors, delayed growth, a need for depopulating broiler breeder flocks and in some cases, litigation. Increased mortality associated with tumors, increased condemnations and decreased egg production have been the most relevant detrimental effects, as it occurred in one of the most recent natural outbreaks of RE in commercial turkeys.[26] Producers of SPF eggs and chickens, vaccine manufacturing companies and producers of meat and egg type breeding stock must invest in costly REV surveillance, as required by law and by importers of breeding stock such as Israel.

In an attempt to further define the economic impact of REV infection, a disease model was pursued in Japanese quail. The effects of RE were studied in two consecutive generations of quail. Delayed growth and increased mortality with tumors were detected by 6-8 weeks of age. Egg production, hatchability and fertility rates were reduced in REV-infected quail in comparison with uninfected quail. Body weight gain was significantly reduced by 8 weeks of age in the first generation of infected quail (quail breeders) and at 3 and 6 weeks of age in the second generation in contrast with non-infected quail (Fig. 6).[128]

Interactions with other Infectious Agents

As indicated above, REV may interact with other immunosuppressive agents, including MDV, CIAV and IBDV, and with non-immunosuppressive viruses, bacteria, fungi and protozoa (see section on Immune responses to avian pathogens).

Diagnosis

Diagnosis of neoplastic diseases can be done in a targeted fashion or by exclusion. That is, by excluding other oncogenic viruses using appropriate diagnostic techniques. REV does not have an endogenous virus counterpart as ALV does and there are no live or killed vaccines against REV that would be detectable by virus isolation, antigen capture ELISA or molecular methods. Antibody ELISA kits are available commercially for detection of seroconversion.

It is easy to target REV specifically using molecular methods such as:

- PCR.
- RT-PCR.
- Real time PCR.
- qPCR.
- Loop-mediated isothermal amplification.[6,10,11,30,33,36,63,77,104,129,130]
- Virus isolation.[50]
- Immunofluorescence.[2,7]
- Immunohistochemical techniques.[110]

Gross and microscopic findings should not be considered diagnostic, as they can be indistinguishable from spontaneous lymphomas and lymphoid leucosis induced by ALV.[43] Serology has limited usefulness in the sense that seroconversion does not prove clinical disease.[50]

In the field, the frequency of infection is much higher than the frequency of clinical disease.

Seroconversion only reflects exposure to virus but it does not always correlate with clinical disease. On the other hand, absence of seroconversion may serve to document absence of exposure to REV. A combined approach may be a more sensible strategy for diagnosis, keeping in mind that in cases of neoplastic disease it is critical to document absence of other oncogenic viruses and spontaneous lymphomas as possible causes.

Vaccination

As with most other retroviral diseases, vaccination against RE is not available at the moment and it is unlikely to become available since attenuation of avian retroviruses has not been accomplished. However, it is important to keep in mind that protection of birds against poxviruses may reduce the opportunity of REV infection associated with poxviruses that may carry almost complete or complete REV genome insertions. Some Asian operations have resorted to deliberate infection with REV after 10 weeks of age with the objective of inducing seroconversion and preventing virus shedding. Results have been at best very disappointing.

THE DEVELOPMENT OF VACCINES AGAINST AVIAN RETROVIRUS HAS A NUMBER OF RISKS

- Reversion to virulence.
- Recombination.
- Possibility of insertional mutagenesis triggering lymphomas.

Treatment

Treatment against RE is not available. Should valuable breeding stock become infected and should virus shedding be documented, it may become necessary to test every elite bird individually to eliminate any virus shedders, thereby preventing the perpetuation of the infection from one generation to the next. Part of the strategy for eradication may be the elimination of virus positive hens, and retaining only virus negative/antibody negative individuals, or at least keeping virus negative/antibody positive hens. Valuable immunosuppressed birds that cannot be readily euthanatized may receive non-specific support treatment with vitamins and antibacterial drugs, although the benefits of this practice are unpredictable.

References

1. Aulisio, C.G., and Shelokov, A. Prevalence of reticuloendotheliosis in chickens: immunofluorescence studies. Proceedings of the Society for Experimental Biology and Medicine. 130:178-181. 1969.
2. Bagust, T.J., and D.P. Dennett Reticuloendotheliosis virus: experimental infection of poultry and immunofluorescent identification of Australian isolates. Australian veterinary journal 53:506-508. 1977.
3. Bagust, T.J., and T.M. Grimes Experimental infection of chickens with an Australian strain of reticuloendotheliosis virus. 2. Serological responses and pathogenesis. Avian pathology : journal of the W.V.P.A 8:375-389. 1979.
4. Bagust, T.J., T.M. Grimes, and D.P. Dennett Infection studies on a reticuloendotheliosis virus contaminant of a commercial Marek's disease vaccine. Australian veterinary journal 55:153-157. 1979.
5. Bagust, T.J., T.M. Grimes, and N. Ratnamohan Experimental infection of chickens with an Australian strain of reticuloendotheliosis virus 3. persistent infection and transmission by the adult hen. Avian pathology : journal of the W.V.P.A 10:375-385. 1981.
6. Barbosa, T., G. Zavala, and S. Cheng Molecular characterization of three recombinant isolates of avian leukosis virus obtained from contaminated Marek's disease vaccines. Avian diseases 52:245-252. 2008.
7. Barbosa, T., G. Zavala, S. Cheng, and P. Villegas Full genome sequence and some biological properties of reticuloendotheliosis virus strain APC-566 isolated from endangered Attwater's prairie chickens. Virus research 124:68-77. 2007.
8. Barbosa, T., G. Zavala, S. Cheng, and P. Villegas Pathogenicity and transmission of reticuloendotheliosis virus isolated from endangered prairie chickens. Avian Dis 51:33-39. 2007.
9. Barth CF, E.D., Olson WC, Humphries EH. Reticuloendotheliosis virus REV-T(REV-A)-induced neoplasia: development of tumors within the T-lymphoid and myeloid lineages. J Virol. 64:6054-6062. 1990.
10. Biswas, S.K., C. Jana, K. Chand, W. Rehman, and B. Mondal Detection of fowl poxvirus integrated with reticuloendotheliosis virus sequences from an outbreak in backyard chickens in India. Veterinaria italiana 47:147-153. 2011.
11. Borenshtein, R., and I. Davidson Development of the hot spot-combined PCR assay for detection of retroviral insertions into Marek's disease virus. Journal of virological methods 82:119-127. 1999.
12. Bose, H.R., Jr. Reticuloendotheliosis virus and disturbance in immune regulation. Microbiological sciences 1:107-112. 1984.
13. Bose, H.R.J. The rel family - models for transcriptional regulation and oncogenic transformation. Biochim. Biophys. Acta 1114:1-17. 1992.
14. Buchen-Osmond, C. Reticuloendotheliosis virus (strain T, A). In: The Universal Virus Database, version 3. ICTV dB- Management. C. Buchen-Osmond, ed., Columbia University, New York. pp 421-440. 2004.
15. Bulow, V.V. Immunological effects of reticuloendotheliosis virus as potential contaminant of Marek's disease vaccines. Avian pathology : journal of the W.V.P.A 6:383-393. 1977.
16. Buscaglia, C., B.W. Calnek, and K.A. Schat Effect of reticuloendotheliosis virus and infectious bursal disease virus on Marek's disease herpesvirus latency. Avian pathology : journal of the W.V.P.A 18:265-281. 1989.
17. Cadman HF, K.P., Zhou R, Davelaar F, Mason PR. A serosurvey using enzyme-linked immunosorbent assay for antibodies against poultry pathogens in ostriches (Struthio camelus) from Zimbabwe. Avian Dis. 38:621-625. 1994.
18. Carlson, H.G., G.L. Seawright, and J. Pettit Reticuloendotheliosis in Japanese quail. Avian pathology : journal of the W.V.P.A 3:169-175. 1974.
19. Carpenter, C.R., A.S. Rubin, and H.R. Bose, Jr. Suppression of the mitogen-stimulated blastogenic response during reticuloendotheliosis virus-induced tumorigenesis: investigations into the mechanism of action of the suppressor. Journal of immunology 120:1313-1320. 1978.
20. Cheng, Z., Y. Shi, L. Zhang, G. Zhu, X. Diao, and Z. Cui Occurrence of reticuloendotheliosis in Chinese partridge. J Vet Med Sci 69:1295-1298. 2007.
21. Cianciolo, G.J., H.P. Bogerd, R.J. Kipnis, T.D. Copeland, S. Oroszlan, and R. Snyderman Inhibition of lymphocyte proliferation by a synthetic peptide homologous to envelope proteins of human and animal retroviruses. Transactions of the Association of American Physicians 98:30-41. 1985.
22. Cianciolo, G.J., T.D. Copeland, S. Oroszlan, and R. Snyderman Inhibition of lymphocyte proliferation by a synthetic peptide homologous to retroviral envelope proteins. Science 230:453-455. 1985.
23. Cianciolo, G.J., M.E. Lostrom, M. Tam, and R. Snyderman Murine malignant cells synthesize a 19,000-dalton protein that is physicochemically and antigenically related to the immunosuppressive retroviral protein, P15E. The Journal of experimental medicine 158:885-900. 1983.
24. Coffin, J.M., B.N. Fields, D.M. Knipe, and P.M. Howley Retroviridae: The viruses and their replication. In: Fields Virology. D.M. Fields, ed. Lippincott-Raven Publishers, Philadelphia, PA. pp 1767-1846. 1996.
25. Coffin, J.M., R. Weiss, N. Teich, and H. Varmus Structure of the retroviral genome. In: RNA Tumor Viruses. D.M. Fields, ed. Cold Spring Harbor Laboratory, Cold Spring Harbor, NY. pp 261-368. 1996.

26. Crespo, R., P.R. Woolcock, A.M. Fadly, C. Hall, and H.L. Shivaprasad Characterization of T-cell lymphomas associated with an outbreak of reticuloendotheliosis in turkeys. Avian Pathol. 31:355-361. 2002.
27. Cui, Z., S. Sun, Z. Zhang, and S. Meng Simultaneous endemic infections with subgroup J avian leukosis virus and reticuloendotheliosis virus in commercial and local breeds of chickens. Avian pathology : journal of the W.V.P.A 38:443-448. 2009.
28. Cui, Z., G. Zhuang, X. Xu, A. Sun, and S. Su Molecular and biological characterization of a Marek's disease virus field strain with reticuloendotheliosis virus LTR insert. Virus genes 40:236-243. 2010.
29. Davidson I, a.B.R. Multiple infection of chickens and turkeys with avian oncogenic viruses: prevalence and molecular analysis. Acta Virol. 43:136-142. 1999.
30. Davidson, I., A. Borovskaya, S. Perl, and M. Malkinson Use of the polymerase chain reaction for the diagnosis of natural infection of chickens and turkeys with Marek's disease virus and reticuloendotheliosis virus. Avian pathology : journal of the W.V.P.A 24:69-94. 1995.
31. Davidson I, B.R. In vivo events of retroviral long terminal repeat integration into Marek's disease virus in commercial poultry: detection of chimeric molecules as a marker. Avian Dis. 45:102-121. 2001.
32. Davidson, I., and Y. Braverman Insect contribution to horizontal transmission of Reticuloendotheliosis virus. Journal of medical entomology 42:128-133. 2005.
33. Davidson, I., and M. Malkinson A non-radioactive method for identifying enzyme-amplified products of the reticuloendotheliosis proviral env and LTR genes using psoralen-biotin labelled probes. Journal of virological methods 59:113-119. 1996.
34. Davidson, I., I. Shkoda, and S. Perk Integration of the reticuloendotheliosis virus envelope gene into the poultry fowlpox virus genome is not universal. The Journal of general virology 89:2456-2460. 2008.
35. De Boer, G.F. Methods for the control of avian tumor virus diseases. Tijdschr-Diergeneeskd. (Dutch, non-English) 102:239-246. 1977.
36. Deng, X., X. Qi, Y. Gao, Y. Wang, L. Qin, H. Gao, L. Gao, and X. Wang Development of a loop-mediated isothermal amplification method for rapid detection of reticuloendotheliosis virus. Journal of virological methods 168:82-86. 2010.
37. Drew ML, W.W., Graham DL, Griffin CP, Silvy NJ, Fadly AM, Witter RL. Reticuloendotheliosis in captive greater and Attwater's prairie chickens. J Wildl Dis. 34:783-791. 1998.
38. Emsley, A. Layer industry experience with ALV eradication in North America. In: 1992 Biannual Meeting of the Poultry Veterinary Study Group for the E.E.C. Lyon, France. pp 52-54. 1993.
39. Eterradossi, N., and Y.M. Saif Infectious Bursal Disease. In: Diseases of Poultry. Y.M. Saif, ed. Blackwell Publishing, Ames, IA. pp 185-208. 2008.
40. Fadly, A.M. Avian leukosis virus (ALV) infection, shedding, and tumors in maternal ALV antibody-positive and -negative chickens exposed to virus at hatching. Avian diseases 32:89-95. 1988.
41. Fadly, A.M. Avian retroviruses. The Veterinary clinics of North America. Food animal practice 13:71-85. 1997.
42. Fadly, A.M. Neoplastic Diseases. In: Diseases of Poultry, 12th ed. Y.M. Saif, ed. Blackwell Publishing, Ames, IA. pp 449-451. 2008.
43. Fadly, A.M. Reticuloendotheliosis and other related tumor virus infections in turkeys. In: 2nd International Symposium on Turkey Diseases. Berlin, Germany. p Electronic proceedings. 1999.
44. Fadly, A.M., and W. Okazaki Studies of avian leukosis virus infection in chickens from a commercial breeder flock. Poultry science 61:1055-1060. 1982.
45. Fadly, A.M., W. Okazaki, and R.L. Witter Hatchery-related contact transmission and short-term small-group-rearing as related to lymphoid leukosis virus eradication programs. Avian diseases 25:667-677. 1981.
46. Fadly, A.M., and E.J. Smith Role of contact and genetic transmission of endogenous virus-21 in the susceptibility of chickens to avian leukosis virus infection and tumors. Ppoultry Science 76:968-973. 1997.
47. Fadly, A.M., R.L. Witter, and L.F. Lee Effects of chemically or virus-induced immunodepression on response of chickens to avian leukosis virus. Avian diseases 29:12-25. 1985.
48. Fadly AM, W.R. Comparative evaluation of in vitro and in vivo assays for the detection of reticuloendotheliosis virus as a contaminant in a live virus vaccine of poultry. Avian Dis. 41:695-701. 1997.
49. Fadly AM, W.R., Smith EJ, Silva RF, Reed WM, Hoerr FJ, and Putnam MR An outbreak of lymphomas in commercial broiler breeder chickens vaccinated with a fowlpox vaccine contaminated with reticuloendotheliosis virus. Avian Pathol. 25:35-47. 1996.
50. Fadly, A.M., G. Zavala, and R.L. Witter Reticuloendotheliosis. In: Diseases of Poultry, 12th ed. Y.M. Saif, ed. Blackwell Publishing, Ames, IA. pp 568-588. 2008.
51. Fitzgerald, S.D. Adenovirus Infections. In: Diseases of Poultry, 12th ed. Y.M. Saif, ed. Blackwell Publishing, Ames, IA. pp 449-451251-451290. 2008.
52. Gabriel, G., K. Klingel, O. Planz, K. Bier, A. Herwig, M. Sauter, and H.D. Klenk Spread of infection and lymphocyte depletion in mice depends on polymerase of influenza virus. The American journal of pathology 175:1178-1186. 2009.
53. Garcia M, N.N., Reed WM, Fadly AM. Molecular characterization of reticuloendotheliosis virus insertions in the genome of field and vaccine strains of fowl poxvirus. Avian Dis. 47:343-354. 2003.
54. Hafez, H. Serological investigations on reticuloendotheliosis in turkey flocks. J Vet Med B Infect Dis Vet Public Health. 48:547-550. 2001.

55. Haraguchi, S., R.A. Good, G.J. Cianciolo, and N.K. Day A synthetic peptide homologous to retroviral envelope protein down-regulates TNF-alpha and IFN-gamma mRNA expression. Journal of leukocyte biology 52:469-472. 1992.
56. Haraguchi, S., R.A. Good, G.J. Cianciolo, R.W. Engelman, and N.K. Day Immunosuppressive retroviral peptides: immunopathological implications for immunosuppressive influences of retroviral infections. Journal of leukocyte biology 61:654-666. 1997.
57. Haraguchi, S., R.A. Good, M. James-Yarish, G.J. Cianciolo, and N.K. Day Differential modulation of Th1- and Th2-related cytokine mRNA expression by a synthetic peptide homologous to a conserved domain within retroviral envelope protein. Proceedings of the National Academy of Sciences of the United States of America 92:3611-3615. 1995.
58. Haraguchi, S., R.A. Good, M. James-Yarish, G.J. Cianciolo, and N.K. Day Induction of intracellular cAMP by a synthetic retroviral envelope peptide: a possible mechanism of immunopathogenesis in retroviral infections. Proceedings of the National Academy of Sciences of the United States of America 92:5568-5571. 1995.
59. Hayes LE, L.K., Witter RL. Reticuloendotheliosis in a wild turkey (Meleagris gallopavo) from coastal Georgia. J Wildl Dis. 28:154-158. 1992.
60. Hertig C, C.B., Gould AR, Boyle DB. Field and vaccine strains of fowlpox virus carry integrated sequences from the avian retrovirus, reticuloendotheliosis virus. Virology 235:367-376. 1997.
61. Isfort, R., R.L. Witter, and H.J. Kung C-myc activation in an unusual retrovirus-induced avian T-lymphoma resembling Marek's disease: proviral insertion 5' of exon one enhances the expression of an intron promoter. Oncogene research 2:81-94. 1987.
62. Jackson, C.A., S.E. Dunn, D.I. Smith, P.T. Gilchrist, and P.A. Macqueen Proventriculitis, "nakanuke" and reticuloendotheliosis in chickens following vaccination with herpesvirus of turkeys (HVT). Australian veterinary journal 53:457-459. 1977.
63. Jiang, L., X. Qi, Y. Gao, Y. Hua, K. Li, X. Deng, Q. Wang, L. Zhang, H. Chai, Y. Chen, C. Yin, H. Gao, L. Qin, Y. Wang, Y. Qu, Q. Chen, Z. Fan, and X. Wang Molecular characterization and phylogenetic analysis of the reticuloendotheliosis virus isolated from wild birds in Northeast China. Veterinary microbiology 166:68-75. 2013.
64. Jiang, T., X. Lu, Y. Yuan, L. Zheng, J. Shi, and D. Zhang Complete genomic sequence of a Muscovy duck-origin reticuloendotheliosis virus from China. Journal of virology 86:13140-13141. 2012.
65. Johnson, E. Poultry oncogenic retroviruses and humans. Cancer Detect Prev. 18:9-30. 1994.
66. Johnson ES, G.C. Oncogenic retroviruses of cattle, chickens and turkeys: potential infectivity and oncogenicity for humans. Med Hypotheses. 46:354-356. 1996.
67. Johnson ES, N.L., Durack DT. Detection of antibodies to avian leukosis/sarcoma viruses (ALSV) and reticuloendotheliosis viruses (REV) in humans by ELISA. Cancer Detect Prev. 19:394-404. 1995.
68. Jones , R.C. Reovirus Infections. In: Diseases of Poultry, 12th ed. Y.M. Saif, ed. Blackwell Publishing, Ames, IA. pp 309-328. 2008.
69. Kawamura, H.T., S. Wakabayashi, and N. Yamaguchi Inoculation experiment of Marek's disease vaccine contaminated with reticuloendotheliosis virus. Nat Inst Anim Health Quarterly 16:135-140. 1976.
70. Kewalramani VN, P.A., Emerman M. Spleen necrosis virus, an avian immunosuppressive retrovirus, shares a receptor with the type D simian retroviruses. J Virol. 66:3026-3031. 1992.
71. Koyama, H., T. Hodatsu, T. Sasaki, Y. Ohwada, Y. Saito, and H. Saito Continuous cell culture from chick embryos inoculated with REV strain T. Avian pathology : journal of the W.V.P.A 10:151-162. 1981.
72. Koyama, H., T. Sasaki, Y. Ohwada, and Y. Saito The relationship between feathering abnormalities ("nakanuke") and tumour production in chickens inoculated with reticuloendotheliosis virus. Avian pathology : journal of the W.V.P.A 9:331-340. 1980.
73. Koyama, H., Y. Suzuki, Y. Ohwada, and Y. Saito Reticuloendotheliosis group virus pathogenic to chicken isolated from material infected with turkey herpesvirus (HVT). Avian diseases 20:429-434. 1976.
74. Landman, W.J., J. Post, A. G. Boonstra-Blom, J. Buuyse, A. R. Elbers, and G. Koch Effect of an in ovo infection with a Dutch avian leukosis virus subgroup J isolate on the growth and immunological performance of SPF broiler chickens. Avian Pathol. 31:59-72. 2002.
75. Ley DH, F.M., Cobb DT, Witter RL. Histomoniasis and reticuloendotheliosis in a wild turkey (Meleagris gallopavo) in North Carolina. J Wildl Dis. 25:262-265. 1989.
76. Li, J., B.W. Calnek, K.A. Schat, and D.L. Graham. Pathogenesis of reticuloendotheliosis virus infection in ducks. Avian Dis. 27:1090-1105. 1983.
77. Li, K., H. Gao, L. Gao, X. Qi, L. Qin, Y. Gao, Y. Xu, and X. Wang Development of TaqMan real-time PCR assay for detection and quantitation of reticuloendotheliosis virus. Journal of virological methods 179:402-408. 2012.
78. Lin, F., C. Gao, S. Chen, X. Zhu, X. Cheng, S. Wang, S. Chen, X. Cai, Z. Li, C. Ma, and J. Zhao [Immunosuppression effect of co-infection with MDRV and H9 AIV on thymus in muscovy ducks]. Wei sheng wu xue bao = Acta microbiologica Sinica 51:1407-1412. 2011.
79. Liu, Q., J. Zhao, J. Su, J. Pu, G. Zhang, and J. Liu Full genome sequences of two reticuloendotheliosis viruses contaminating commercial vaccines. Avian diseases 53:341-346. 2009.
80. Markowski-Grimsrud, C.J., and K.A. Schat Infection with chicken anemia virus impairs the generation of pathogen-specific cytotoxic T lymphocytes. Immunology 109:283-294. 2003.

81. Martinez I, D.R. Mapping of receptor binding domains in the envelope protein of spleen necrosis virus. J Virol. 69:4339-4346. 1995.
82. McDougall, J.S., P.M. Biggs, and R.W. Shilleto A leukosis in turkeys associated with infection with reticuloendotheliosis virus. Avian pathology : journal of the W.V.P.A 7:557-568. 1978.
83. McDougall, J.S., R.W. Shilleto, and P.M. Biggs Experimental infection and vertical transmission of reticuloendotheliosis virus in the turkey. Avian pathology : journal of the W.V.P.A 9:445-454. 1980.
84. McDougall, J.S., R.W. Shilleto, and P.M. Biggs Further studies on vertical transmission of reticuloendotheliosis virus in turkeys. Avian pathology : journal of the W.V.P.A 10:163-169. 1981.
85. Meroz, M. Reticuloendotheliosis and 'pullet disease' in Israel. Vet Rec. 130:107-108. 1992.
86. Moore KM, D.J., Sato T, Yasuda A. Reticuloendotheliosis virus (REV) long terminal repeats incorporated in the genomes of commercial fowl poxvirus vaccines and pigeon poxviruses without indication of the presence of infectious REV. Avian Dis. 44:827-841. 2000.
87. Motha, M.X. Distribution of virus and tumour formation in ducks experimentally infected with reticuloendotheliosis virus. Avian pathology : journal of the W.V.P.A 13:303-319. 1984.
88. Motha, M.X., and J.R. Egerton Effect of reticuloendotheliosis virus on the response of chickens to Salmonella typhimurium infection. Research in veterinary science 34:188-192. 1983.
89. Motha, M.X., and J.R. Egerton Influence of reticuloendotheliosis on the severity of Eimeria tenella infection in broiler chickens. Veterinary microbiology 9:121-129. 1984.
90. Motha, M.X., and J.R. Egerton Outbreak of atypical fowlpox in chickens with persistent reticuloendotheliosis viraemia. Avian pathology : journal of the W.V.P.A 16:177-182. 1987.
91. Motha, M.X., J.R. Egerton, and A.W. Sweeney Some evidence of mechanical transmission of reticuloendotheliosis virus by mosquitoes. Avian diseases 28:858-867. 1984.
92. Mussman, H.C., and M.J. Twiehaus Pathogenesis of reticuloendothelial virus disease in chicks - an acute runting syndrome. Avian diseases 15:483-502. 1971.
93. Nazerian, K., A. Elmubarak, and J.M. Sharma Establishment of B-lymphoblastoid cell lines from Marek's disease virus-induced tumors in turkeys. International journal of cancer. Journal international du cancer 29:63-68. 1982.
94. Nazerian, K., R.L. Witter, L.B. Crittenden, M.R. Noori-Dalloii, and H.J. Kung An IgM-producing B lymphoblastoid cell line established from lymphomas induced by a non-defective reticuloendotheliosis virus. The Journal of general virology 58:351-360. 1982.
95. Neimanis, A.S., and F.A. Leighton Health risk assessment for the introduction of Eastern wild turkeys (Meleagris gallopavo silvestris) into Nova Scotia. In. C.C.W.H. Centre, ed. Department of Veterinary Pathology, Western College of Veterinary Medicine, University of Saskatchewan, Saskatoon, SK, Canada S7N 5B4. 2004.
96. Paul, P.S., K.H. Johnson, K.A. Pomeroy, B.S. Pomeroy, and P.S. Sarma Experimental transmission of reticuloendotheliosis in turkeys with the cell-culture-propagated reticuloendotheliosis viruses of turkey origin. Journal of the National Cancer Institute 58:1819-1824. 1977.
97. Paul, P.S., R.E. Werdin, and B.S. Pomeroy Spontaneously occurring lymphoproliferative disease in ducks. Avian diseases 22:191-195. 1978.
98. Payne, L. Retrovirus-induced disease in poultry. Poult Sci. 77:1204-1212. 1998.
99. Payne, L.N., and K. Howes Eradication of exogenous avian leukosis virus from commercial layer breeder lines. Veterinary Record 128:8-11. 1991.
100. Payne, L.N., K. Howes, L.M. Smith, and N. Venugopal Current status of diagnosis, epidemiology and control of ALV-J. In: Avian Tumor Virus Symposium. A.A.o.A. Pathologists, ed. American Association of Avian Pathologists, Reno, Nevada (U.S.A.). pp 58-62. 1997.
101. Payne LN, V.K. Neoplastic diseases: Marek's disease, avian leukosis and reticuloendotheliosis. Rev Sci Tech. 19:544-564. 2000.
102. Pierson, F.W., and S.D. Fizgerald Hemorrhagic enteritis and related infections. In: Diseases of Poultry, 12th ed. Y.M. Saif, ed. Blackwell Publishing, Ames, IA. pp 276-286. 2008.
103. Ratnamohan, N., T.M. Grimes, Bagust, and P.B. Spradbrow A transmissible chicken tumour associated with reticuloendotheliosis virus infection. Australian veterinary journal 56:34-38. 1980.
104. Reimann I, W.O. Use of the polymerase chain reaction for the detection of reticuloendotheliosis virus in Marek's disease vaccines and chicken tissues. Zentralbl Veterinarmed B. 43:75-84. 1996.
105. Ridgway, A.A., R.A. Swift, H.J. Kung, and D.J. Fujita In vitro transcription analysis of the viral promoter involved in c-myc activation in chicken B lymphomas: detection and mapping of two RNA initiation sites within the reticuloendotheliosis virus long terminal repeat. Journal of virology 54:161-170. 1985.
106. Rispens, B.H., G.F. De Boer, A. Hoogerbrugge, and J. Van Vloten A method for the control of lymphoid leukosis in chickens. Journal of the National Cancer Institute 57:1151-1156. 1976.
107. Rombout, J.H., B.T. van Rens, S.R. Sijtsma, M.C. van der Weide, and C.E. West Effects of vitamin A deficiency and Newcastle disease virus infection on lymphocyte subpopulations in chicken blood. Veterinary immunology and immunopathology 31:155-166. 1992.
108. Saif, Y.M. Infectious bursal disease and hemorrhagic enteritis. Poultry science 77:1186-1189. 1998.
109. Sandelin, K., and T. Estola Testing and Management of a Specific Pathogen Free Chicken Flock with Special Reference to

Avian Leukosis Virus Infections. Acta vet. scand. 16:341-356. 1975.
110. Santos, V.L., S.M. Williams, G. Zavala, T. Barbosa, J. Zhang, S. Cheng, H.L. Shivaprasad, S. Hafner, A. Fadly, R.L. Santos, and C.C. Brown Detection of reticuloendotheliosis virus by immunohistochemistry and in situ hybridization in experimentally infected Japanese quail embryos and archived formalin-fixed and paraffin-embedded tumours. Avian pathology : journal of the W.V.P.A 37:451-456. 2008.
111. Sasaki T, S.S., Koyama H. A survey of an antibody to reticuloendotheliosis virus in sera of chickens and other avian species in Japan. J Vet Med Sci. 55:885-888. 1993.
112. Schat, K.A., and V. Nair Marek's Disease. In: Diseases of Poultry. Y.M. Saif, ed. Blackwell Publishing, Ames, IA. pp 452-514. 2008.
113. Schat, K.A., and M.A. Skinner Avian Immunosuppressive Diseases and Immune Evasion. In: Avian Immunology. F. Davison, B. Kaspers, K.A. Schat and P. Kaiser, eds. Academic Press, London, U.K. pp 299-322. 2008.
114. Schat, K.A., and V.L. van Santen Chicken Infectious Anemia. In: Diseases of Poultry. Y.M. Saif, ed. Blackwell Publishing, Ames, IA. pp 209-249. 2008.
115. Scofield, V.L., and H.R. Bose, Jr. Depression of mitogen response in spleen cells from reticuloendotheliosis virus-infected chickens and their suppressive effect on normal lymphocyte response. Journal of immunology 120:1321-1325. 1978.
116. Sharma, J.M., K. Karaca, and T. Pertile Virus-induced immunosuppression in chickens. Poultry science 73:1082-1086. 1994.
117. Sidorova, E.V., M.G. Agadzhanian, L.A. Mazhul, I. Biladi, M. Bakai, and K. Berenchi [Immunosuppression induced by respiratory viruses (influenza virus, adenovirus) in mice]. Biulleten' eksperimental'noi biologii i meditsiny 111:510-512. 1991.
118. Sijtsma, S.R., J.H. Rombout, A. Kiepurski, C.E. West, and A.J. van der Zijpp Changes in lymphoid organs and blood lymphocytes induced by vitamin A deficiency and Newcastle disease virus infection in chickens. Developmental and comparative immunology 15:349-356. 1991.
119. Singh, P., W.M. Schnitzlein, and D.N. Tripathy Construction and characterization of a fowlpox virus field isolate whose genome lacks reticuloendotheliosis provirus nucleotide sequences. Avian diseases 49:401-408. 2005.
120. Singh, P., W.M. Schnitzlein, and D.N. Tripathy Reticuloendotheliosis virus sequences within the genomes of field strains of fowlpox virus display variability. Journal of virology 77:5855-5862. 2003.
121. Singh P, S.W., Tripathy DN. Reticuloendotheliosis virus sequences within the genomes of field strains of fowlpox virus display variability. J Virol. 77:5855-5862. 2003.
122. Spencer, J.L. Laboratory diagnostic procedures for detecting for detecting avian leukosis virus infections. In: Avian Leukosis. d. BOER, ed. Martinus Nijhoff, Boston, MA. pp 213-240. 1987.
123. Spencer, J.L. An overview of problems and progress in control of avian leukosis. In: Avian Tumor Virus Symposium. A.A.o.A. Pathologists, ed. American Association of Avian Pathologists, Reno, Nevada (U.S.A.). pp 48-53. 1977.
124. Su, S., N. Cui, Z. Cui, P. Zhao, Y. Li, J. Ding, and X. Dong Complete genome sequence of a recombinant Marek's disease virus field strain with one reticuloendotheliosis virus long terminal repeat insert. Journal of virology 86:13818-13819. 2012.
125. Sun, A.J., X.Y. Xu, L. Petherbridge, Y.G. Zhao, V. Nair, and Z.Z. Cui Functional evaluation of the role of reticuloendotheliosis virus long terminal repeat (LTR) integrated into the genome of a field strain of Marek's disease virus. Virology 397:270-276. 2010.
126. Swayne, D.E., and D.A. Halvorson Influenza. In: Diseases of Poultry, 12th ed. Y.M. Saif, ed. Blackwell Publishing, Ames, IA. pp 153-184. 2008.
127. Swift RA, B.C., Ridgway A, Fujita DJ, Dodgson JB, Kung HJ. B-lymphoma induction by reticuloendotheliosis virus: characterization of a mutated chicken syncytial virus provirus involved in c-myc activation. J Virol. 61:2084-2090. 1987.
128. T., B., Z. G., S. Cheng, T. Lourenco, and P. Villegas Effects of reticuloendotheliosis virus on the viability and reproductive performance of Japanese quail. J. Appl. Poult. Res. 15:558-563. 2006.
129. Tadese T, R.W. Detection of specific reticuloendotheliosis virus sequence and protein from REV-integrated fowlpox virus strains. J Virol Methods. 110:99-104. 2003.
130. Takagi, M., K. Ishikawa, H. Nagai, T. Sasaki, K. Gotoh, and H. Koyama Detection of contamination of vaccines with the reticuloendotheliosis virus by reverse transcriptase polymerase chain reaction (RT-PCR). Virus research 40:113-121. 1996.
131. Taniguchi, T., N. Yuasa, S. Sato, and T. Horiuchi Pathological changes in chickens inoculated with reticuloendotheliosis-virus-contaminated Marek's disease vaccine. National Institute of Animal Health quarterly 17:141-150. 1977.
132. Thompson, K.D., R.G. Fischer, and D.H. Luecke Determination of the viremic period of avian reticuloendotheliosis virus (strain T) in chicks and virus viability in Triatoma infestans (Klug) [Hemiptera: Reduviidae]. Avian diseases 12:354-360. 1968.
133. Thompson, K.D., R.G. Fischer, and D.H. Luecke Quantitative infectivity studies of avian reticuloendotheliosis virus (strain T) in certain hematophagous arthropods. Journal of medical entomology 8:486-490. 1971.
134. Trampel DW, P.T., Witter RL. Reticuloendotheliosis in Hungarian partridge. J Wildl Dis. 38:438-442. 2002.
135. Tripathy, D.N., and W.M. Reed Pox. In: Diseases of Poultry, 12th ed. Y.M. Saif, ed. Blackwell Publishing, Ames, IA. pp 291-307. 2008.
136. Turner, P.C., and R.W. Moyer Poxvirus immune modulators: functional insights from animal models. Virus research 88:35-53. 2002.

137. Walker, M.H., B.J. Rup, A.S. Rubin, and H.R. Bose, Jr. Specificity in the immunosuppression induced by avian reticuloendotheliosis virus. Infection and immunity 40:225-235. 1983.
138. Wang, G., Y. Wang, L. Yu, Y. Jiang, J. Liu, and Z. Cheng New pathogenetic characters of reticuloendotheliosis virus isolated from Chinese partridge in specific-pathogen-free chickens. Microbial pathogenesis 53:57-63. 2012.
139. Wang, J., J. Meers, P.B. Spradbrow, and W.F. Robinson Evaluation of immune effects of fowlpox vaccine strains and field isolates. Veterinary microbiology 116:106-119. 2006.
140. Wang, Y., Z. Cui, and S. Jiang Sequence analysis for the complete proviral genome of reticuloendotheliosis virus Chinese strain HA9901. Science in China. Series C, Life sciences / Chinese Academy of Sciences 49:149-157. 2006.
141. Wei, K., Z. Sun, S. Zhu, W. Guo, P. Sheng, Z. Wang, C. Zhao, Q. Zhao, and R. Zhu Probable congenital transmission of reticuloendotheliosis virus caused by vaccination with contaminated vaccines. PloS one 7:e43422. 2012.
142. Witter, R. Avian tumor viruses: persistent and evolving pathogens. Acta Vet Hung. 45:251-266. 1997.
143. Witter, R.L., and L.B. Crittenden Lymphomas resembling lymphoid leukosis in chickens inoculated with reticuloendotheliosis virus. International journal of cancer. Journal international du cancer 23:673-678. 1979.
144. Witter, R.L., and D.C. Johnson Epidemiology of reticuloendotheliosis virus in broiler breeder flocks. Avian Dis. 29:1140-1154. 1985.
145. Witter, R.L., L.F. Lee, L.D. Bacon, and E.J. Smith Depression of vaccinal immunity to Marek's disease by infection with reticuloendotheliosis virus. . Infection and immunity 26:90-98. 1979.
146. Witter, R.L., D. Li, D. Jones, L.F. Lee, and H.J. Kung Retroviral insertional mutagenesis of a herpesvirus: a Marek's disease virus mutant attenuated for oncogenicity but not for immunosuppression or in vivo replication. Avian diseases 41:407-421. 1997.
147. Witter RL, P.I., Smith EJ, and Johnson DC Serologic evidence in commercial chicken and turkey flocks of infection with reticuloendotheliosis virus. Avian Dis. 26:753-762. 1982.
148. Witter, R.L., H.G. Purchase, and G.H. Burgone Peripheral nerve lesions siilar to those of Marek's disease in chickens inoculated with reticuloendotheliosis virus. J of the National Cancer Inst 45:567-577. 1970.
149. Witter RL, S.D. Vertical transmission of reticuloendotheliosis virus in breeder turkeys. Avian Dis. 33:226-235. 1989.
150. Witter, R.L., E.J. Smith, and L.B. Crittenden Tolerance, viral shedding, and neoplasia in chickens infected with non-defective reticuloendotheliosis viruses. Avian diseases 25:374-394. 1981.
151. Wong, T.C., and M.M. Lai Avian reticuloendotheliosis virus contains a new class of oncogene of turkey origin. Virology 111:289-293. 1981.
152. Woodruff, J.F., and J.J. Woodruff Virus-induced alterations of lymphoid tissues. I. Modification of the recirculating pool of small lymphocytes by Newcastle disease virus. Cellular immunology 1:333-354. 1970.
153. Xu, X., A. Sun, Y. Cui, and Z. Cui [Comparision of pathogenicity and horizontal transmission ability between recombinant Marek's disease virus field strain with REV-LTR and a very virulent reference strain]. Wei sheng wu xue bao = Acta microbiologica Sinica 49:540-543. 2009.
154. Yoshida, I., M. Sakata, K. Fujita, T. Noguchi, and N. Yuasa Modification of low virulent Newcastle disease virus infection in chickens infected with reticuloendotheliosis virus. National Institute of Animal Health quarterly 21:1-6. 1981.
155. Yu, L.J., and Z.Z. Cui [Sequence analysis of integration sites of reticuloendotheliosis virus LTR in fowlpox vaccine virus genomes]. Wei sheng wu xue bao = Acta microbiologica Sinica 46:660-662. 2006.
156. Yuasa, N., I. Yoshida, and T. Taniguchi Isolation of a reticuloendotheiosis virus from chickens inoculated with Marek's disease vaccine. Natl Anim Health Q (Tokyo) 16:141-151. 1976.
157. Zavala, G. Immunosuppression induced by reticuloendotheliosis virus. In: Impact of subclinical immunosuppression on poultry production. American Association of Avian Pathologists, Honolulu, HI. 2006.
158. Zavala, G. Myeloid leukosis: a new challenge for the poultry industry. Vineland Update 61:1-4. 1998.
159. Zavala, G. An overview of myeloid leukosis in meat-type chickens. The Poultry Informed Professional. Published by The University of Georgia. 1998.
160. Zavala, G., S. Cheng, T. Barbosa, and H. Haefele Enzootic reticuloendotheliosis in the endangered Attwater's and greater prairie chickens. Avian Dis 50:520-525. 2006.

This work published by Servet has just finished printing
in Grupo Milán in November 2013.